WEBSTER'S

MEDICAL SPELLER

Second Edition

Webster's
MEDICAL
SPELLER

Second Edition

A Merriam-Webster

MERRIAM-WEBSTER INC.

Springfield, Massachusetts

A GENUINE MERRIAM-WEBSTER

The name *Webster* alone is no guarantee of excellence. It is used by a number of publishers and may serve mainly to mislead an unwary buyer.

A Merriam-Webster® is the registered trademark you should look for when you consider the purchase of dictionaries or other fine reference books. It carries the reputation of a company that has been publishing since 1831 and is your assurance of quality and authority.

Library of Congress Cataloging in Publication

Webster's medical speller.
    p.   cm.
  ISBN 0-87779-137-6
  1. Medicine—Terminology.   2. Spellers.
R123.W35   1987
610′.14—dc19   87-26947

MADE IN THE UNITED STATES OF AMERICA

18IP02

CONTENTS

PREFACE

Webster's Medical Speller, Second Edition, is a pocket-size guide to the spelling and division of 35,000 medical words and words with special medical meanings. In addition, special sections contain more than 1,000 medical abbreviations, a list of medical symbols, and a table of weights and measures. The words and abbreviations are drawn from the vocabulary entries of Webster's Medical Desk Dictionary, published by Merriam-Webster Inc. The word divisions follow the principles of end-of-line division embodied in Webster's Ninth New Collegiate Dictionary and Webster's Medical Desk Dictionary.

Anyone who prepares or processes written matter with medical content frequently needs to know whether a medical word is spelled with one *l* or two, whether a compound term is written as one word or two words or with a hyphen, which of several variant spellings or plurals is most widely used, and where a word is divided at the end of a line. Webster's Medical Speller, Second Edition, provides a ready and authoritative answer to such questions.

The 35,000 word corpus was selected from the boldface vocabulary entries in Webster's Medical Desk Dictionary. Usage was the final arbiter in making the selection. Vocabulary entries in Webster's Medical Desk Dictionary were rated according to a scale of frequency and importance based on citational evidence in the Merriam-Webster files. Terms with lower frequency ratings have been omitted from this speller to keep it within the range of a pocket-size guide. The vocabulary files on which this edition of the speller is based contained approximately 13,400,000 citations of words in context kept on 3 x 5 slips.

Open compound terms, such as **rectal venous plexus,** are not included if each of the component elements appears at its own place in alphabetical sequence, except for a few (as **beta globulin**) about which a question often arises as to whether they are open or hyphenated. Elements of a compound that occur only in compounds and do not have independent use are not entered at their own alphabetical place. For example, **obliterans** occurs only as part of compound terms such as **endarteritis obliterans** and **thromboangiitis obliterans** and is not entered at its own place in alphabetical sequence.

Inflected forms of nouns, verbs, and adjectives are entered in Webster's Medical Speller, Second Edition, according to the criteria used for entry in Webster's Medical Desk Dictionary except that in this book they are always spelled out in full. In general, inflected forms are shown in the following cases: when they are irregular (as the plural **lice**); when addition of the inflectional suffix requires a change in a letter (as in the plural **appendectomies**), the dropping of a letter (as in the present participle **operating**), or the doubling of a letter (as in the past participle **embedded**); and when the user might have doubts about the inflected form even though it is regular (as the plural **helminths**, which might be expected to assume the form "helminthes" by analogy with the plural used in the name of the phylum **Platyhelminthes**).

Not only are base words like **laparoscope** entered, but derivatives like **laparoscopic, laparoscopist,** and **laparoscopy** also appear in alphabetical sequence. If a verbal noun, like **teething,** does not appear at its own alphabetical place, one should look for it at the parent verb (**teethe**). Terms that are frequently confused, like **perineal, peritoneal,** and **peroneal,** are given short definitions.

When a main entry is followed by the word *or* and another spelling (as **tendinitis** *or* **tendonitis**), the two spellings are equal variants. If two variants joined by *or* are out of alphabetical order (as **physiological** *or* **physiologic**), they remain equal variants, but the first is slightly more common than the second. When another spelling is joined to the main entry by the word *also* (as **lipid** *also* **lipide**), the spelling after *also* is a secondary variant and occurs less frequently than the first. If there are two secondary variants, the second is joined to the first by *or*. Once the word *also* is used to signal a secondary variant, all following secondary variants are joined by *or* (as **cesarean** *or* **caesarean** *also* **cesarian** *or* **caesarian**).

The Merriam-Webster vocabulary files are constantly updated, and they reflect numerous changes in medical usage since publication of the first edition of Webster's Medical Speller. Changes in this edition include not only additions to and deletions from the vocabulary but occasional changes in the relationships of variants. For example, **Saint Vitus' dance** is found now consistently with greater frequency than the form **Saint Vitus's dance** so that the two variants are shown in this book separated by *also* rather than *or*. On the other hand, the first edition of Webster's Medical Speller contained an entry **Gram stain** *also* **Gram's stain** indicating that the first form had far more currency than the second. In this edition the entry has been revised to **Gram's stain** *or* **Gram stain** indicating that both forms are now commonly encountered with the first slightly more frequent.

Some special rules of alphabetization have been used to accommodate the numbers and the Greek or Roman letters that are sometimes used as prefixes or infixes in chemical terms. If a number or letter appears within a term, it is used in determining alphabetical place: **alpha-1-antitrypsin** is alphabetized as if spelled *alphaoneantitrypsin* and thus comes after **alpha-ketogularic acid** and ahead of **alpha-receptor.** If a prefix is spelled out, it too is used for alphabetizing: **beta globulin** and **beta-lipotropin** are found in the *B*'s. However, if the prefix is a number or is an abbreviation set off by a hyphen, it is ignored in determining alphabetical place: **N-allylnormorphine** is in the *A*'s, **5-hydroxytryptamine** is in the *H*'s, and β_2**-microglobulin** is in the *M*'s.

Scientific names of genera and higher taxonomic categories in biological nomenclature are included if they are of medical significance. In scientific and medical writing, names of genera (as *Neisseria*) begin with a capital letter and are written in italics while the names of families (as Babesiidae) and higher taxonomic categories (as the class or subclass Cestoda) begin with a capital letter but are not italicized. Many genus names (*Bacterium, Chlamydia, Penicillium*) are also used as common names which take a plural (bacteria, chlamydiae, penicillia), and when used in this way they are not capitalized or italicized in either the singular or plural forms. For example, if the context reads "a sample of members of the genus *Chlamydia*," both a capital letter and italic type are used. On the other hand, in such a context as "a sample of chlamydiae," a lowercase initial letter and roman type are used. In this book, usually only the common name is given when there is evidence in the Merriam-Webster citation files for use of the same word as both a genus and a common name. Therefore, a writer who wants to use a genus name when only the common name is given in the speller should take particular care to use the singular form, to begin with a capital letter, and to indicate italics.

The word divisions indicated by centered dots do not necessarily separate words into syllables. They are intended only to show points at which words may be divided at the end of a line of typing or writing. Common sense and the appearance of the printed page are important considerations in end-of-line division. The easiest principle to remember is that a single letter of a word should not end or begin a line. This principle is extended in the speller to include words that occur as part of a solid compound. For example, **cat·e·chol· amine** is not divided *cat·e·chol·a·mine* because the element *amine* is a word in its own right and the initial letter *a* should not stand alone even when *amine* is part of a larger word. Although many people prefer not to divide a hyphenated compound (as *glucose-6-phosphate*) anywhere but at the hyphen, divisions are indicated for the benefit of those who wish to divide elsewhere.

Since this speller is based on Webster's Medical Desk Dictionary, its content depends heavily on the work of those who edited the larger book. However, several people have contributed directly to Webster's Medical Speller, Second Edition. Eileen M. Haraty and Peter D. Haraty, Assistant Editors, edited the computer printout and made the initial selection of words, with help from Kelly L. Tierney, Editorial Assistant. Proofreading was done largely by Daniel J. Hopkins, Assistant Editor, with help from Eileen M. Haraty. The abbreviations section was edited by Kathleen M. Doherty, Associate Editor. Thomas L. Coopee, Secretary/Treasurer, and Michael Alaimo, Assistant to the Treasurer, were responsible for computer programming. Keyboarding was done by Barbara A. Winkler under the general supervision of Gloria J. Afflitto, Supervisor of the Typing Room. Additional manuscript typing was done by Helene Gingold, Department Secretary. John M. Morse, Manager of Editorial Operations and Planning, contributed to the initial stages of the book. Robert Copeland, Senior Editor, in his capacity as Editorial Production Coordinator, made numerous useful suggestions, contributed to the data processing, and guided the manuscript through its various stages.

Roger W. Pease, Jr.
Editor

A

abac·te·ri·al
aba·sia
aba·sic
ab·ax·i·al
Ab·be con·dens·er
Ab·be-Est·lan·der
    op·er·a·tion
Ab·der·hal·den re·
    ac·tion
ab·do·men
ab·dom·i·nal
ab·dom·i·nal·ly
ab·dom·i·no·pel·
    vic
ab·dom·i·no·per·i·
    ne·al
ab·dom·i·nous
ab·du·cens
    pl ab·du·cen·tes

ab·du·cent
ab·duct
ab·duc·tion
ab·duc·tor
    pl ab·duc·to·res
    or ab·duc·tors

ab·duc·tor di·gi·ti
    mi·ni·mi
ab·duc·tor hal·lu·
    cis
ab·duc·tor pol·li·
    cis brev·is
ab·duc·tor pol·li·
    cis lon·gus
Abegg's rule
ab·em·bry·on·ic

ab·er·rant
ab·er·ra·tion
ab·er·ra·tion·al
abey·ance
ab·i·ence
ab·i·ent
abio·gen·e·sis
    pl abio·gen·e·ses

abio·gen·ic
abi·o·log·i·cal
abi·ot·ic
abi·ot·i·cal·ly
abio·tro·phic
abi·ot·ro·phy
    pl abi·ot·ro·phies

ablas·te·mic
ablas·tin
ab·late
    ab·lat·ed
    ab·lat·ing
ab·la·tion
ab·la·tio pla·cen·
    tae
ab·lu·tion
ab·lu·tion·ary
ab·nor·mal
ab·nor·mal·i·ty
    pl ab·nor·mal·i·ties

ab·oma·sal
ab·oma·si·tis
ab·oma·sum
    pl ab·oma·sa

ab·orad
ab·oral
abort
abort·er
abor·ti·cide

abor·ti·fa·cient
abor·tion
abor·tion·ist
abor·tive
abor·tus
ABO sys·tem
abou·lia
    var of abulia

abra·chia
abrad·ant
abrade
    abrad·ed
    abrad·ing
abra·sion
abra·sive
ab·re·act
ab·re·ac·tion
ab·re·ac·tive
abro·sia
ab·rup·tio pla·cen·
    tae
    pl ab·rup·tio pla·cen·
        ta·rum
    or ab·rup·ti·o·nes pla·
        cen·ta·rum

Abrus
ab·scess
    pl ab·scess·es

ab·scessed
ab·scis·sion
ab·sco·pal
ab·sence
ab·sinthe
    also ab·sinth

ab·sin·thin
ab·sin·thism

ab·sin·thi·um
pl ab·sin·thi·um

ab·sin·thol

ab·sorb

ab·sorb·able

ab·sor·bance

ab·sor·be·fa·cient

ab·sor·ben·cy
or ab·sor·ban·cy
pl ab·sor·ben·cies
or ab·sor·ban·cies

ab·sor·bent
also ab·sor·bant

ab·sorb·er

ab·sorp·ti·om·e·ter

ab·sorp·tion

ab·sorp·tive

ab·sorp·tiv·i·ty
pl ab·sorp·tiv·i·ties

ab·stain

ab·stain·er

ab·ster·gent

ab·sti·nence

ab·sti·nent

ab·stract

ab·strac·tor
or ab·stract·er

abu·lia
or abou·lia

abu·lic
also abou·lic

abus·able

abuse
abused
abus·ing

abus·er

abut·ment

aca·cia

acal·cu·lia

acan·thi·on

Acan·tho·ceph·a·la

acan·tho·ceph·a·lan

Acan·tho·chei·lo·ne·ma

acan·tho·cyte

ac·an·thol·y·sis
pl ac·an·thol·y·ses

ac·an·tho·ma
pl ac·an·tho·mas
or ac·an·tho·ma·ta

ac·an·tho·sis
pl ac·an·tho·ses

ac·an·tho·sis ni·gri·cans

ac·an·thot·ic

acap·nia

acap·ni·al

acar·dius

ac·a·ri·a·sis
pl ac·a·ri·a·ses

acar·i·cid·al

acar·i·cide

ac·a·rid

Acar·i·dae

Ac·a·ri·na

ac·a·ri·no·sis
pl ac·a·ri·no·ses

ac·aro·der·ma·ti·tis

ac·a·rol·o·gist

ac·a·rol·o·gy
pl ac·a·rol·o·gies

ac·a·ro·pho·bia

ac·a·rus
pl aca·ri

acau·dal
or acau·date

ac·cel·er·ate
ac·cel·er·at·ed
ac·cel·er·at·ing

ac·cel·er·a·tion

ac·cel·er·a·tive

ac·cel·er·a·tor

ac·cel·e·ra·to·ry

ac·cel·e·rin

ac·cel·er·om·e·ter

ac·cep·tor

ac·ces·so·ri·us
pl ac·ces·so·rii

ac·ces·so·ry

ac·ci·dent

ac·ci·den·tal

ac·ci·dent-prone

ac·cli·mate
ac·cli·mat·ed
ac·cli·mat·ing

ac·cli·ma·tion

ac·cli·ma·ti·za·tion

ac·cli·ma·tize
ac·cli·ma·tized
ac·cli·ma·tiz·ing

ac·com·mo·date
ac·com·mo·dat·ed
ac·com·mo·dat·ing

ac·com·mo·da·tion

ac·com·mo·da·tive

ac·couche·ment

acholous

ac·couche·ment
for·cé
  pl ac·couche·ments
  for·cé
ac·cre·tion
ac·cre·tion·ary
acel·lu·lar
ace·nes·the·sia
acen·tric
ace·pha·lia
aceph·a·lo·cyst
aceph·a·lo·cyst·ic
aceph·a·lous
aceph·a·lus
  pl aceph·a·li
acer·vu·lus
  pl acer·vu·li
acer·vu·lus ce·re·
bri
aces·o·dyne
ace·ta
  pl of acetum
ac·e·tab·u·lar
ac·e·tab·u·lar
ac·e·tab·u·lo·plas·
ty
  pl ac·e·tab·u·lo·plas·
  ties
ac·e·tab·u·lum
  pl ac·e·tab·u·lums
  or ac·e·tab·u·la
ac·et·al·de·hyde
acet·amin·o·phen
ac·et·an·i·lide
  or ac·et·an·i·lid
ac·et·ar·sone
  also ac·et·ar·sol

ac·e·tate
ac·et·azol·amide
ace·tic
ace·ti·fi·ca·tion
ace·ti·fi·er
ace·ti·fy
  ace·ti·fied
  ace·ti·fy·ing
ac·e·tin
ace·to·ac·e·tate
ace·to·ace·tic
ace·to·bac·ter
ace·to·hex·amide
acet·o·in
ac·e·tol·y·sis
  pl ac·e·tol·y·ses
ace·to·me·roc·tol
ac·e·tom·e·ter
ace·to·mor·phine
ace·to·naph·thone
ac·e·tone
ac·e·ton·emia
ac·e·ton·emic
ac·e·ton·ic
ace·to·ni·trile
ac·e·ton·uria
ace·to·phe·net·i·
din
  also ac·et·phe·net·i·
  din
ace·to·phe·none
ace·to·sol·u·ble
ace·tous
ac·e·tract
ace·tum
  pl ace·ta
ace·tyl

acet·y·lase
acet·y·late
  acet·y·lat·ed
  acet·y·lat·ing
acet·y·la·tion
acet·y·la·tive
ace·tyl·cho·line
ace·tyl·cho·lin·es·
ter·ase
ace·tyl·cho·lin·ic
ace·tyl-coA
ace·tyl co·en·zyme
A
ace·tyl·cys·te·ine
acet·y·lene
acet·y·le·nic
ace·tyl·meth·yl·car·
bi·nol
ace·tyl·phe·nyl·hy·
dra·zine
ace·tyl·sa·lic·y·late
ace·tyl·sal·i·cyl·ic
ace·tyl·trans·fer·
ase
Ac-glob·u·lin
acha·la·sia
ache
  ached
  ach·ing
Achil·lea
achil·le·ine
Achil·les ten·don
achlor·hy·dria
achlor·hy·dric
acho·lia
achol·ic
  or acho·lous

achol·uria
achol·uric
achon·dro·pla·sia
achon·dro·plas·tic
achroa·cyte
achro·ma·cyte
achro·ma·sia
ach·ro·mat
ach·ro·mat·ic
ach·ro·mat·i·cal·ly
achro·ma·tism
achro·ma·tize
  achro·ma·tized
  achro·ma·tiz·ing
achro·mato·cyte
achro·ma·tol·y·sis
  pl achro·ma·tol·y·ses
achro·ma·to·phil·ia
achro·ma·top·sia
achro·mia
achro·mic
achro·mo·bac·ter
achro·mo·trich·ia
achy
  ach·i·er
  ach·i·est
achy·lia
achy·lia gas·tri·ca
achy·lous
acic·u·lar
acid
ac·i·de·mia
ac·id-fast
acid·ic
acid·i·fi·able
acid·i·fi·ca·tion
acid·i·fi·er

acid·i·fy
  acid·i·fied
  acid·i·fy·ing
ac·i·dim·e·ter
ac·i·di·met·ric
ac·i·dim·e·try
  pl ac·i·dim·e·tries
acid·i·ty
  pl acid·i·ties
acid·o·gen·ic
acid·o·phil
  also acid·o·phile
acid·o·phil·ia
acid·o·phil·ic
ac·i·doph·i·lus
ac·i·do·sis
  pl ac·i·do·ses
ac·i·dot·ic
acid·u·late
  acid·u·lat·ed
  acid·u·lat·ing
acid·u·la·tion
acid·u·lous
ac·id·uria
ac·id·uric
ac·i·nar
acin·ic
ac·i·nous
aci·nus
  pl aci·ni
ac·la·sis
  pl ac·la·ses
aclas·tic
ac·me
ac·ne
ac·ned

ac·ne·form
  or ac·ne·iform
ac·ne·gen·ic
ac·ne ro·sa·cea
  pl ac·nae ro·sa·ce·ae
ac·ne ur·ti·ca·ta
ac·ne vul·gar·is
  pl ac·nae vul·gar·es
ac·ni·tis
acoe·lo·mate
ac·o·ine
acon·i·tase
ac·o·nite
ac·o·nit·ic
acon·i·tine
Ac·o·ni·tum
acou·me·ter
acous·ma
  pl acous·mas
  or acous·ma·ta
acous·tic
  or acous·ti·cal
acous·tics
ac·quire
  ac·quired
  ac·quir·ing
ac·ral
acra·nia
  absence of the skull (see
  Acrania)
Acra·nia
  a division of the chor-
  dates (see acrania)
ac·rid
ac·ri·dine
ac·ri·fla·vine
ac·ro·blast

ac·ro·cen·tric
ac·ro·ce·pha·lia
ac·ro·ce·phal·ic
ac·ro·ceph·a·lo·
　syn·dac·ty·ly
　pl ac·ro·ceph·a·lo·
　　syn·dac·ty·lies
ac·ro·ceph·a·ly
　pl ac·ro·ceph·a·lies
ac·ro·chor·don
ac·ro·cy·a·no·sis
　pl ac·ro·cy·a·no·ses
ac·ro·cy·a·not·ic
ac·ro·der·ma·ti·tis
ac·ro·der·ma·ti·tis
　en·tero·path·i·ca
ac·ro·dyn·ia
ac·ro·ge·ria
ac·ro·ker·a·to·sis
　pl ac·ro·ker·a·to·ses
acro·le·in
ac·ro·me·gal·ic
ac·ro·meg·a·loid
ac·ro·meg·a·ly
　pl ac·ro·meg·a·lies
acro·mi·al
ac·ro·mi·cria
acro·mio·cla·vic·u·
　lar
acro·mi·on
acro·mi·on·ec·to·
　my
　pl acro·mi·on·ec·to·
　　mies
acro·pa·chy
　pl acro·pa·chies
ac·ro·par·es·the·sia

acrop·a·thy
　pl acrop·a·thies
ac·ro·phobe
ac·ro·pho·bia
ac·ro·sclero·der·
　ma
ac·ro·scle·ro·sis
　pl ac·ro·scle·ro·ses
ac·ro·so·mal
ac·ro·some
ac·ry·late
acryl·ic
ac·ry·lo·ni·trile
Ac·taea
ac·tin
ac·tin·ic
ac·ti·nism
ac·tin·i·um
ac·ti·no·bac·il·lo·
　sis
　pl ac·ti·no·bac·il·lo·
　　ses
ac·ti·no·ba·cil·lus
　pl ac·ti·no·ba·cil·li
ac·ti·no·der·ma·ti·
　tis
　pl ac·ti·no·der·ma·ti·
　　tis·es
　or ac·ti·no·der·ma·tit·
　　i·des
ac·ti·nom·e·ter
ac·ti·nom·e·try
　pl ac·ti·nom·e·tries
ac·ti·no·my·ces
　pl ac·ti·no·my·ces
Ac·ti·no·my·ce·ta·
　ce·ae

ac·ti·no·my·ce·tal
Ac·ti·no·my·ce·ta·
　les
ac·ti·no·my·cete
ac·ti·no·my·ce·tin
ac·ti·no·my·ce·
　tous
ac·ti·no·my·cin
ac·ti·no·my·co·ma
　pl ac·ti·no·my·co·mas
　or ac·ti·no·my·co·ma·
　　ta
ac·ti·no·my·co·sis
　pl ac·ti·no·my·co·ses
ac·ti·no·my·cot·ic
ac·ti·non
ac·tin·o·phage
ac·ti·no·phy·to·sis
　pl ac·ti·no·phy·to·ses
ac·ti·no·spec·ta·
　cin
ac·ti·no·ther·a·py
　pl ac·ti·no·ther·a·pies
ac·tion
ac·ti·va·tor
ac·tive
ac·tiv·i·ty
　pl ac·tiv·i·ties
ac·to·my·o·sin
Ac·u·ar·ia
acu·ity
　pl acu·ities
acu·le·ate
acu·mi·nate
acu·pres·sure
acu·pres·sur·ist
acu·punc·ture

acu·punc·tur·ist
acu·sec·tor
acute
acy·a·not·ic
acy·clic
acy·clo·vir
ac·yl
ac·yl·ase
ac·yl·ate
　ac·yl·at·ed
　ac·yl·at·ing
ac·y·la·tion
acys·tic
adac·tyl·ia
ad·a·man·tine
ad·a·man·ti·no·ma
　pl ad·a·man·ti·no·
　　mas
　also ad·a·man·ti·no·
　　ma·ta
ad·a·man·ti·no·ma·
　tous
ad·a·man·to·blast
ad·a·man·to·blas·
　to·ma
　pl ad·a·man·to·blas·
　　to·mas
　or ad·a·man·to·blas·
　　to·ma·ta
Ad·am's ap·ple
ad·ams·ite
Ad·ams-Stokes
　syn·drome
Ad·an·so·nia
ad·ap·ta·tion
ad·ap·ta·tion·al
adapt·er
　also adap·tor

adap·tive
ad·ap·tom·e·ter
ad·ap·tom·e·try
　pl ad·ap·tom·e·tries
ad·ax·i·al
ad·der
ad·dict
ad·dic·tion
ad·dic·tive
Ad·dis count
Ad·di·so·ni·an
Ad·di·son's dis·
　ease
ad·di·tive
ad·di·tiv·i·ty
　pl ad·di·tiv·i·ties
ad·du·cent
ad·duct
ad·duc·tion
ad·duc·tive
ad·duc·tor
ad·duc·tor brev·
　is
ad·duc·tor hal·lu·
　cis
ad·duc·tor lon·
　gus
ad·duc·tor mag·
　nus
ad·duc·tor pol·li·
　cis
ad·e·nase
aden·drit·ic
aden·i·form
ad·e·nine
ad·e·ni·tis

ad·e·no·ac·an·tho·
　ma
　pl ad·e·no·ac·an·tho·
　　mas
　or ad·e·no·ac·an·tho·
　　ma·ta
ad·e·no·car·ci·no·
　ma
　pl ad·e·no·car·ci·no·
　　mas
　or ad·e·no·car·ci·no·
　　ma·ta
ad·e·no·car·ci·no·
　ma·tous
ad·e·no·cys·to·ma
　pl ad·e·no·cys·to·mas
　or ad·e·no·cys·to·ma·
　　ta
ad·e·no·fi·bro·ma
　pl ad·e·no·fi·bro·mas
　or ad·e·no·fi·bro·ma·
　　ta
ad·e·no·hy·poph·y·
　se·al
　or ad·e·no·hy·po·
　　phys·i·al
ad·e·no·hy·poph·y·
　sis
　pl ad·e·no·hy·poph·y·
　　ses
ad·e·noid
ad·e·noi·dal
ad·e·noid·ec·to·my
　pl ad·e·noid·ec·to·
　　mies
ad·e·noid·ism
ad·e·noid·itis
ad·e·no·lym·pho·
　cele

ad·e·no·lym·pho·ma
  pl ad·e·no·lym·pho·mas
  or ad·e·no·lym·pho·ma·ta

ad·e·no·ma
  pl ad·e·no·mas
  or ad·e·no·ma·ta

ad·e·no·ma·toid
ad·e·no·ma·to·sis
  pl ad·e·no·ma·to·ses

ad·e·no·ma·tous
ad·e·no·mere
ad·e·no·my·o·ma
  pl ad·e·no·my·o·mas
  or ad·e·no·my·o·ma·ta

ad·e·no·my·o·sis
  pl ad·e·no·my·o·ses

ad·e·no·neu·ral
ad·e·nop·a·thy
  pl ad·e·nop·a·thies

aden·o·sine
aden·o·sine mo·no·phos·phate
aden·o·sine 3′,5′-mo·no·phos·phate
aden·o·sine tri·phos·pha·tase
aden·o·sine tri·phos·phate
ad·e·no·sis
  pl ad·e·no·ses

S-aden·o·syl·me·thi·o·nine
ad·e·no·tome

ad·e·not·o·my
  pl ad·e·not·o·mies

ad·e·no·vi·ral
ad·e·no·vi·rus
ad·e·nyl
ade·nyl·ate cy·clase
ad·e·nyl·ic
ad·eps
  pl ad·i·pes

ad·eps la·nae
  pl adi·pes la·nae

ad·here
  ad·hered
  ad·her·ing
ad·her·ence
ad·he·sion
ad·he·sion·al
ad·he·sive
adi·a·do·ko·ki·ne·sis
  or adi·a·do·cho·ki·ne·sis
  pl adi·a·do·ko·ki·ne·ses
  or adi·a·do·cho·ki·ne·ses

Ad·i·an·tum
adi·a·ther·man·cy
  pl adi·a·ther·man·cies

ad·i·ence
ad·i·ent
ad·i·pes
  pl of adeps

ad·i·phen·ine
adip·ic
ad·i·po·cere
ad·i·po·cyte

ad·i·po·gen·e·sis
  pl ad·i·po·gen·e·ses

ad·i·po·ge·net·ic
ad·i·pose
ad·i·po·sis
  pl ad·i·po·ses

ad·i·po·sis do·lo·ro·sa
ad·i·pos·i·ty
  pl ad·i·pos·i·ties

ad·i·po·so·gen·i·tal
adip·sia
ad·i·tus
  pl ad·i·tus
  or ad·i·tus·es

ad·junct
ad·junc·tive
ad·just
ad·just·abil·i·ty
  pl ad·just·abil·i·ties

ad·just·able
ad·just·ed
ad·jus·tive
ad·just·ment
ad·just·men·tal
ad·ju·vant
Ad·le·ri·an
ad-lib
  adjective
    not controlled by
    schedule

ad lib
  adverb
    without limit

ad li·bi·tum
ad·max·il·lary

ad·mi·nic·u·lum
lin·e·ae al·bae
ad·min·is·ter
  ad·min·is·tered
  ad·min·is·ter·ing
ad·min·is·tra·tion
ad·nexa
ad·nex·al
ad·nex·i·tis
ad·o·les·cence
ad·o·les·cent
ad·oral
ad·re·nal
ad·re·nal·ec·to·
  mized
ad·re·nal·ec·to·my
  pl ad·re·nal·ec·to·
  mies

adren·a·line
adren·a·lin·emia
adren·a·lone
ad·ren·ar·che
adren·er·gen
ad·ren·er·gic
ad·ren·er·gi·cal·ly
ad·re·no·chrome
ad·re·no·cor·ti·cal
ad·re·no·cor·ti·coid
ad·re·no·cor·ti·co·
  mi·met·ic
ad·re·no·cor·ti·co·
  ste·roid
ad·re·no·cor·ti·co·
  tro·pic
  or ad·re·no·cor·ti·co·
  tro·phic

ad·re·no·cor·ti·co·
  tro·pin
  or ad·re·no·cor·ti·co·
  tro·phin
adre·no·gen·i·tal
adre·no·glo·mer·u·
  lo·tro·pin
adre·no·lyt·ic
adre·no·med·ul·
  lary
adre·no·pause
adre·no·re·cep·tor
adre·no·ste·rone
adre·no·sym·pa·
  thet·ic
adre·no·tro·pic
  or adre·no·tro·phic
adria·my·cin
ad·sorb
ad·sorb·abil·i·ty
  pl ad·sorb·abil·i·ties
ad·sorb·able
ad·sor·bate
ad·sor·bent
ad·sorp·tion
ad·sorp·tive
adult
adul·ter·ant
adul·ter·ate
  adul·ter·at·ed
  adul·ter·at·ing
adul·ter·a·tion
adul·ter·a·tor
adult·hood
ad·vance·ment
ad·ven·ti·tia
ad·ven·ti·tial

ad·ven·ti·tious
ady·na·mia
ady·nam·ic
ae·des
  pl ae·des
ae·dine
ae·lu·ro·phobe
  var of ailurophobe
ae·lu·ro·pho·bia
  var of ailurophobia
aer·ate
  aer·at·ed
  aer·at·ing
aer·a·tion
aer·a·tor
aero·bac·ter
aer·obe
aer·o·bic
aer·o·bi·cal·ly
aer·o·bics
aero·bi·o·log·i·cal
aero·bi·ol·o·gy
  pl aero·bi·ol·o·gies
aero·bi·o·sis
  pl aero·bi·o·ses
aero·bi·ot·ic
aero·cele
aer·odon·tal·gia
aer·odon·tal·gic
aer·odon·tia
aero·dy·nam·ic
  or aero·dy·nam·i·cal
aero·dy·nam·i·cist
aero·dy·nam·ics
aero·em·bo·lism
aero·em·phy·se·ma
aero·gel

ae·rog·e·nous
aero·med·i·cal
aero·med·i·cine
aer·om·e·ter
aero·neu·ro·sis
  pl aero·neu·ro·ses
aero-oti·tis me·dia
aero·pause
aero·pha·gia
aer·oph·a·gy
  pl aer·oph·a·gies
aero·pho·bia
aero·pho·bic
aero·plank·ton
aero·scope
aero·si·nus·itis
aero·sol
aero·sol·iza·tion
aero·sol·ize
  aero·sol·ized
  aero·sol·iz·ing
aero·ther·a·peu·
  tics
aer·oti·tis
aero·to·nom·e·ter
aer·ot·ro·pism
Aes·cu·la·pi·an
Aes·cu·la·pi·us
aes·cu·le·tin
  var of esculetin
aes·cu·lin
  var of esculin
afe·brile
af·fect
af·fec·tion
af·fec·tive

af·fec·tiv·i·ty
  pl af·fec·tiv·i·ties
af·fer·ent
  conducting toward a
  nerve center (see
  efferent)
af·fin·i·ty
  pl af·fin·i·ties
af·flux
afi·brin·o·gen·emia
af·la·tox·in
af·ter·birth
af·ter·care
af·ter·cat·a·ract
af·ter·damp
af·ter·dis·charge
af·ter·ef·fect
af·ter·im·age
af·ter·load
af·ter·pain
af·ter·po·ten·tial
af·ter·sen·sa·tion
af·ter·taste
af·to·sa
aga·lac·tia
aga·lac·tic
aga·mete
agam·ic
agam·ma·glob·u·
  lin·emia
Aga·mo·mer·mis
agam·ont
agan·gli·on·ic
agar
agar-agar
aga·ric
Agar·i·ca·ce·ae

agar·i·cin
Agar·i·cus
aga·rose
agas·tric
aga·ve
agen·e·sis
  pl agen·e·ses
agen·i·tal·ism
Agent Or·ange
ageu·sia
ageu·sic
ag·ger
ag·glom·er·ate
  ag·glom·er·at·ed
  ag·glom·er·at·ing
ag·glom·er·a·tion
ag·glu·ti·na·bil·i·ty
  pl ag·glu·ti·na·bil·i·
  ties
ag·glu·ti·na·ble
ag·glu·ti·nate
  ag·glu·ti·nat·ed
  ag·glu·ti·nat·ing
ag·glu·ti·na·tion
ag·glu·ti·na·tive
ag·glu·ti·nin
ag·glu·ti·no·gen
ag·glu·ti·no·gen·ic
ag·glu·ti·noid
ag·glu·ti·no·scope
ag·gre·gate
  ag·gre·gat·ed
  ag·gre·gat·ing
ag·gres·sin
ag·gres·sion
ag·gres·sive
ag·gres·sor

ag·i·to·pha·sia
aglu·con
  or aglu·cone
agly·cone
  also agly·con
ag·mi·nate
  or ag·mi·nat·ed
ag·nail
ag·na·thia
ag·na·thus
ag·no·gen·ic
ag·no·sia
ag·o·nal
ag·o·nist
ag·o·nis·tic
ag·o·ny
  pl ag·o·nies
ag·o·ra·phobe
ag·o·ra·pho·bia
ag·o·ra·pho·bi·ac
ag·o·ra·pho·bic
agou·ti
agram·ma·tism
agran·u·lo·cyte
agran·u·lo·cyt·ic
agran·u·lo·cy·to·sis
  pl agran·u·lo·cy·to·ses
agraph·ia
agraph·ic
agryp·nia
ague
aich·mo·pho·bia
aid·man
  pl aid·men
AIDS-re·lat·ed
  com·plex
ail·ment

ai·lu·ro·phobe
  or ae·lu·ro·phobe
ai·lu·ro·pho·bia
  or ae·lu·ro·pho·bia
ai·nhum
air·sick
air·way
aj·o·wan
akar·y·ote
aka·thi·sia
  also aca·thi·sia
aki·ne·sia
aki·ne·sis
  pl aki·ne·ses
aki·net·ic
ala
  pl alae
ala na·si
  pl alae na·si
al·a·nine
al·a·nyl
alar
alas·trim
al·ba
al·be·do
  pl al·be·dos
Al·bers-Schön·berg
  dis·ease
al·bin·ic
al·bi·nism
al·bi·nis·tic
al·bi·no
  pl al·bi·nos
al·bi·not·ic
al·bo·ci·ne·re·ous
al·bu·gin·ea
al·bu·men

al·bu·min
al·bu·mi·nate
al·bu·min·oid
al·bu·mi·nom·e·ter
al·bu·min·ous
al·bu·min·uria
al·bu·min·uric
al·bu·mose
al·bu·mos·uria
al·ca·lig·e·nes
  pl al·ca·lig·e·nes
al·cap·ton
  var of alkapton
al·cap·ton·uria
  var of alkaptonuria
al·cap·ton·uric
  var of alkaptonuric
Al·cock's ca·nal
al·co·gel
al·co·hol
al·co·hol·ate
al·co·hol·ic
al·co·hol·i·cal·ly
al·co·hol·ism
al·co·hol·iza·tion
al·co·hol·ize
al·co·hol·ized
al·co·hol·iz·ing
al·co·hol·om·e·ter
al·co·hol·om·e·try
  pl al·co·hol·om·e·tries
al·co·hol·ophil·ia
al·co·hol·y·sis
  pl al·co·hol·y·ses
al·co·sol
al·de·hyde
al·de·hy·dic

al·do·bi·uron·ic
al·do·hex·ose
al·dol
al·dol·ase
al·don·ic
al·dose
al·do·side
al·do·ste·rone
al·do·ste·ron·ism
al·dox·ime
al·drin
alec·i·thal
alem·bic
alem·mal
Al·e·tris
aleu·ke·mia
aleu·ke·mic
al·eu·rone
alex·ia
alex·ic
alex·in
al·ga
    pl al·gae
    also al·gas

Al·gae
al·gal
al·ge·do·nic
al·ge·sia
al·ge·sic
al·ge·sim·e·ter
al·ge·sim·e·try
    pl al·ge·sim·e·tries
al·get·ic
al·gi·cid·al
al·gi·cide
    or al·gae·cide
al·gid

al·gin
al·gi·nate
al·gin·ic
al·go·lag·nia
al·go·lag·ni·ac
al·go·lag·nic
al·go·lag·nist
al·gol·o·gy
    pl al·gol·o·gies
al·gom·e·ter
al·gom·e·try
    pl al·gom·e·tries

al·go·phil·ia
al·goph·i·list
al·go·pho·bia
al·gor
al·gor mor·tis
alien·ate
    alien·at·ed
    alien·at·ing
alien·ation
alien·ist
ali·es·ter·ase
ali·form
al·i·ment
al·i·men·ta·ry
al·i·men·ta·tion
al·i·men·to·ther·a·
    py
    pl al·i·men·to·ther·a·
    pies
ali·na·sal
al·i·phat·ic
al·i·quot
ali·sphe·noid
aliz·a·rin
    also aliz·a·rine

al·ka·le·mia
al·ka·les·cence
al·ka·les·cent
al·ka·li
    pl al·ka·lies
    or al·ka·lis
al·ka·lim·e·ter
al·ka·lim·e·try
    pl al·ka·lim·e·tries
al·ka·line
al·ka·lin·i·ty
    pl al·ka·lin·i·ties
al·ka·lin·iza·tion
al·ka·lin·ize
    al·ka·lin·ized
    al·ka·lin·iz·ing
al·ka·li·za·tion
al·ka·lize
    al·ka·lized
    al·ka·liz·ing
al·ka·loid
al·ka·loi·dal
al·ka·lo·sis
    pl al·ka·lo·ses
al·ka·lot·ic
al·kane
al·kan·nin
al·kap·ton
    or al·cap·ton
al·kap·ton·uria
    or al·cap·ton·uria
al·kap·ton·uric
    or al·cap·ton·uric
al·ka·ver·vir
al·kene
alky
al·kyl

al·kyl·amine
al·kyl·ate
 al·kyl·at·ed
 al·kyl·at·ing
al·kyl·ation
al·lan·to·ic
al·lan·to·in
al·lan·to·is
 pl al·lan·to·ides
al·lele
al·le·lic
al·lel·ism
al·le·lo·morph
al·le·lo·mor·phic
al·le·lo·mor·phism
al·ler·gen
al·ler·gen·ic
al·ler·ge·nic·i·ty
 pl al·ler·ge·nic·i·ties
al·ler·gic
al·ler·gist
al·ler·gol·o·gy
 pl al·ler·gol·o·gies
al·ler·gy
 pl al·ler·gies
al·le·vi·ate
 al·le·vi·at·ed
 al·le·vi·at·ing
al·le·vi·a·tion
al·le·vi·a·tive
al·li·cin
al·li·ga·tion
al·li·um
al·lo·an·ti·body
 pl al·lo·an·ti·bod·ies
al·lo·an·ti·gen
al·lo·an·ti·gen·ic

al·lo·bar·bi·tal
al·lo·chi·ria
 also al·lo·chei·ria
al·lo·cor·tex
Al·lo·der·ma·nys·sus
al·lo·erot·ic
al·lo·er·o·tism
 also al·lo·erot·i·cism
al·lo·ge·ne·ic
 also al·lo·gen·ic
al·lo·graft
al·lo·im·mune
al·lo·me·tric
al·lom·e·try
 pl al·lom·e·tries
al·lo·morph
al·lo·mor·phic
al·lo·mor·phism
al·lo·path
al·lo·path·ic
al·lo·path·i·cal·ly
al·lop·a·thy
 pl al·lop·a·thies
al·lo·plas·tic·i·ty
 pl al·lo·plas·tic·i·ties
al·lo·plas·ty
 pl al·lo·plas·ties
al·lo·poly·ploid
al·lo·poly·ploi·dy
 pl al·lo·poly·ploi·dies
al·lo·psy·chic
al·lo·pu·ri·nol
all-or-none
all-or-noth·ing
al·lose
al·lo·some

al·lo·ste·ric
al·lo·ste·ri·cal·ly
al·lo·ste·ry
 pl al·lo·ste·ries
al·lo·te·tra·ploid
al·lo·te·tra·ploi·dy
 pl al·lo·te·tra·ploi·dies
al·lo·trans·plant
al·lo·trans·plan·ta·
 tion
al·lo·trope
al·lo·tro·phic
al·lo·trop·ic
al·lo·trop·i·cal·ly
al·lot·ro·py
 pl al·lot·ro·pies
al·lo·type
al·lo·typ·ic
al·lo·typ·i·cal·ly
al·lo·typy
 pl al·lo·typies
al·lox·an
al·lox·azine
al·loy
al·lo·zyme
al·lo·zy·mic
al·lyl
al·lyl·amine
N-al·lyl·nor·mor·
 phine
al·mond
al·oe
al·oe-em·o·din
alo·et·ic
alo·gia
al·o·in

al·o·pe·cia
al·o·pe·cia ar·e·a·ta
al·o·pe·cic
al·pha
al·pha-ad·ren·er·
gic
al·pha-ad·re·no·
cep·tor
   also al·pha-ad·re·no·
   re·cep·tor
al·pha-fe·to·pro·
tein
   or α-fe·to·pro·tein
al·pha-he·li·cal
al·pha-he·lix
   or α-he·lix
al·pha-ke·to·glu·
tar·ic ac·id
al·pha-1-an·ti·tryp·
sin
al·pha-re·cep·tor
al·pha-to·coph·er·
ol
al·pren·o·lol
al·ser·ox·y·lon
Al·sto·nia
al·sto·nine
al·ter
   al·tered
   al·ter·ing
al·ter·ant
al·ter·ative
al·ter·nate
al·ter·nat·ing
al·ter·na·tion
al·thaea
   or al·thea

al·ti·tude
Alt·mann's gran·
ules
al·tri·gen·der·ism
al·trose
al·um
alu·men
   pl alu·mens
   or alu·mi·na
alu·mi·na
alu·mi·num
al·ve·o·lar
al·ve·o·late
al·ve·o·la·tion
al·ve·o·lec·to·my
   pl al·ve·o·lec·to·mies
al·ve·o·li·tis
al·ve·o·lo·con·dyl·
e·an
al·ve·o·lo·na·sal
al·ve·o·lo·plas·ty
   or al·veo·o·lo·plas·ty
   pl al·ve·o·lo·plas·ties
   or al·veo·plas·ties
al·ve·o·lus
   pl al·ve·o·li
al·ve·us
   pl al·vei
Alz·hei·mer's dis·
ease
amaas
am·a·cri·nal
   or am·a·crine
amal·gam
amal·gam·ate
   amal·gam·at·ed
   amal·gam·at·ing

amal·gam·ation
amal·gam·ator
am·an·din
am·a·ni·ta
am·a·ni·tin
aman·ta·dine
am·a·ranth
am·a·roid
amas·tia
ama·tho·pho·bia
am·au·ro·sis
   pl am·au·ro·ses
am·au·ro·sis fu·
gax
am·au·rot·ic
amax·o·pho·bia
am·ber
am·ber·gris
am·bi·dex·ter·i·ty
   pl am·bi·dex·ter·i·ties
am·bi·dex·trous
am·bi·ent
am·bi·lat·er·al
am·bi·lat·er·al·i·ty
   pl am·bi·lat·er·al·i·
   ties
am·bi·o·pia
am·bi·sex·u·al
am·bi·sex·u·al·i·ty
   pl am·bi·sex·u·al·i·
   ties
am·bi·tend·en·cy
   pl am·bi·tend·en·cies
am·biv·a·lence
am·biv·a·len·cy
   pl am·biv·a·len·cies
am·biv·a·lent

am·bi·ver·sion
am·bi·ver·sive
am·bi·vert
am·bly·chro·mat·ic
am·bly·om·ma
am·bly·ope
am·bly·opia
am·bly·opic
am·bly·o·scope
am·bo·cep·tor
am·bon
   also am·bo
   pl am·bo·nes

am·bos
Am·bro·sia
am·bu·lance
am·bu·lant
am·bu·late
   am·bu·lat·ed
   am·bu·lat·ing
am·bu·la·tion
am·bu·la·to·ri·ly
am·bu·la·to·ry
ame·ba
   also amoe·ba
   pl ame·bas
   or ame·bae
   also amoe·bas
   or amoe·bae

am·e·bi·a·sis
   also am·oe·bi·a·sis
   pl am·e·bi·a·ses
   also am·oe·bi·a·ses

ame·bic
   also amoe·bic
ame·bi·cid·al
   also amoe·bi·cid·al

ame·bi·cide
   also amoe·bi·cide
ame·bi·form
   also amoe·bi·form
ame·bo·cyte
   also amoe·bo·cyte
ame·boid
   also amoe·boid
amel·a·not·ic
am·e·lo·blast
am·e·lo·blas·tic
am·e·lo·blas·to·ma
   pl am·e·lo·blas·to·
     mas
   or am·e·lo·blas·to·
     ma·ta

am·e·lo·den·tin·al
am·e·lo·gen·e·sis
   pl am·e·lo·gen·e·ses

am·e·lo·gen·e·sis
   im·per·fec·ta
am·e·lus
   pl am·e·li
amen·or·rhea
amen·or·rhe·ic
amen·tia
am·er·i·ci·um
ameth·o·caine
am·e·thop·ter·in
am·e·trope
am·e·tro·pia
am·e·tro·pic
am·i·an·thoid
ami·cron
am·i·dase
am·ide
amid·ic

am·i·dine
ami·do
am·i·done
ami·do·py·rine
amil·o·ride
amim·ia
am·i·nate
   am·i·nat·ed
   am·i·nat·ing
amin·azine
   or amin·azin
amine
ami·no
ami·no·ace·tic
ami·no·ac·i·de·mia
ami·no·ac·id·uria
ami·no·ben·zo·ate
ami·no·ben·zo·ic
γ-ami·no·bu·tyr·ic
   ac·id
   var of gamma-amino-
     butyric acid

ami·no·glu·teth·i·
   mide
am·i·nol·y·sis
   pl am·i·nol·y·ses

ami·no·lyt·ic
ami·no·pep·ti·dase
am·i·noph·yl·line
am·i·nop·ter·in
ami·no·py·rine
ami·no·sal·i·cyl·ic
ami·no·thi·a·zole
ami·no·trans·fer·
   ase
ami·to·sis
   pl ami·to·ses

ami·tot·ic
ami·tot·i·cal·ly
am·i·trip·ty·line
am·me·ter
am·mo·nia
am·mo·ni·ac
am·mo·ni·a·cal
   am·mo·ni·at·ed
   am·mo·ni·at·ing
am·mo·ni·fi·ca·tion
am·mo·ni·fy
   am·mo·ni·fied
   am·mo·ni·fy·ing
am·mo·ni·um
am·ne·sia
am·ne·si·ac
   also am·ne·sic
   noun
am·ne·sic
   also am·ne·si·ac
   adjective
am·nes·tic
am·nio·cen·te·sis
   pl am·nio·cen·te·ses
am·nio·gen·e·sis
   pl am·nio·gen·e·ses
am·ni·og·ra·phy
   pl am·ni·og·ra·phies
am·ni·on
   pl am·ni·ons
   or am·nia
am·nio·scope
am·ni·os·co·py
   pl am·ni·os·co·pies
Am·ni·o·ta
am·ni·ote
am·ni·ot·ic

am·ni·ot·o·my
   pl am·ni·ot·o·mies
amo·bar·bi·tal
amo·di·a·quine
   or amo·di·a·quin
amoe·ba
   var of ameba
Amoe·ba
am·oe·bi·a·sis
   var of amebiasis
amoe·bic
   var of amebic
amoe·bi·cid·al
   var of amebicidal
amoe·bi·cide
   var of amebicide
amoe·bi·form
   var of amebiform
amoe·bo·cyte
   var of amebocyte
amoe·boid
   var of ameboid
Amoe·bo·tae·nia
amor·phin·ism
amor·phous
amor·phus
   pl amor·phi
   or amor·phus·es
amox·i·cil·lin
am·per·age
am·pere
am·phet·amine
am·phi·ar·thro·di·al
am·phi·ar·thro·sis
   pl am·phi·ar·thro·ses
Am·phib·ia

am·phib·i·an
am·phi·bol·ic
am·phi·cen·tric
am·phi·cra·nia
am·phi·mix·is
   pl am·phi·mix·es
am·phi·ox·us
   pl am·phi·oxi
   or am·phi·ox·us·es
am·phi·phile
am·phi·phil·ic
Am·phi·sto·ma·ta
am·phi·stome
am·phit·ri·chous
am·pho·lyte
am·pho·lyt·ic
am·pho·phil
am·pho·phil·ic
am·phor·ic
am·pho·ter·ic
am·pho·ter·i·cin
am·pho·ter·ism
am·pi·cil·lin
am·pli·fi·ca·tion
am·pli·fi·er
am·pli·fy
   am·pli·fied
   am·pli·fy·ing
am·pli·tude
am·pule
   or am·poule
   or am·pul
am·pul·la
   pl am·pul·lae
am·pul·la of Va·ter
am·pul·la·ry
   also am·pul·lar

am·pul·lu·la
pl am·pul·lu·lae

am·pu·tate
am·pu·tat·ed
am·pu·tat·ing

am·pu·ta·tion

am·pu·tee

amu·sia

amy·e·lia

amy·e·lin·ic

amy·e·lon·ic

amyg·da·la
pl amyg·da·lae

amyg·da·lase

amyg·da·lec·to·mized

amyg·da·lec·to·my
pl amyg·da·lec·to·mies

amyg·da·lin

amyg·da·line

amyg·da·loid

amyg·da·lot·o·my
pl amyg·da·lot·o·mies

am·yl

am·y·la·ceous

am·y·lase

am·y·lene

am·y·lo·dex·trin

am·y·loid

am·y·loid·osis
pl am·y·loid·oses

am·y·lol·y·sis
pl am·y·lol·y·ses

am·y·lo·lyt·ic

am·y·lo·pec·tin

am·y·lop·sin

amy·lose

am·y·lum

amyo·to·nia

amyo·to·nia con·gen·i·ta

amyo·tro·phia

amyo·tro·phic

amy·ot·ro·phy
pl amy·ot·ro·phies

ana

an·a·bae·na

ana·bi·o·sis
pl ana·bi·o·ses

ana·bi·ot·ic

an·a·bol·ic

anab·o·lism

anab·o·lite

an·acid·i·ty
pl an·acid·i·ties

an·a·clit·ic

an·a·crot·ic

anac·ro·tism

ana·cul·ture

anae·mia
var of anemia

anae·mic
var of anemic

an·aer·obe

an·aer·o·bic

an·aer·o·bi·cal·ly

an·aero·bi·o·sis
pl an·aero·bi·o·ses

an·a·gen

anal

an·a·lep·tic

an·al·ge·sia

an·al·ge·sic

an·al·get·ic

anal·i·ty
pl anal·i·ties

anal·ly

an·al·o·gous

an·a·logue
or an·a·log

anal·o·gy
pl anal·o·gies

anal·y·sand

anal·y·sis
pl anal·y·ses

an·a·lyst

an·a·lyt·ic
or an·a·lyt·i·cal

an·a·lyze
an·a·lyzed
an·a·lyz·ing
an·a·lyz·er

an·am·ne·sis
pl an·am·ne·ses

an·am·nes·tic

an·am·ni·on·ic

an·an·kas·tic
or an·an·cas·tic

ana·phase

ana·pha·sic

anaph·o·ret·ic

an·aph·ro·di·sia

an·aph·ro·dis·i·ac

ana·phy·lac·tic

ana·phy·lac·ti·cal·ly

ana·phy·lac·to·gen

an·a·phy·lac·to·gen·ic

ana·phy·lac·toid

an·a·phyl·a·tox·in
ana·phy·lax·is
  pl ana·phy·lax·es
an·a·pla·sia
an·a·plas·ma
  pl an·a·plas·ma·ta
  or an·a·plas·mas
an·a·plas·mo·sis
  pl an·a·plas·mo·ses
an·a·plas·tic
an·a·rith·mia
an·ar·thria
an·a·sar·ca
an·a·sar·cous
an·a·stal·sis
  pl an·a·stal·ses
anas·to·mose
  anas·to·mosed
  anas·to·mos·ing
anas·to·mo·sis
  pl anas·to·mo·ses
anas·to·mot·ic
an·a·tom·ic
  or an·a·tom·i·cal
an·a·tom·i·co·path·
  o·log·ic
  or an·a·tom·i·co·path·
  o·log·i·cal
anat·o·mist
anat·o·mize
  anat·o·mized
  anat·o·miz·ing
anat·o·my
  pl anat·o·mies
ana·tox·in
an·au·dia
an·chor·age

an·cil·lary
  pl an·cil·lar·ies
an·co·nal
  also an·co·ne·al
an·co·ne·us
  pl an·co·nei
An·cy·los·to·ma
An·cy·lo·sto·mat·i·
  dae
an·cyl·o·stome
  or an·kyl·o·stome
an·cy·lo·sto·mi·a·
  sis
  or an·ky·lo·sto·mi·a·
  sis
  also an·chy·lo·sto·mi·
  a·sis
  pl an·cy·lo·sto·mi·a·
  ses
  or an·ky·lo·sto·mi·a·
  ses
  also an·chy·lo·sto·mi·
  a·ses
an·dro·gen
an·dro·gen·e·sis
  pl an·dro·gen·e·ses
an·dro·ge·net·ic
an·dro·gen·ic
an·drog·e·nize
  an·drog·e·nized
  an·drog·e·niz·ing
an·dro·gyne
an·drog·y·nism
an·drog·y·nous
an·drog·y·ny
  pl an·drog·y·nies
an·droid
an·dro·mi·met·ic
an·dro·pho·bia

an·dro·pho·bic
an·dro·stane
an·dro·stene·di·
  one
an·dros·ter·one
an·elec·tro·ton·ic
an·elec·trot·o·nus
ane·mia
  also anae·mia
ane·mic
  also anae·mic
ane·mi·cal·ly
anem·o·ne
anem·o·nin
an·en·ce·pha·lia
an·en·ce·phal·ic
an·en·ceph·a·lus
  pl an·en·ceph·a·li
an·en·ceph·a·ly
  pl an·en·ceph·a·lies
an·en·ter·ous
aneph·ric
an·er·gic
an·er·gy
  pl an·er·gies
an·er·oid
an·es·the·sia
an·es·the·si·ol·o·
  gist
an·es·the·si·ol·o·gy
  pl an·es·the·si·ol·o·
  gies
an·es·thet·ic
an·es·thet·i·cal·ly
anes·the·tist
anes·the·ti·za·tion

anes·the·tize
 anes·the·tized
 anes·the·tiz·ing
an·es·trous
an·es·trus
ane·thum
 pl ane·tha
 or ane·thums
an·eu·ploid
an·eu·ploi·dy
 pl an·eu·ploi·dies
an·eu·rine
 also an·eu·rin
aneu·ro·gen·ic
an·eu·rysm
 also an·eu·rism
an·eu·rys·mal
 also an·eu·ris·mal
an·eu·rys·mal·ly
an·gel·i·ca
an·gen·e·sis
 pl an·gen·e·ses
an·gi·i·tis
 pl an·gi·it·i·des
an·gi·na
an·gi·nal
an·gi·na pec·to·ris
an·gi·noid
an·gi·nose
 or an·gi·nous
an·gio·blast
an·gio·blas·tic
an·gio·car·dio·gram
an·gio·car·dio·graph·ic

an·gio·car·di·og·ra·phy
 pl an·gio·car·di·og·ra·phies
an·gio·cho·li·tis
an·gio·cyst
an·gio·ede·ma
 pl an·gio·ede·mas
 or an·gio·ede·ma·ta
an·gio·gen·e·sis
 pl an·gio·gen·e·ses
an·gio·gen·ic
an·gio·gram
an·gio·graph·ic
an·gio·graph·i·cal·ly
an·gi·og·ra·phy
 pl an·gi·og·ra·phies
an·gi·oid
an·gio·ker·a·to·ma
 pl an·gio·ker·a·to·mas
 or an·gio·ker·a·to·ma·ta
an·gi·ol·o·gy
 pl an·gi·ol·o·gies
an·gi·o·ma
 pl an·gi·o·mas
 or an·gi·o·ma·ta
an·gi·o·ma·to·sis
 pl an·gi·o·ma·to·ses
an·gi·o·ma·tous
an·gio·neu·rot·ic
an·gi·op·a·thy
 pl an·gi·op·a·thies
an·gio·plas·ty
 pl an·gio·plas·ties

an·gio·sar·co·ma
 pl an·gio·sar·co·mas
 or an·gio·sar·co·ma·ta
an·gio·sco·to·ma
 pl an·gio·sco·to·mas
 or an·gio·sco·to·ma·ta
an·gio·sco·tom·e·try
 pl an·gio·sco·tom·e·tries
an·gio·spasm
an·gio·spas·tic
an·gio·sperm
an·gio·sper·mous
an·gi·os·to·my
 pl an·gi·os·to·mies
an·gio·ten·sin
an·gio·ten·sin·ase
an·gio·ten·sin·o·gen
an·gio·ton·ic
an·gio·to·nin
an·gle·ber·ry
 pl an·gle·ber·ries
an·gos·tu·ra
ang·strom
an·gu·late
 an·gu·lat·ed
 an·gu·lat·ing
an·gu·la·tion
an·gu·lus
 pl an·gu·li
an·he·do·nia
an·he·don·ic
an·hi·dro·sis
 pl an·hi·dro·ses
an·hi·drot·ic

an·hy·drase
  an·hy·drat·ed
  an·hy·drat·ing
an·hy·dra·tion
an·hy·dre·mia
an·hy·dre·mic
an·hy·dride
an·hy·dro·hy·
  droxy·pro·ges·
  ter·one
an·hy·drous
ani
  pl of anus
an·ic·ter·ic
anile
an·i·lide
an·i·line
ani·lin·gus
  or ani·linc·tus
an·i·lin·ism
anil·i·ty
  pl anil·i·ties
an·i·ma
an·i·mal
an·i·mal·cule
  also an·i·mal·cu·lum
  pl an·i·mal·cules
  also an·i·mal·cu·la
an·i·mate
an·i·mat·ed
an·i·ma·tion
an·i·mism
an·i·mist
an·i·mis·tic
an·i·mus
an·ion
an·ion·ic

an·ion·i·cal·ly
an·ion·ot·ro·py
  pl an·ion·ot·ro·pies
an·irid·ia
ani·seed
  also an·ise·seed
an·is·ei·ko·nia
an·is·ei·kon·ic
an·iso·co·ria
an·iso·cy·to·sis
  pl an·iso·cy·to·ses
an·iso·cy·tot·ic
an·isog·a·mous
an·isog·a·my
  pl an·isog·a·mies
an·iso·me·tro·pia
an·iso·me·tro·pic
an·iso·trop·ic
an·isot·ro·py
  pl an·isot·ro·pies
an·kle
an·kle·bone
an·ky·lose
  an·ky·losed
  an·ky·los·ing
an·ky·lo·sis
  pl an·ky·lo·ses
An·ky·los·to·ma
an·kyl·o·stome
  var of ancylostome
an·ky·lo·sto·mi·a·
  sis
  var of ancylostomiasis
an·ky·lot·ic
an·la·ge
  pl an·la·gen
  also an·la·ges

an·nat·to
an·neal
an·ne·lid
An·nel·i·da
an·nel·i·dan
an·nu·lar
an·nu·lus
  pl an·nu·li
  also an·nu·lus·es
ano·ci·as·so·ci·a·
  tion
ano·ci·a·tion
an·od·al
an·ode
an·od·ic
an·od·i·cal·ly
an·odon·tia
an·o·dyne
an·o·dy·nia
an·o·e·sis
  pl an·o·e·ses
an·o·et·ic
ano·gen·i·tal
anoia
anom·a·lo·scope
anom·a·lous
anom·a·ly
  pl anom·a·lies
an·o·mer
ano·mia
ano·mic
an·onych·ia
anon·y·ma
  pl anon·y·mae
  or anon·y·mas
ano·op·sia
  or an·op·sia

anoph·e·les

anoph·e·li·cide

anoph·e·line

anoph·e·lism

an·oph·thal·mia

an·oph·thal·mic

an·oph·thal·mos

ano·plas·ty
  pl ano·plas·ties

An·op·lo·ceph·a·la

An·o·plu·ra

an·or·chism

ano·rec·tal

an·o·rec·tic

an·o·ret·ic

an·orex·ia

an·orex·ia ner·vo·sa

ano·rex·i·ant

ano·rex·ic

ano·rex·i·gen·ic

an·or·tho·pia

ano·scope

ano·sco·py
  pl ano·sco·pies

an·os·mia

an·os·mic

an·os·phre·sia

an·otia

ano·vag·i·nal

an·ovu·lant

an·ovu·la·tion

an·ovu·la·to·ry

an·ox·emia

an·ox·emic

an·ox·ia

an·ox·ic

an·sa
  pl an·sae

an·sa cer·vi·ca·lis

an·sa hy·po·glos·si

an·sa sub·cla·via

an·si·form

ant·ac·id
  also an·ti·ac·id

an·tag·o·nism

an·tag·o·nist

an·tag·o·nis·tic

an·tag·o·nis·ti·cal·ly

an·tag·o·nize

an·tag·o·nized

an·tag·o·niz·ing

an·te·bra·chi·al
  or an·ti·bra·chi·al

an·te·bra·chi·um
  or an·ti·bra·chi·um
  pl an·te·bra·chia
  or an·ti·bra·chia

an·te·car·di·um
  var of anticardium

an·te·cor·nu
  pl an·te·cor·nua

an·te·cu·bi·tal

an·te·flex·ion

an·te·grade

an·te·hy·poph·y·sis
  pl an·te·hy·poph·y·ses

an·te·mor·tem

an·te·na·tal

an·te·par·tum

an·te·ri·or

an·tero·grade

an·tero·in·fe·ri·or

an·tero·lat·er·al

an·tero·me·di·al

an·tero·pos·te·ri·or

an·tero·su·pe·ri·or

an·te·ver·sion

an·te·vert

ant·he·lix
  var of antihelix

an·thel·min·tic
  also an·thel·min·thic

an·tho·cy·a·nin
  also an·tho·cy·an

an·thra·cene

an·thra·coid

an·thra·co·sil·i·co·sis
  pl an·thra·co·sil·i·co·ses

an·thra·co·sis
  pl an·thra·co·ses

an·thra·cot·ic

an·thra·lin

an·thra·ni·late

an·thra·nil·ic

an·thrax
  pl an·thra·ces

an·throne

an·thro·po·gen·ic

an·thro·pog·ra·phy
  pl an·thro·pog·ra·phies

an·thro·poid

An·thro·poi·dea

an·thro·poi·de·an

an·thro·po·log·i·cal

an·thro·pol·o·gist

an·thro·pol·o·gy
  pl an·thro·pol·o·gies

an·thro·pom·e·ter

an·thro·po·met·ric

an·thro·pom·e·try
  pl an·thro·pom·e·tries

an·thro·poph·a·
  gous

an·thro·poph·a·gy
  pl an·thro·poph·a·gies

an·thro·po·phil·ic

an·ti·abor·tion

an·ti·ac·id
  var of antacid

an·ti·al·ler·gic
  also an·ti·al·ler·gen·ic

an·ti·an·a·phy·lax·
  is
  also an·ti·an·a·phy·
    lax·es

an·ti·an·dro·gen

an·ti·ane·mic

an·ti·an·gi·nal

an·ti·an·ti·body
  pl an·ti·an·ti·bod·ies

an·ti·anx·i·ety

an·ti·ar·rhyth·mic

an·ti·ar·thrit·ic

an·ti·bac·te·ri·al

an·ti·bi·o·sis
  pl an·ti·bi·o·ses

an·ti·bi·ot·ic

an·ti·bi·ot·i·cal·ly

an·ti·body
  pl an·ti·bod·ies

an·ti·bra·chi·al
  var of antebrachial

an·ti·bra·chi·um
  var of antebrachium

an·ti·can·cer

an·ti·car·cin·o·gen

an·ti·car·ci·no·gen·
  ic

an·ti·car·di·um
  or an·te·car·di·um
  pl an·ti·car·dia
  or an·te·car·dia

an·ti·car·ies

an·ti·cat·a·lyst

an·ti·cho·lin·er·gic

an·ti·cho·lin·es·ter·
  ase

an·ti·clot·ting

an·tic·ne·mi·on

an·ti·co·ag·u·lant

an·ti·co·ag·u·late

  an·ti·co·ag·u·lat·
    ed

  an·ti·co·ag·u·lat·
    ing

an·ti·co·ag·u·la·
  tion

an·ti·co·ag·u·lat·ive

an·ti·co·ag·u·la·to·
  ry

an·ti·co·ag·u·lin

an·ti·co·don

an·ti·com·ple·ment

an·ti·com·ple·men·
  ta·ry

an·ti·con·vul·sant
  also an·ti·con·vul·sive

an·ti·cus

an·ti·de·pres·sant
  also an·ti·de·pres·sive

an·ti·di·a·bet·ic

an·ti·di·ar·rhe·al

an·ti·di·ure·sis
  pl an·ti·di·ure·ses

an·ti·di·uret·ic

an·ti·dot·al

an·ti·dote

an·ti·dro·mic

an·ti·dro·mi·cal·ly

an·ti·dys·en·ter·ic

an·ti·emet·ic

an·ti·en·zyme

an·ti·ep·i·lep·tic

an·ti·es·tro·gen

an·ti·fer·til·i·ty

an·ti·fi·bril·la·to·ry

an·ti·fi·bri·no·ly·
  sin

an·ti·fi·bri·no·ly·sis
  pl an·ti·fi·bri·no·ly·
    ses

an·ti·fi·bri·no·lyt·ic

an·ti·flat·u·lent

an·ti·flu·o·ri·da·
  tion·ist

an·ti·fun·gal

an·ti·gen

an·ti·gen·emia

an·ti·gen·ic

an·ti·gen·i·cal·ly

an·ti·gen·ic·i·ty
  pl an·ti·gen·ic·i·ties

an·ti·glob·u·lin

an·ti·go·nad·o·trop·
  ic

an·ti·go·nad·o·tro·
pin
an·ti·he·lix
also ant·he·lix
pl an·ti·he·li·ces
or an·ti·he·lix·es
also ant·he·li·ces
or ant·he·lix·es
an·ti·he·mo·phil·ic
an·ti·hem·or·rhag·
ic
an·ti·hi·drot·ic
an·ti·his·ta·mine
an·ti·his·ta·min·ic
an·ti·hor·mone
an·ti·hu·man
an·ti·hy·per·lip·id·
emic
an·ti·hy·per·ten·
sive
also an·ti·hy·per·ten·
sion
an·ti·im·mu·no·
glob·u·lin
an·ti·in·fec·tive
an·ti·in·flam·ma·
to·ry
pl an·ti·in·flam·ma·
to·ries
an·ti·in·su·lin
an·ti·ke·to·gen·ic
an·ti·leu·ke·mic
also an·ti·leu·ke·mia
an·ti·lu·et·ic
an·ti·lym·pho·cyte
an·ti·lym·pho·cyt·
ic
an·ti·ly·sin

an·ti·ly·sis
pl an·ti·ly·ses
an·ti·lyt·ic
an·ti·ma·lar·i·al
an·ti·me·tab·o·lite
an·ti·mi·cro·bi·al
also an·ti·mi·cro·bic
an·ti·mi·tot·ic
an·ti·mo·ni·al
an·ti·mo·ny
pl an·ti·mo·nies
an·ti·mo·nyl
an·ti·mus·ca·rin·ic
an·ti·mu·ta·gen·ic
an·ti·my·cin A
an·ti·my·cot·ic
an·ti·neo·plas·tic
an·ti·neu·rit·ic
an·tin·i·on
an·ti·nu·cle·ar
an·ti·ox·i·dant
an·ti·par·a·sit·ic
an·ti·par·kin·so·
nian
also an·ti·par·kin·son
an·ti·path·ic
an·tip·a·thy
pl an·tip·a·thies
an·ti·pe·ri·od·ic
an·ti·peri·stal·sis
pl an·ti·peri·stal·ses
an·ti·peri·stal·tic
an·ti·per·spi·rant
an·ti·phlo·gis·tic
an·ti·plas·min
an·ti·plas·tic
an·ti·plate·let

an·ti·pneu·mo·coc·
cal
or an·ti·pneu·mo·coc·
cic
or an·ti·pneu·mo·coc·
cus
an·ti·pode
pl an·tip·o·des
an·ti·pol·lu·tion
an·ti·pol·lu·tion·ist
an·ti·pro·te·ase
an·ti·pro·throm·
bin
an·ti·pro·to·zo·al
an·ti·pru·rit·ic
an·ti·pseu·do·mo·
nal
an·ti·psy·chot·ic
an·ti·py·re·sis
pl an·ti·py·re·ses
an·ti·py·ret·ic
an·ti·py·rine
also an·ti·py·rin
an·ti·ra·chit·ic
an·ti·re·tic·u·lar
an·ti·rheu·mat·ic
an·ti·schis·to·so·
mal
an·ti·schizo·phren·
ic
an·ti·scor·bu·tic
an·ti·se·cre·to·ry
an·ti·sep·sis
pl an·ti·sep·ses
an·ti·sep·tic
an·ti·sep·ti·cal·ly

an·ti·sep·ti·cize
  an·ti·sep·ti·cized
  an·ti·sep·ti·ciz·ing
an·ti·se·rum
an·ti·si·al·a·go·gic
an·ti·si·der·ic
an·ti·so·cial
an·ti·spas·mod·ic
an·ti·strep·to·coc·cal
  or an·ti·strep·to·coc·cic
an·ti·strep·to·ki·nase
an·ti·strep·to·ly·sin
an·ti·syph·i·lit·ic
an·ti·the·nar
an·ti·throm·bic
an·ti·throm·bin
an·ti·throm·bo·plas·tin
an·ti·throm·bot·ic
an·ti·thy·roid
an·ti·tox·ic
an·ti·tox·in
an·ti·tox·i·no·gen·ic
an·ti·trag·i·cus
  pl an·ti·trag·i·ci
an·ti·tra·gus
  pl an·ti·tra·gi
an·ti·try·pano·som·al
  or an·ti·try·pano·some
an·ti·tryp·sin

an·ti·tryp·tic
an·ti·tu·ber·cu·lous
  or an·ti·tu·ber·cu·lo·sis
  also an·ti·tu·ber·cu·lar
an·ti·tu·mor
  also an·ti·tu·mor·al
an·ti·tus·sive
an·ti·ty·phoid
an·ti·ul·cer
an·ti·ven·in
an·ti·vi·ral
an·ti·vi·ta·min
an·ti·vivi·sec·tion
an·ti·xe·roph·thal·mic
an·tral
an·trec·to·my
  pl an·trec·to·mies
an·trorse
an·tro·scope
an·tros·to·my
  pl an·tros·to·mies
an·trot·o·my
  pl an·trot·o·mies
an·trum
  pl an·tra
an·trum of High·more
anu·cle·ate
  also anu·cle·at·ed
an·u·re·sis
  pl an·u·re·ses
an·u·ret·ic
an·uria
an·uric

anus
  pl anus·es
  or ani
an·vil
anx·i·ety
  pl anx·i·eties
anx·io·lyt·ic
anx·ious
aor·ta
  pl aor·tas
  or aor·tae
aor·tic
aor·tico·pul·mo·nary
aor·tico·re·nal
aor·ti·tis
aor·to·cor·o·nary
aor·to·gram
aor·to·graph·ic
aor·tog·ra·phy
  pl aor·tog·ra·phies
aor·to·il·i·ac
aor·to·pul·mo·nary
aor·to·sub·cla·vi·an
apar·a·lyt·ic
ap·a·thet·ic
ap·a·thet·i·cal·ly
ap·a·thy
  pl ap·a·thies
ap·a·tite
ape·ri·ent
ape·ri·od·ic
aper·i·tive
ap·er·tu·ra
  pl ap·er·tu·rae
ap·er·ture

apex
pl apex·es
or api·ces

apex·car·di·og·ra·
phy
pl apex·car·di·og·ra·
phies

Ap·gar score
apha·gia
apha·kia
apha·kic
apha·sia
apha·si·ac
apha·sic
apha·si·ol·o·gist
apha·si·ol·o·gy
pl apha·si·ol·o·gies

aphe·mia
apho·nia
apho·nic
aphos·pho·ro·sis
pl aphos·pho·ro·ses

aphra·sia
aphra·sic
aph·ro·di·sia
aph·ro·di·si·ac
also aph·ro·di·si·a·cal

aph·tha
also ap·tha
pl aph·thae
also ap·thae

aph·thic
aph·thoid
aph·thon·gia
aph·tho·sis
pl aph·tho·ses

aph·thous

api·cal
apic·ec·to·my
pl apic·ec·to·mies

api·ces
pl of apex

api·ci·tis
pl api·ci·tes

api·co·ec·to·my
pl api·co·ec·to·mies

api·col·y·sis
pl api·col·y·ses

Api·um
apla·cen·tal
ap·la·nat·ic
aplan·a·tism
apla·sia
aplas·tic
ap·nea
ap·ne·ic
ap·neu·sis
pl ap·neu·ses

ap·neus·tic
apo·chro·mat·ic
apo·crine
Apoc·y·num
ap·o·dal
or ap·o·dus

apo·en·zyme
ap·o·fer·ri·tin
apo·lar
apo·li·po·pro·tein
apo·mor·phine
apo·neu·ro·sis
pl apo·neu·ro·ses

apo·neu·rot·ic
apoph·y·se·al

apoph·y·sis
pl apoph·y·ses

apoph·y·si·tis
ap·o·plec·tic
ap·o·plec·ti·cal·ly
ap·o·plec·ti·form
ap·o·plexy
pl ap·o·plex·ies

apo·pro·tein
apoth·e·car·ies'
mea·sure
apoth·e·cary
pl apoth·e·car·ies

ap·ox·e·sis
apo·zy·mase
ap·pa·ra·tus
pl ap·pa·ra·tus·es
or ap·pa·ra·tus

ap·par·ent
ap·pear·ance
ap·pend·age
ap·pen·dec·to·my
pl ap·pen·dec·to·mies

ap·pen·di·ceal
also ap·pen·di·cal
or ap·pen·di·cial

ap·pen·di·cec·to·
my
pl ap·pen·di·cec·to·
mies

ap·pen·di·ces epi·
ploi·cae
ap·pen·di·ci·tis
ap·pen·di·cos·to·
my
pl ap·pen·di·cos·to·
mies

ap·pen·dic·u·lar

ap·pen·dix
 pl ap·pen·dix·es
 or ap·pen·di·ces

ap·per·ceive
 ap·per·ceived
 ap·per·ceiv·ing
ap·per·cep·tion
ap·per·cep·tive
ap·per·son·a·tion
ap·pe·tite
ap·pe·ti·tion
ap·pe·ti·tive
ap·pla·nate
ap·pla·na·tion
ap·pli·ance
ap·pli·ca·tion
ap·pli·ca·tor
ap·pose
 ap·posed
 ap·pos·ing
ap·po·si·tion
ap·prox·i·mal
ap·prox·i·mate
 ap·prox·i·mat·ed
 ap·prox·i·mat·
  ing
ap·prox·i·ma·tion
aprac·tic
 or aprax·ic

aprax·ia
apron
apros·ex·ia
apro·ti·nin
ap·tha
 var of aphtha

ap·ti·tude

apty·a·lism
ap·y·rase
apy·ret·ic
apy·rex·ia
apy·rex·i·al
aqua
 pl aquae
 or aquas

aqua pu·ra
aqua re·gia
aquat·ic
aqua vi·tae
aq·ue·duct
aq·ue·duct of Syl·
  vi·us
aque·ous
arab·i·nose
ara·bi·no·side
arab·i·tol
ar·a·chid·ic
ar·a·chi·don·ic
arach·nid
Arach·ni·da
arach·nid·ism
ar·ach·ni·tis
arach·no·dac·ty·ly
 pl arach·no·dac·ty·lies

arach·noid
arach·noi·dal
arach·noi·dea
arach·noid·ism
arach·noid·itis
ara·lia
ar·a·ro·ba
ar·bo·res·cent
ar·bo·ri·za·tion

ar·bor·ize
 ar·bor·ized
 ar·bor·iz·ing
ar·bo·vi·rol·o·gy
 pl ar·bo·vi·rol·o·gies

ar·bo·vi·rus
ar·bu·tin
arc
ar·cade
ar·cha·ic
arch·en·ter·on
 pl arch·en·tera

ar·che·typ·al
ar·che·type
ar·chil
 also or·chil

ar·chi·pal·li·um
ar·chi·tec·ton·ic
ar·chi·tec·ton·ics
ar·chi·tec·tur·al
ar·chi·tec·ture
arch of Cor·ti
ar·ci·form
arc·to·staph·y·los
ar·cu·a·le
 pl ar·cu·a·lia

ar·cu·ate
ar·cus
 pl ar·cus

ar·cus se·nil·is
ar·dor uri·nae
ar·ea pla·cen·ta·lis
ar·ea po·stre·ma
ar·e·ca
arec·o·line
are·flex·ia
are·flex·ic

are·gen·er·a·tive
ar·e·na·ceous
ar·e·na·tion
ar·e·na·vi·rus
are·o·la
 pl are·o·lae
 or are·o·las

are·o·lar
are·o·late
are·o·la·tion
ar·e·om·e·ter
ar·gen·taf·fin
 or ar·gen·taf·fine

ar·gen·taf·fin·i·ty
 pl ar·gen·taf·fin·i·ties

ar·gen·taf·fin·o·ma
 pl ar·gen·taf·fin·o·
 mas
 or ar·gen·taf·fin·o·
 ma·ta

ar·gen·to·phil
 or ar·gen·to·phile
 or ar·gen·to·phil·ic

ar·gen·tum
ar·gi·nase
ar·gi·nine
ar·gon
Ar·gyll Rob·ert·son
 pu·pil
ar·gyr·ia
ar·gyr·o·phil
 or ar·gyr·o·phile
 or ar·gyr·o·phil·ic

ar·gyr·o·phil·ia
ar·gy·ro·sis
 pl ar·gy·ro·ses

ari·bo·fla·vin·osis
 pl ari·bo·fla·vin·oses

arith·mo·ma·nia
ar·ma·men·tar·i·
 um
 pl ar·ma·men·tar·ia

arm·pit
Ar·neth in·dex
ar·ni·ca
ar·o·mat·ic
aro·ma·ti·za·tion
aro·ma·tize
 aro·ma·tized
 aro·ma·tiz·ing

arous·al
ar·rec·tor
 pl ar·rec·to·res
 or ar·rec·tors

ar·rec·tor pi·li
 mus·cle
ar·rest
ar·rest·ment
ar·rhe·no·blas·to·
 ma
 pl ar·rhe·no·blas·to·
 mas
 also ar·rhe·no·blas·to·
 ma·ta

ar·rhe·not·o·ky
 pl ar·rhe·not·o·kies

ar·rhyth·mia
ar·rhyth·mic
ar·row·root
ar·sa·nil·ic
ar·se·nate
ar·se·nic
 noun

ar·sen·ic
 adjective

ar·sen·i·cal
ar·sen·i·cal·ism
ar·se·nide
ar·se·ni·ous
 also ar·se·nous

ar·se·ni·um
ar·se·no·ther·a·py
 pl ar·se·no·ther·a·pies

ar·sen·ox·ide
ar·sine
ars·phen·a·mine
ar·te·mis·ia
ar·te·re·nol
ar·te·ria
 pl ar·te·ri·ae

ar·te·ri·al
ar·te·ri·al·iza·tion
ar·te·ri·al·ize
 ar·te·ri·al·ized
 ar·te·ri·al·iz·ing

ar·te·rio·cap·il·lary
ar·te·rio·gram
ar·te·rio·graph·ic
ar·te·rio·graph·i·
 cal·ly
ar·te·ri·og·ra·phy
 pl ar·te·ri·og·ra·phies

ar·te·ri·o·la
 pl ar·te·ri·o·lae

ar·te·ri·o·lar
ar·te·ri·ole
ar·te·rio·li·tis
ar·te·rio·lop·a·thy
 pl ar·te·rio·lop·a·thies

ar·te·rio·lo·scle·ro·sis
   pl ar·te·rio·lo·scle·ro·ses
ar·te·rio·lu·mi·nal
ar·te·rio·mes·en·ter·ic
ar·te·ri·op·a·thy
   pl ar·te·ri·op·a·thies
ar·te·ri·or·rha·phy
   pl ar·te·ri·or·rha·phies
ar·te·rio·scle·ro·sis
   pl ar·te·rio·scle·ro·ses
ar·te·rio·scle·rot·ic
ar·te·rio·si·nu·soi·dal
ar·te·rio·spasm
ar·te·rio·spas·tic
ar·te·ri·ot·o·my
   pl ar·te·ri·ot·o·mies
ar·te·rio·ve·nous
ar·ter·it·ic
ar·ter·i·tis
ar·tery
   or ar·ter·ies
ar·thral
ar·thral·gia
ar·thral·gic
ar·threc·to·my
   pl ar·threc·to·mies
ar·thrit·ic
ar·thrit·i·cal·ly
ar·thri·tis
   pl ar·thrit·i·des
ar·thri·tis de·for·mans

ar·thro·cen·te·sis
   pl ar·thro·cen·te·ses
ar·throd·e·sis
   pl ar·throd·e·ses
ar·thro·dia
   pl ar·thro·di·ae
ar·thro·di·al
ar·throd·ic
ar·thro·gram
ar·thro·graph·ic
ar·throg·ra·phy
   pl ar·throg·ra·phies
ar·thro·gry·po·sis
ar·thro·gry·po·sis
   mul·ti·plex con·gen·i·ta
ar·throl·o·gy
   pl ar·throl·o·gies
ar·throl·y·sis
   pl ar·throl·y·ses
ar·throm·e·ter
ar·throp·a·thy
   pl ar·throp·a·thies
ar·thro·plas·ty
   pl ar·thro·plas·ties
ar·thro·pod
Ar·throp·o·da
ar·throp·o·dan
ar·thro·scope
ar·thro·scop·ic
ar·thros·co·py
   pl ar·thros·co·pies
ar·thro·sis
   pl ar·thro·ses
ar·thro·spore
ar·throt·o·my
   pl ar·throt·o·mies

Ar·thus phe·nom·e·non
ar·tic·u·lar
ar·tic·u·late
   ar·tic·u·lat·ed
   ar·tic·u·lat·ing
ar·tic·u·la·tion
ar·tic·u·la·tor
ar·tic·u·la·to·ry
ar·ti·fact
ar·ti·fac·tu·al
ar·ti·fi·cial
ar·tio·dac·tyl
Ar·tio·dac·ty·la
ar·tio·dac·ty·lous
ary·ep·i·glot·tic
ary·te·noid
ary·te·noi·dec·to·my
   pl ary·te·noi·dec·to·mies
ary·te·noi·do·pexy
   pl ary·te·noi·do·pex·ies
asa·fet·i·da
   or asa·foet·i·da
as·a·rum
as·bes·tos
   also as·bes·tus
as·bes·to·sis
   pl as·bes·to·ses
as·ca·ri·a·sis
   pl as·ca·ri·a·ses
as·car·i·cid·al
as·car·i·cide
as·ca·rid
As·car·i·dae

as·car·i·di·a·sis
or as·ca·rid·i·o·sis
pl as·car·i·di·a·ses
or as·ca·rid·i·o·ses

as·car·i·do·sis
pl as·car·i·do·ses

as·ca·ris
pl as·car·i·des

As·ca·rops

as·cend

Asch·heim-Zon·dek test

Asch·off body

as·ci·tes
pl as·ci·tes

as·cit·ic

as·cle·pi·as

as·co·carp

as·co·carp·ic

as·co·my·cete

As·co·my·ce·tes

as·co·my·ce·tous

ascor·bate

ascor·bic

as·co·spore

as·co·spor·ic

as·cus
pl as·ci

asep·sis
pl asep·ses

asep·tic

asep·ti·cal·ly

asex·u·al

asex·u·al·i·ty
pl asex·u·al·i·ties

asex·u·al·i·za·tion

Asi·at·ic chol·era

asleep

aso·cial

as·pa·rag·i·nase

L-as·pa·rag·i·nase

as·par·a·gine

as·par·a·gus

as·par·tame

as·par·tase

as·par·tate

as·par·tic

as·par·to·ki·nase

as·pect

as·per·gil·lin

as·per·gil·lo·sis
pl as·per·gil·lo·ses

as·per·gil·lus
pl as·per·gil·li

asper·ma·tism

asper·mia

asper·mic

aspher·ic
or aspher·i·cal

as·phyx·ia

as·phyx·i·al

as·phyx·i·ant

as·phyx·i·ate
as·phyx·i·at·ed
as·phyx·i·at·ing

as·phyx·i·a·tion

as·phyx·i·a·tor

as·pid·i·nol

as·pid·i·um
pl as·pid·ia

as·pi·do·sper·ma

as·pi·do·sper·mine

as·pi·rate

as·pi·rat·ed

as·pi·rat·ing

as·pi·ra·tion

as·pi·ra·tor

as·pi·rin
pl as·pi·rin
or as·pi·rins

aspo·rog·e·nous

aspor·ous

aspor·u·late

as·say

as·sim·i·la·ble

as·sim·i·late
as·sim·i·lat·ed
as·sim·i·lat·ing

as·sim·i·la·tion

as·sim·i·la·tive

as·sist

as·so·ci·ate
verb
as·so·ci·at·ed
as·so·ci·at·ing

as·so·ci·ate
adjective or noun

as·so·ci·a·tion

as·so·ci·a·tion·ism

as·so·ci·a·tion·is·tic

as·so·cia·tive

as·sor·ta·tive

as·sort·ment

asta·sia

asta·sia-aba·sia

astat·ic

as·ta·tine

as·ter

astere·og·no·sis
  pl astere·og·no·ses

as·te·ri·on
  pl as·te·ria

as·te·ri·on·ic

aster·nal

as·tero·coc·cus
  pl as·tero·coc·ci

as·ter·oid

as·the·nia

as·then·ic

as·the·no·pia

as·the·no·pic

asth·ma

asth·mat·ic

asth·mat·i·cal·ly

asth·mo·gen·ic

as·tig·mat·ic

astig·ma·tism

astig·mia

as·tig·mom·e·ter
  or as·tig·ma·tom·e·ter

asto·ma·tous

as·trag·a·lar

astrag·a·lec·to·my
  pl astrag·a·lec·to·mies

as·trag·a·lus
  pl as·trag·a·li

as·tral

as·trin·gen·cy
  pl as·trin·gen·cies

as·trin·gent

as·tro·bi·o·log·i·cal

as·tro·bi·ol·o·gy
  pl as·tro·bi·ol·o·gies

as·tro·blast

as·tro·blas·to·ma
  pl as·tro·blas·to·mas
  or as·tro·blas·to·ma·ta

as·tro·cyte

as·tro·cyt·ic

as·tro·cy·to·ma
  pl as·tro·cy·to·mas
  or as·tro·cy·to·ma·ta

as·tro·glia

as·troid

asyl·la·bia

asy·lum

asym·bo·lia

asym·met·ri·cal
  or asym·met·ric

asym·me·try
  pl asym·me·tries

asymp·tom·at·ic

asymp·tom·at·i·cal·ly

asyn·ap·sis
  pl asyn·ap·ses

asyn·clit·ism

asy·ner·gia

asy·ner·gic

asyn·er·gy
  pl asyn·er·gies

asys·to·le

asys·to·lia

asys·tol·ic

asys·to·lism

atac·tic

at·a·rac·tic
  or at·a·rax·ic

at·a·rax·ia

at·a·raxy
  pl at·a·rax·ies

at·a·vism

at·a·vis·tic

atax·apha·sia
  or ataxi·apha·sia

atax·ia

atax·ia·gram

atax·ia·graph

atax·i·am·e·ter

atax·ic

at·el·ec·ta·sis
  pl at·el·ec·ta·ses

at·el·ec·tat·ic

ate·li·o·sis
  pl ate·li·o·ses

ate·li·ot·ic

at·e·lo·my·elia

ather·mic

ath·ero·gen·e·sis
  pl ath·ero·gen·e·ses

ath·ero·gen·ic

ath·er·o·ma
  pl ath·er·o·mas
  also ath·er·o·ma·ta

ath·er·o·ma·to·sis
  pl ath·er·o·ma·to·ses

ath·er·o·ma·tous

ath·ero·scle·ro·sis
  pl ath·ero·scle·ro·ses

ath·ero·scle·rot·ic

ath·ero·scle·rot·i·cal·ly

ath·e·toid

ath·e·to·sis
  pl ath·e·to·ses

ath·e·tot·ic
  or ath·e·to·sic

ath·lete's foot

ath·let·ic
athrep·sia
athrep·tic
ath·ro·cyte
ath·ro·cy·to·sis
pl ath·ro·cy·to·ses
athy·mic
athy·re·o·sis
pl athy·re·o·ses
athy·re·ot·ic
at·lan·tad
at·lan·tal
at·lan·to·ax·i·al
at·lan·to·oc·cip·i·
tal
at·las
at·mol·y·sis
pl at·mol·y·ses
at·mom·e·ter
at·mo·sphere
at·mo·spher·ic
at·om
atom·ic
atom·i·cal·ly
at·om·ism
at·om·is·tic
at·om·iza·tion
at·om·ize
at·om·ized
at·om·iz·ing
at·om·iz·er
ato·nia
aton·ic
ato·nic·i·ty
pl ato·nic·i·ties
at·o·ny
pl at·o·nies

ato·pen
ato·pic
ato·pog·no·sis
pl ato·pog·no·ses
at·o·py
pl at·o·pies
atox·ic
ATPase
atre·sia
atre·sic
atret·ic
atria
pl of atrium
atri·al
atrich·ia
at·ri·cho·sis
pl at·ri·cho·ses
atri·chous
atrio·ven·tric·u·lar
atri·um
pl atria
also atri·ums
At·ro·pa
atro·phia
atro·phic
at·ro·phy
noun
pl at·ro·phies
at·ro·phy
verb
at·ro·phied
at·ro·phy·ing
at·ro·pine
at·ro·pin·iza·tion
at·ro·pin·ize
at·ro·pin·ized
at·ro·pin·iz·ing

at·ro·scine
at·tach·ment
at·tack
at·tar
at·tend
at·ten·dance
at·ten·dant
at·tend·ing
at·ten·tion
at·ten·tion·al
at·ten·u·ate
at·ten·u·at·ed
at·ten·u·at·ing
at·ten·u·a·tion
at·tic
at·ti·co·mas·toid
at·ti·co·to·my
pl at·ti·co·to·mies
at·ti·tude
at·ti·tu·di·nal
at·tract
at·trac·tion
at·tri·tion
at·tri·tion·al
atyp·ia
atyp·i·cal
atyp·ism
au·di·bil·i·ty
pl au·di·bil·i·ties
au·di·ble
au·di·bly
au·dile
au·dio·gen·ic
au·dio·gram
au·di·o·log·i·cal
also au·di·o·log·ic
au·di·ol·o·gist

au·di·ol·o·gy
  pl au·di·ol·o·gies

au·di·om·e·ter

au·dio·met·ric

au·di·om·e·trist

au·di·om·e·try
  pl au·di·om·e·tries

au·dio·vi·su·al

au·di·tion

au·di·to·ry

Auer·bach's plex·
  us

au·la
  pl au·las
  or au·lae

au·ra
  pl au·ras
  also au·rae

au·ral
  of the ear or hearing
    (*see* oral)

au·ric

au·ri·cle

au·ric·u·la
  pl au·ric·u·lae

au·ric·u·lar

au·ric·u·lar·is
  pl au·ric·u·lar·es

au·ric·u·late

au·ric·u·lo·tem·po·
  ral

au·ric·u·lo·ven·tric·
  u·lar

au·rin

au·rist

au·ro·ther·a·py
  pl au·ro·ther·a·pies

au·ro·thio·glu·cose

au·rum

aus·cul·tate
  aus·cul·tat·ed
  aus·cul·tat·ing

aus·cul·ta·tion

aus·cul·ta·tor

aus·cul·ta·to·ry

au·ta·coid

au·te·cious
  var of autoecious

au·tism

au·tis·tic

au·to·ag·glu·ti·na·
  tion

au·to·ag·glu·ti·nin

au·to·anal·y·sis
  pl au·to·anal·y·ses

au·to·an·ti·body
  pl au·to·an·ti·bod·ies

au·to·as·phyx·i·a·
  tion

au·to·ca·tal·y·sis
  pl au·to·ca·tal·y·ses

au·to·cat·a·lyt·ic

au·toch·tho·nous

au·to·clav·abil·i·ty
  pl au·to·clav·abil·i·
    ties

au·to·clav·able

au·to·clave
  au·to·claved
  au·to·clav·ing

au·to·toe·cious
  also au·te·cious

au·to·erot·ic

au·to·erot·i·cal·ly

au·to·er·o·tism
  or au·to·erot·i·cism

au·tog·a·mous

au·tog·a·my
  pl au·tog·a·mies

au·tog·e·nous
  also au·to·gen·ic

au·tog·e·ny
  pl au·tog·e·nies

au·tog·no·sis
  pl au·tog·no·ses

au·to·graft

au·to·he·mo·ly·sin

au·to·he·mo·ly·sis
  pl au·to·he·mo·ly·ses

au·to·he·mo·ther·a·
  py
  pl au·to·he·mo·ther·a·
    pies

au·to·hyp·no·sis
  pl au·to·hyp·no·ses

au·to·hyp·not·ic

au·to·im·mune

au·to·im·mu·ni·ty
  pl au·to·im·mu·ni·
    ties

au·to·im·mu·ni·za·
  tion

au·to·im·mu·nize
  au·to·im·mu·
    nized
  au·to·im·mu·niz·
    ing

au·to·in·fec·tion

au·to·in·oc·u·la·ble

au·to·in·oc·u·la·
  tion

au·to·in·tox·i·ca·
tion
au·to·ki·ne·sis
pl au·to·ki·ne·ses
au·to·ki·net·ic
au·tol·o·gous
au·tol·y·sate
also au·tol·y·zate

au·tol·y·sin
au·tol·y·sis
pl au·tol·y·ses

au·to·lyt·ic
au·to·lyze
au·to·lyzed
au·to·lyz·ing
au·to·ma·nip·u·la·
tion
au·to·ma·nip·u·la·
tive
au·tom·a·tism
au·to·mne·sia
au·to·nom·ic
au·to·nom·i·cal·ly
au·ton·o·mous
au·ton·o·my
pl au·ton·o·mies
au·toph·a·gic
au·toph·a·gy
pl au·toph·a·gies
au·to·pho·bia
au·to·plas·tic
au·to·plas·ty
pl au·to·plas·ties

au·to·poly·ploid
au·to·poly·ploi·dy
pl au·to·poly·ploi·dies

au·top·sy
noun
pl au·top·sies

au·top·sy
verb
au·top·sied
au·top·sy·ing
au·to·psy·chic
au·to·ra·dio·gram
au·to·ra·dio·graph
au·to·ra·dio·graph·
ic
au·to·ra·di·og·ra·
phy
pl au·to·ra·di·og·ra·
phies

au·to·reg·u·la·tion
au·to·reg·u·la·to·ry
au·to·scope
au·tos·co·py
pl au·tos·co·pies

au·to·sen·si·ti·za·
tion
au·to·se·rum
au·to·sex·ing
au·to·so·mal
au·to·some
au·to·sug·gest
au·to·sug·gest·ibil·
i·ty
pl au·to·sug·gest·ibil·
i·ties

au·to·sug·ges·ti·ble
au·to·sug·ges·tion
au·to·ther·a·py
pl au·to·ther·a·pies

au·to·top·ag·no·sia

au·to·tox·emia
au·to·tox·in
au·to·trans·fuse
au·to·trans·fused
au·to·trans·fus·
ing
au·to·trans·fu·sion
au·to·trans·plant
au·to·trans·plan·ta·
tion
au·to·troph
au·to·tro·phic
au·to·tro·phi·cal·ly
au·to·tro·phy
pl au·to·tro·phies

au·to·vac·ci·na·tion
au·tox·i·da·tion
aux·an·o·gram
aux·an·o·graph·ic
aux·a·nog·ra·phy
pl aux·a·nog·ra·phies

aux·e·sis
pl aux·e·ses

aux·et·ic
aux·in
auxo·chrome
auxo·cyte
auxo·drome
auxo·troph
auxo·tro·phic
aux·ot·ro·phy
pl aux·ot·ro·phies

aval·vu·lar
avas·cu·lar
avas·cu·lar·i·ty
pl avas·cu·lar·i·ties

Ave·na

backbone

ave·nin
  or ave·nine

aver·sion

aver·sive

Aves

avi·an

avi·an·ize
  avi·an·ized
  avi·an·iz·ing

av·i·din

avir·u·lent

avi·ta·min·osis
  pl avi·ta·min·oses

avi·ta·min·ot·ic

A-V node
  or AV node

Avo·ga·dro's law

Avo·ga·dro's num·ber
  or Avo·ga·dro num·ber

avoid·ance

avoid·ant

av·oir·du·pois

avulse
  avulsed
  avuls·ing

avul·sion

axe·nic

axe·ni·cal·ly

ax·i·al

ax·ile

ax·il·la
  pl ax·il·lae
  or ax·il·las

ax·il·lary

ax·is
  pl ax·es

axo·ax·o·nal
  or axo·ax·on·ic

axo·den·drit·ic

axo·lem·ma

ax·om·e·ter

ax·on
  also ax·one

ax·o·nal

ax·o·ne·mal

ax·o·neme

ax·on·o·tme·sis
  pl ax·on·o·tme·ses

axo·plasm

axo·plas·mic

axo·so·mat·ic

axo·style

Ayer·za's dis·ease

aza·se·rine

aza·thi·o·prine

azeo·trope

azide

az·i·do

az·i·do·thy·mi·dine

azin·phos·meth·yl

azo

azo·lit·min

azo·osper·mia

azo·osper·mic

azo·pro·tein

azo·sul·fa·mide

azote

azo·te·mia

azo·te·mic

azo·tor·rhea

azo·tu·ria

azure

azy·gog·ra·phy
  pl azy·gog·ra·phies

azy·gos
  noun

azy·gos
  also azy·gous
  adjective

B

Ba·bes-Ernst gran·ule

ba·be·sia

babe·si·a·sis
  pl babe·si·a·ses

Ba·be·si·i·dae

ba·be·si·o·sis
  pl ba·be·si·o·ses

Ba·bin·ski re·flex
  or Ba·bin·ski's re·flex

Bac·il·la·ce·ae

ba·cil·la·ry
  or ba·cil·lar

bac·il·le·mia

bac·il·li·form

bac·il·lo·sis
  pl bac·il·lo·ses

bac·il·lu·ria

bac·il·lu·ric

ba·cil·lus
  pl ba·cil·li

ba·cil·lus Cal·mette-Gué·rin

bac·i·tra·cin

back·ache

back·bone

back·cross
bac·ter·emia
bac·ter·emic
bac·te·ria
   pl of bacterium
Bac·te·ri·a·ce·ae
bac·te·ri·al
bac·te·ri·cid·al
bac·te·ri·cid·al·ly
bac·te·ri·cide
bac·te·ri·cid·in
   or bac·te·ri·o·cid·in

bac·ter·id
bac·ter·in
bac·te·rio·cin
bac·te·rio·gen·ic
   also bac·te·ri·og·e·
   nous

bac·te·ri·o·log·ic
   or bac·te·ri·o·log·i·cal
bac·te·ri·ol·o·gist
bac·te·ri·ol·o·gy
   pl bac·te·ri·ol·o·gies
bac·te·rio·ly·sin
bac·te·ri·ol·y·sis
   pl bac·te·ri·ol·y·ses
bac·te·ri·o·lyt·ic
bac·te·rio·phage
bac·te·ri·oph·a·gy
   pl bac·te·ri·oph·a·gies
bac·te·rio·sta·sis
   pl bac·te·rio·sta·ses
bac·te·rio·stat
bac·te·rio·stat·ic
bac·te·rio·stat·i·cal·
   ly

bac·te·rio·ther·a·
   peu·tic
bac·te·rio·ther·a·py
   pl bac·te·rio·ther·a·
   pies

bac·te·rio·tox·in
bac·te·rio·tro·pic
bac·te·ri·ot·ro·pin
bac·te·ri·um
   sing of bacteria
bac·te·ri·uria
bac·te·ri·uric
bac·te·ri·za·tion
bac·te·rize
  bac·te·rized
  bac·te·riz·ing
bac·te·roid
Bac·te·roi·da·ce·ae
bac·te·roi·des
   pl bac·te·roi·des

bac·u·lum
   pl bac·u·lums
   or bac·u·la

ba·gasse
bag·as·so·sis
   pl bag·as·so·ses

Bain·bridge re·flex
bak·er's itch
bal·ance
bal·anced
ba·lan·ic
bal·a·ni·tis
bal·a·no·pos·thi·tis
ba·lan·tid·i·al
   or ba·lan·tid·ic

bal·an·ti·di·a·sis
   or bal·an·tid·i·o·sis
   pl bal·an·ti·di·a·ses
   or bal·an·tid·i·o·ses

bal·an·tid·i·um
   pl bal·an·tid·ia

bald·ness
ball-and-sock·et
ball·ing iron
bal·ism
   or bal·lis·mus
   pl bal·lisms
   or bal·lis·mus·es

bal·lis·to·car·dio·
   gram
bal·lis·to·car·dio·
   graph
bal·lis·to·car·dio·
   graph·ic
bal·lis·to·car·di·og·
   ra·phy
   pl bal·lis·to·car·di·og·
   ra·phies

bal·lot·ta·ble
bal·lotte·ment
balm
bal·ne·ol·o·gy
   pl bal·ne·ol·o·gies
bal·neo·ther·a·peu·
   tics
bal·neo·ther·a·py
   pl bal·neo·ther·a·pies

bal·sam
bal·sam·ic
bam·boo spine
ba·nal
ba·nana oil

Ban·croft·i·an fil·a·
 ri·a·sis
 or Ban·croft's fil·a·ri·
 a·sis
ban·dage
 ban·daged
 ban·dag·ing
ban·dag·er
ban·dy-leg
ban·dy-leg·ged
bane·ber·ry
 pl bane·ber·ries
Bang's dis·ease
ban·ting
Ban·ti's dis·ease
bar·ag·no·sis
 pl bar·ag·no·ses
Bá·rá·ny chair
barb·al·o·in
bar·ber·ry
 pl bar·ber·ries
bar·ber's itch
bar·bi·tal
bar·bi·tu·rate
bar·bi·tu·ric
bar·bi·tur·ism
bar·bone
bar·bo·tage
bar·iat·ric
bar·ia·tri·cian
bar·iat·rics
bar·ic
bar·i·to·sis
 pl bar·i·to·ses
bar·i·um
Bar·low's dis·ease

bar·og·no·sis
 pl bar·og·no·ses
baro·gram
baro·graph
baro·phil·ic
baro·re·cep·tor
 also baro·cep·tor
bar·o·scope
baro·tac·tic
baro·tax·is
 pl baro·tax·es
baro·trau·ma
 pl baro·trau·ma·ta
Barr body
bar·ren
bar·ren·ness
bar·ri·er
bar·tho·lin·itis
 pl bar·tho·lin·ites
Bar·tho·lin's gland
bar·ton·el·la
Bar·ton·el·la·ce·ae
bar·ton·el·lo·sis
 pl bar·ton·el·lo·ses
bar·ye
ba·ry·ta
ba·sad
ba·sal
ba·sa·lis
 pl ba·sa·les
Ba·se·dow's dis·
 ease
base·ment
base·plate
ba·sic·i·ty
 pl ba·sic·i·ties
ba·si·cra·ni·al

ba·sid·io·my·cete
Ba·sid·io·my·ce·tes
ba·sid·io·my·ce·
 tous
ba·sid·io·spore
ba·sid·i·um
 pl ba·sid·ia
ba·si·fa·cial
ba·si·hy·al
ba·si·hy·oid
bas·i·lar
ba·sil·ic
ba·si·oc·cip·i·tal
ba·si·on
ba·sip·e·tal
ba·si·sphe·noid
ba·si·ver·te·bral
Basle Nom·i·na
 An·a·tom·i·ca
ba·so·cyte
ba·so·phil
 or ba·so·phile
 noun
ba·so·phil·ia
ba·so·phil·ic
 also ba·so·phil
 or ba·so·phile
 adjective
bas·so·rin
bath
bathe
 bathed
 bath·ing
bath·mo·trop·ic
bath·mot·ro·pism
ba·tracho·tox·in
bat·tle fa·tigue

bat·tle-fa·tigued
Bau·mé
  also Bau·me
  or Beau·mé
Baumé scale
B cell
BCG vac·cine
B com·plex
bdel·li·um
Bdel·lo·nys·sus
bdel·lo·vi·brio
  pl bdel·lo·vi·bri·os
bead·ing
bea·ker
Beau·mé
  var of Baumé
be·bee·rine
Bech·te·rew's nu·
  cle·us
  var of Bekhterev's
  nucleus
Bec·que·rel ray
bed·bug
bed·fast
bed·pan
bed·rid·den
  or bed·rid
bed·side
bed·so·nia
  pl bed·so·ni·ae
bed·sore
bed-wet·ter
bed-wet·ting
beef mea·sles
Beer's law
bees·wax
be·hav·ior

be·hav·ior·al
be·hav·ior·ism
be·hav·ior·ist
be·hav·ior·is·tic
Beh·cet's syn·
  drome
bej·el
Bekh·te·rev's nu·
  cle·us
  or Bech·te·rew's nu·
  cle·us
belch
bel·em·noid
bel·la·don·na
Bel·li·ni's duct
Bell-Ma·gen·die
  law
bel·lows
Bell's law
Bell's pal·sy
bel·ly
  pl bel·lies
bel·ly·ache
bel·ly·band
bel·ly but·ton
be·me·gride
Bence-Jones pro·
  tein
Ben·der Ge·stalt
  test
bends
Ben·e·dict's so·lu·
  tion
Ben·e·dict's test
be·nign
be·nig·ni·ty
  pl be·nig·ni·ties

ben·ne
  or bene
ben·ton·ite
ben·ton·it·ic
benz·al·de·hyde
benz·al·ko·ni·um
benz·an·thra·cene
ben·za·thine
ben·zene
ben·ze·noid
ben·zes·trol
ben·zi·dine
benz·imid·azole
ben·zo·[a]·py·rene
ben·zo·ate
ben·zo·caine
ben·zo·di·az·e·pine
ben·zo·ic
ben·zo·in
ben·zol
ben·zol·ism
ben·zo·mor·phan
ben·zo·phe·none
ben·zo·py·rene
  or benz·py·rene
ben·zo·sul·fi·mide
ben·zo·yl
benz·pyr·in·i·um
benz·tro·pine
ben·zyl·pen·i·cil·
  lin
ber·ber·ine
ber·ber·is
beri·beri
berke·li·um
ber·serk

be·ryl·li·o·sis
also ber·yl·lo·sis
pl be·ryl·li·o·ses
also ber·yl·lo·ses

be·ryl·li·um

bes·ti·al·i·ty
pl bes·ti·al·i·ties

be·ta

be·ta-ad·ren·er·gic

be·ta-block·er

be·ta-en·dor·phin
or β-en·dor·phin

be·ta glob·u·lin

be·ta-he·mo·lyt·ic

be·ta-hy·poph·amine

be·ta·ine

be·ta-li·po·pro·tein
or β-li·po·pro·tein

be·ta-li·po·tro·pin

be·ta·meth·a·sone

be·ta-naph·thol

be·ta-ox·i·da·tion

be·ta-re·cep·tor

be·ta-thal·as·se·mia
or β-thal·as·se·mia

be·ta·tron

be·tel

be·tha·ne·chol

Bet·u·la

bet·u·la oil

be·tween·brain

Betz cell

be·zoar

bhang

bi·ar·tic·u·lar

bi·au·ri·cu·lar

bib·lio·clast

bib·lio·klep·to·ma·nia

bib·lio·ma·nia

bib·lio·ma·ni·ac

bib·lio·ma·ni·a·cal

bib·lio·ther·a·peu·tic

bib·lio·ther·a·pist

bib·li·o·ther·a·py
pl bib·li·o·ther·a·pies

bib·u·lous

bi·cam·er·al

bi·cap·su·lar

bi·carb

bi·car·bon·ate

bi·cel·lu·lar

bi·ceps

bi·ceps bra·chii

bi·ceps fe·mo·ris

bi·ceps flex·or cu·bi·ti

bi·chlo·ride

bi·chro·mate

bi·cip·i·tal

bi·con·cave

bi·con·cav·i·ty
pl bi·con·cav·i·ties

bi·con·vex

bi·con·vex·i·ty
pl bi·con·vex·i·ties

bi·cor·nate

bi·cor·nu·ate

bi·cor·nu·ous

bi·cu·cul·line

bi·cus·pid

bi·det

bi·di·rec·tion·al

Bie·brich scar·let

bi·fid

bi·fla·gel·late

bi·fo·cal

bi·func·tion·al

bi·fur·cate

bi·fur·cat·ed

bi·fur·cat·ing

bi·fur·ca·tion

bi·gem·i·nal

bi·gem·i·ny
pl bi·gem·i·nies

bi·ge·ner·ic

big·head

bi·gua·nide

bi·la·bi·al

bi·lat·er·al

bi·lat·er·al·ism

bi·lat·er·al·i·ty
pl bi·lat·er·al·i·ties

bi·lay·er

bile

bil·har·zia

bil·har·zi·al

bil·har·zi·a·sis
pl bil·har·zi·a·ses

bil·i·ary

bili·cy·a·nin

bil·i·fi·ca·tion

bili·fus·cin

bil·ious

bil·i·ru·bin

bil·i·ru·bi·ne·mia
also bil·i·ru·bi·nae·mia

bil·i·ru·bi·nu·ria
bil·i·ver·din
bi·lo·bate
bi·lobed
bi·lob·u·lar
bi·loc·u·lar
  or bi·loc·u·late
bi·man·u·al
bi·mas·toid
bi·mo·lec·u·lar
bi·na·ry
bin·au·ral
bind·er
Bi·net age
Bi·net-Si·mon
  scale
bin·oc·u·lar
bi·no·mi·al
bin·ovu·lar
bi·nu·cle·ate
  also bi·nu·cle·at·ed
bi·nu·cle·o·late
bio·ac·cu·mu·la·
  tion
bio·ac·ous·ti·cian
bio·acous·tics
bio·ac·tive
bio·ac·tiv·i·ty
  pl bio·ac·tiv·i·ties
bio·as·say
bio·as·tro·nau·ti·
  cal
bio·as·tro·nau·tics
bio·au·to·graph
bio·au·tog·ra·phy
  pl bio·au·tog·ra·phies

bio·avail·abil·i·ty
  pl bio·avail·abil·i·ties
bio·cat·a·lyst
bio·chem·i·cal
bio·chem·ist
bio·chem·is·try
  pl bio·chem·is·tries
bio·chem·or·phol·
  o·gy
  pl bio·chem·or·phol·
    o·gies
bio·cid·al
bio·cide
bio·clean
bio·cli·mat·ics
bio·cli·ma·tol·o·gy
  pl bio·cli·ma·tol·o·
    gies
bio·com·pat·i·bil·i·
  ty
  pl bio·com·pat·i·bil·i·
    ties
bio·com·pat·i·ble
bio·de·grad·abil·i·
  ty
  pl bio·de·grad·abil·i·
    ties
bio·de·grad·able
bio·deg·ra·da·tion
bio·de·grade
  bio·de·grad·ed
  bio·de·grad·ing
bio·dy·nam·ics
bio·elec·tric
  or bio·elec·tri·cal
bio·elec·tric·i·ty
  pl bio·elec·tric·i·ties

bio·elec·tro·gen·e·
  sis
  pl bio·elec·tro·gen·e·
    ses
bio·elec·tron·ics
bio·en·er·get·ics
bio·en·gi·neer·ing
bio·en·vi·ron·men·
  tal
bio·eth·i·cal
bio·eth·i·cist
bio·eth·ics
bio·feed·back
bio·fla·vo·noid
bio·gen·e·sis
  pl bio·gen·e·ses
bio·ge·net·ic
bio·gen·ic
bio·geo·chem·is·try
  pl bio·geo·chem·is·
    tries
bio·geo·graph·ic
  or bio·geo·graph·i·cal
bio·ge·og·ra·phy
  pl bio·ge·og·ra·phies
bio·haz·ard
bio·haz·ard·ous
bio·in·stru·men·ta·
  tion
bi·o·log·ic
bi·o·log·i·cal
bi·ol·o·gist
bi·ol·o·gy
  pl bi·ol·o·gies
bio·lu·mi·nes·
  cence
bio·lu·mi·nes·cent

bi·ol·y·sis
  pl bi·ol·y·ses

bi·o·lyt·ic

bio·ma·te·ri·al

bio·math·e·mat·ics

bio·me·chan·i·cal

bio·me·chan·ics

bio·med·i·cal

bio·med·i·cine

bio·mem·brane

bi·om·e·ter

bio·met·ric
  or bio·met·ri·cal

bio·me·tri·cian

bio·met·rics

bi·om·e·try
  pl bi·om·e·tries

bio·mi·cro·scope

bio·mi·cros·co·py
  pl bio·mi·cros·co·pies

bio·mo·lec·u·lar

bi·on·ics

bi·o·nom·ics

bio·or·gan·ic

bio·phar·ma·ceu·ti·cal

bio·phar·ma·ceu·tics

bi·o·phore

bio·pho·tom·e·ter

bio·phys·i·cal

bio·phys·i·cist

bio·phys·ics

bio·poly·mer

bi·op·sy
  pl bi·op·sies

bi·op·sy

bi·op·sied

bi·op·sy·ing

bio·psy·chol·o·gist

bio·psy·chol·o·gy
  pl bio·psy·chol·o·gies

bi·or·bit·al

bio·re·search

bio·rhythm

bio·rhyth·mic

bio·rhyth·mic·i·ty
  pl bio·rhyth·mic·i·ties

bio·sci·ence

bio·sci·en·tif·ic

bio·sci·en·tist

bi·ose

bio·stat·is·ti·cian

bio·sta·tis·tics

bio·syn·the·sis
  pl bio·syn·the·ses

bio·syn·the·size

bio·syn·the·sized

bio·syn·the·siz·ing

bio·syn·thet·ic

bio·syn·thet·i·cal·ly

bio·tech·no·log·i·cal

bio·tech·nol·o·gy
  pl bio·tech·nol·o·gies

bio·tel·e·met·ric

bio·te·lem·e·try
  pl bio·te·lem·e·tries

bi·o·tin

bio·trans·for·ma·tion

bi·ovu·lar

bi·pa·ren·tal

bi·pa·ri·etal

bip·a·rous

bi·par·tite

bi·ped
  noun

bi·ped
  or bi·ped·al
  adjective

bi·pen·nate

bi·pen·ni·form

bi·phe·nyl

bi·po·lar

bi·po·ten·ti·al·i·ty
  pl bi·po·ten·ti·al·i·ties

bi·ra·mous

bi·re·frin·gence

bi·re·frin·gent

birth con·trol

birth·mark

birth pang

birth·rate

bis·cuit

bi·sex·u·al

bi·sex·u·al·i·ty
  pl bi·sex·u·al·i·ties

bis·muth

bis·mu·thic

bis·tou·ry
  pl bis·tou·ries

bi·sul·fate

bi·sul·fide

bi·sul·fite

bi·tem·po·ral

bite·wing

Bi·tot's spots

bit·ters
bit·ter·sweet
bi·uret
bi·va·lent
bi·valve
  also bi·valved
bi·ven·ter
bi·ven·tral
bi·zy·go·mat·ic
black-and-blue
black·damp
black eye
black·fly
  pl black·flies
black·head
black·leg
black lung
black·out
black·tongue
black·wa·ter
blad·der
blain
Bla·lock-Taus·sig
  op·er·a·tion
blast
  noun or verb
blas·te·ma
  pl blas·te·mas
  or blas·te·ma·ta
blas·te·mat·ic
  or blas·te·mic
blas·tic
  or blast
  adjective
blas·to·coel
  or blas·to·coele
blas·to·coe·lic

blas·to·cyst
blas·to·cyte
blas·to·derm
blas·to·disc
  or blas·to·disk
blas·to·gen·e·sis
  pl blas·to·gen·e·ses
blas·to·gen·ic
blas·to·mere
blas·to·mer·ic
blas·to·my·cete
Blas·to·my·ce·tes
blas·to·my·ce·tic
blas·to·my·cin
blas·to·my·co·sis
  pl blas·to·my·co·ses
blas·to·my·cot·ic
blas·toph·tho·ria
blas·toph·tho·ric
blas·to·por·al
  or blas·to·por·ic
blas·to·pore
blas·to·sphere
blas·to·spher·ic
blas·to·spore
blas·tot·o·my
  pl blas·tot·o·mies
blas·tu·la
  pl blas·tu·las
  or blas·tu·lae
blas·tu·lar
blas·tu·la·tion
Blat·ta
Blat·tel·la
Blaud's pill
bleb
bleb·by

bleed
  bled
  bleed·ing
bleed·er
blem·ish
blen·noid
blen·nor·rhea
blen·nor·rheal
bleo·my·cin
bleph·a·ral
bleph·a·rism
bleph·a·ri·tis
  pl bleph·a·rit·i·des
bleph·a·ro·con·
  junc·ti·vi·tis
bleph·a·ro·plast
bleph·a·ro·plas·ty
  pl bleph·a·ro·plas·ties
bleph·a·rop·to·sis
  pl bleph·a·rop·to·ses
bleph·a·ro·spasm
bleph·a·ro·stat
bleph·a·rot·o·my
  pl bleph·a·rot·o·mies
blind gut
blind spot
blis·ter
  blis·tered
  blis·ter·ing
blis·tery
block·ade
  block·ad·ed
  block·ad·ing
block·age
block·er
blood bank
blood cell

blood count
blood fluke
blood group
blood heat
blood·i·ly
blood·i·ness
blood is·land
blood·less
blood·let·ting
blood·mo·bile
blood poi·son·ing
blood pres·sure
blood·root
blood se·rum
blood·shot
blood·stain
blood·stained
blood·stream
blood·suck·er
blood·suck·ing
blood sug·ar
blood test
blood type
blood·typ·ing
blood ves·sel
bloody
  blood·i·er
  blood·i·est
blotch
blotchy
  blotch·i·er
  blotch·i·est
blow·fish
blow·fly
  pl blow·flies
blow·pipe
blue ba·by

blue·bot·tle
blue comb
blue mold
blue ne·vus
blue·tongue
B lym·pho·cyte
Bo·dan·sky unit
bodi·ly
body
  pl bod·ies
body louse
body odor
body snatch·er
body wall
Boeck's dis·ease
  or Boeck's sar·coid
Bohr ef·fect
Bohr the·o·ry
bo·lom·e·ter
bo·lo·met·ric
bo·lus
bone·let
bone·set·ter
boney
  var of bony
bont tick
bony
  or bon·ey
  bon·i·er
  bon·i·est
Bo·oph·i·lus
boost·er
bo·rac·ic
bo·rate
bo·rat·ed
bo·rax
bor·bo·ryg·mic

bor·bo·ryg·mus
  pl bor·bo·ryg·mi
Bor·de·tel·la
Bor·det-Gen·gou
  ba·cil·lus
bo·ric
bor·ne·ol
bo·ron
bo·ron·ic
Bor·rel body
bor·re·lia
boss
bos·se·lat·ed
bot
  also bott
bo·tan·i·cal
bot·a·nist
bot·a·ny
  pl bot·a·nies
botch
bot·fly
  pl bot·flies
bo·thrid·i·um
  pl bo·thrid·ia
  or bo·thrid·i·ums
Both·rio·ceph·a·lus
both·ri·um
  pl both·ria
  or both·ri·ums
bot·ry·oid
bot·ry·o·my·co·ma
  pl bot·ry·o·my·co·mas
  or bot·ry·o·my·co·ma·ta
bot·ry·o·my·co·sis
  pl bot·ry·o·my·co·ses
bot·ry·o·my·cot·ic

bot·tle
bot·tle-feed
  bot·tle-fed
  bot·tle-feed·ing
bot·u·lin
bo·tu·li·nal
bot·u·li·num
  also bot·u·li·nus
bot·u·lism
bou·gie
bou·gi·nage
  or bou·gie·nage
bouil·lon
Bou·in's flu·id
bou·lim·ia
  var of bulimia
bour·tree
bou·ton
Bo·vic·o·la
bo·vine
bow·el
Bow·en's dis·ease
bow·leg
bow·legged
Bow·man's cap·
  sule
Bow·man's gland
Bow·man's mem·
  brane
Boyle's law
bra·chi·al
bra·chi·alis
bra·chio·ce·phal·ic
bra·chio·ra·di·alis
  pl bra·chio·ra·di·ales
bra·chi·um
  pl bra·chia

bra·chi·um con·
  junc·ti·vum
bra·chi·um pon·tis
brachy·ce·phal·ic
brachy·ceph·a·ly
  pl brachy·ceph·a·lies
brachy·dac·ty·lous
brachy·dac·ty·ly
  pl brachy·dac·ty·lies
brachy·fa·cial
brachy·ther·a·py
  pl brachy·ther·a·pies
brachy·uran·ic
Brad·ford frame
brad·sot
bra·dy·car·dia
  slow heart action
  (see tachycardia*)*
bra·dy·crot·ic
bra·dy·ki·ne·sia
bra·dy·ki·nin
bra·dy·lex·ia
bra·dy·pha·sia
bra·dy·phre·nia
bra·dy·pnea
bra·dy·rhyth·mia
braille
braille·writ·er
brain·case
brain-dead
brain death
brain·pan
brain sand
brain stem
brain·wash
brain·wash·ing
brain wave

bran
bran·chia
  pl bran·chi·ae
bran·chi·al
bran·chi·og·e·nous
bran·chi·oma
  pl bran·chi·omas
  or bran·chi·oma·ta
bran·chio·mere
bran·chi·om·er·
  ism
brash
braxy
  pl brax·ies
bra·yera
break
  broke
  bro·ken
  break·ing
break·bone fe·ver
break·down
breast
breast·bone
breast-feed
breath
breathe
  breathed
  breath·ing
breath·er
breath·less
breech
breed
  bred
  breed·ing
breed·er
breg·ma
  pl breg·ma·ta

breg·mat·ic
brei
bridge·work
bright·ness
Bright's dis·ease
Brill's dis·ease
brim·stone
Bri·nell hard·ness
Bri·nell num·ber
bris·ket
bris·tle
Brit·ish anti·lew·is·
  ite
broad-spec·trum
Bro·ca's apha·sia
Bro·ca's ar·ea
Bro·ca scale
Brod·mann ar·ea
  or Brod·mann's ar·ea
broke
  past of break
bro·ken
bro·ken-wind·ed
bro·mate
  bro·mat·ed
  bro·mat·ing
bro·me·lain
  also bro·me·lin
bro·mic
bro·mide
bro·mi·dro·sis
  also brom·hi·dro·sis
  pl bro·mi·dro·ses
  also brom·hi·dro·ses
bro·mi·nate
  bro·mi·nat·ed
  bro·mi·nat·ing

bro·mi·na·tion
bro·mine
bro·min·ism
bro·mism
bro·mo
  pl bro·mos
bro·mo·crip·tine
bro·mo·de·oxy·ur·i·
  dine
  or 5-bro·mo·de·oxy·
  ur·i·dine
bro·mo·der·ma
bro·mo·phe·nol
  also brom·phe·nol
bro·mo·ura·cil
bron·chi·al
bron·chi·ec·ta·sia
bron·chi·ec·ta·sis
  pl bron·chi·ec·ta·ses
bron·chi·ec·tat·ic
bron·chio·gen·ic
bron·chi·o·lar
bron·chi·ole
bron·chi·ol·ec·ta·
  sis
  pl bron·chi·ol·ec·ta·
  ses
bron·chi·ol·itis
bron·chi·o·lus
  pl bron·chi·o·li
bron·chit·ic
bron·chi·tis
bron·chi·um
  pl bron·chia
bron·cho·con·stric·
  tion

bron·cho·con·stric·
  tor
bron·cho·di·la·ta·
  tion
bron·cho·di·la·tion
bron·cho·di·la·tor
  also bron·cho·di·la·to·
  ry
  adjective
bron·cho·di·la·tor
  noun
bron·cho·gen·ic
bron·cho·gram
bron·cho·graph·ic
bron·chog·ra·phy
  pl bron·chog·ra·phies
bron·cho·li·thi·a·
  sis
  pl bron·cho·li·thi·a·
  ses
bron·cho·mo·ni·li·
  a·sis
  pl bron·cho·mo·ni·li·
  a·ses
bron·cho·mo·tor
bron·cho·my·co·sis
  pl bron·cho·my·co·ses
bron·choph·o·ny
  pl bron·choph·o·nies
bron·cho·plas·ty
  pl bron·cho·plas·ties
bron·cho·pleu·ral
bron·cho·pneu·mo·
  nia
bron·cho·pneu·
  mon·ic

bron·cho·pul·mo·
nary
bron·chor·rhea
bron·cho·scope
bron·cho·scop·ic
bron·chos·co·pist
bron·chos·co·py
pl bron·chos·co·pies
bron·cho·spasm
bron·cho·spas·tic
bron·cho·spi·rom·
e·ter
bron·cho·spi·ro·
met·ric
bron·cho·spi·rom·
e·try
pl bron·cho·spi·rom·
e·tries
bron·cho·ste·no·sis
pl bron·cho·ste·no·ses
bron·chus
pl bron·chi
bron·to·pho·bia
broth
pl broths
Brown·ian move·
ment
brow·ridge
bru·cel·la
pl bru·cel·lae
or bru·cel·las
Bru·cel·la·ce·ae
bru·cel·lo·sis
pl bru·cel·lo·ses
bru·cine
Brud·zin·ski sign
or Brud·zin·ski's sign

bruise
bruised
bruis·ing
bruit
Brun·ner's gland
Brunn's mem·
brane
brush bor·der
brux·ism
bry·o·nia
bu·bo
pl bu·boes
bu·bon·ic
bu·bon·o·cele
buc·ca
pl buc·cae
buc·cal
buc·ci·na·tor
buc·co·lin·gual
buc·co·pha·ryn·
geal
Büch·ner fun·nel
bu·chu
buck·thorn
buck·tooth
pl buck·teeth
buck-toothed
Buer·ger's dis·ease
buff·er
buffy coat
bu·fo
bu·fo·ta·lin
bu·fo·ten·ine
or bu·fo·ten·in
bu·fo·tox·in
bug·gery
pl bug·ger·ies

bul·bar
bul·bo·cap·nine
bul·bo·cav·er·no·
sus
pl bul·bo·cav·er·no·si
bul·bo·cav·er·nous
bul·bo·spi·nal
bul·bo·spon·gi·o·
sus
bul·bo·ure·thral
bul·bous
bul·bus
pl bul·bi
bu·lim·ia
also bou·lim·ia
bu·lim·ic
bul·la
pl bul·lae
bul·late
bull neck
bull·necked
bul·lous
bun·dle
bun·dle of His
bun·ga·ro·tox·in
Bun·ga·rus
bun·ion
bu·no·dont
Bu·nos·to·mum
Bun·sen burn·er
buph·thal·mia
buph·thal·mos
pl buph·thal·mos·es
bur
or burr
bur·dock

bu·rette
or bu·ret

Bur·kitt's lym·pho·ma
also Bur·kitt lym·pho·ma

burr
var of bur

Bur·row's so·lu·tion

bur·sa
pl bur·sas
or bur·sae

bur·sal

bur·sa of Fa·bri·cius

bur·sec·to·mize
bur·sec·to·mized
bur·sec·to·miz·ing

bur·sec·to·my
pl bur·sec·to·mies

bur·si·tis

bush·mas·ter

bu·sul·fan

bu·to·py·ro·nox·yl

but·ter

but·ter·fat

but·ter·fly
pl but·ter·flies

but·ter·milk

but·tock

bu·tyl·at·ed hy·droxy·an·i·sole

bu·tyl·at·ed hy·droxy·tol·u·ene

bu·tyl·ene

bu·ty·rate

bu·tyr·ic

bu·tyr·in

bu·ty·ro·phe·none

by·pass

bys·si·no·sis
pl bys·si·no·ses

C

Cab·ot's ring
or Cab·ot ring

ca·cao
pl ca·caos

ca·chec·tic

ca·chet

ca·chex·ia
also ca·chexy
pl ca·chex·ias
also ca·chex·ies

caco·de·mo·nia
or caco·de·mo·no·ma·nia

cac·o·dyl

cac·o·dyl·ate

cac·o·dyl·ic

ca·cos·mia

ca·dav·er

ca·dav·er·ic

ca·dav·er·ine

ca·dav·er·ous

cade

cad·mi·um

ca·du·ceus
pl ca·du·cei

cae·sar·e·an, cae·sar·i·an
vars of cesarean

caf·feine

caf·fein·ic

caf·fein·ism

ca·hin·ca

cais·son dis·ease

caj·e·put
also caj·u·put

caj·e·put·ol
or caj·u·put·ol

Cal·a·bar swell·ing

cal·a·mine

cal·a·mus
pl cal·a·mi

cal·ca·ne·al
also cal·ca·ne·an

cal·ca·neo·cu·boid

cal·ca·ne·um
pl cal·ca·nea

cal·ca·ne·us
pl cal·ca·nei

cal·car
pl cal·car·ia

cal·car avis
pl cal·car·ia avi·um

cal·car·e·ous

cal·ca·rine

cal·ces
pl of calx

cal·cic

cal·ci·co·sis
pl cal·ci·co·ses

cal·cif·er·ol

cal·cif·er·ous

cal·cif·ic

cal·ci·fi·ca·tion
cal·ci·fy
  cal·ci·fied
  cal·ci·fy·ing
cal·cim·e·ter
cal·ci·na·tion
cal·cine
  cal·cined
  cal·cin·ing
cal·ci·no·sis
  pl cal·ci·no·ses
cal·ci·phy·lac·tic
cal·ci·phy·lac·ti·
  cal·ly
cal·ci·phy·lax·is
  pl cal·ci·phy·lax·es
cal·cite
cal·cit·ic
cal·ci·to·nin
cal·ci·um
cal·co·sphe·rite
cal·cu·lo·sis
  pl cal·cu·lo·ses
cal·cu·lous
cal·cu·lus
  pl cal·cu·li
  also cal·cu·lus·es
cal·e·fa·cient
ca·len·du·la
ca·len·du·lin
cal·en·ture
calf
  pl calves
cal·i·ber
cal·i·brate
  cal·i·brat·ed
  cal·i·brat·ing

cal·i·bra·tion
cal·i·bra·tor
ca·li·ce·al
  var of calyceal
ca·li·ces
  pl of calix
cal·i·for·ni·um
cal·i·per
  or cal·li·per
  cal·i·pered
  or cal·li·pered
  cal·i·per·ing
  or cal·li·per·ing
cal·is·then·ic
cal·is·then·ics
ca·lix
  var of calyx
Cal·liph·o·ra
cal·liph·o·rid
Cal·li·phor·i·dae
cal·liph·o·rine
Cal·li·tro·ga
cal·lo·sal
cal·los·i·ty
  pl cal·los·i·ties
cal·lous
cal·loused
  or cal·lused
cal·lus
calm·ant
calm·ative
cal·o·mel
cal·or
ca·lo·ric
ca·lo·ri·cal·ly

cal·o·rie
  also cal·o·ry
  pl cal·o·ries
ca·lor·i·fa·cient
cal·o·rif·ic
ca·lor·i·gen·ic
cal·o·rim·e·ter
ca·lo·ri·met·ric
ca·lo·ri·met·ri·cal·
  ly
cal·o·rim·e·try
  pl cal·o·rim·e·tries
ca·lum·ba
  or co·lom·bo
cal·va
  pl cal·vas
  or cal·vae
cal·var·ia
  pl cal·var·i·ae
cal·var·i·al
cal·var·i·um
  pl cal·var·ia
calves
  pl of calf
cal·vi·ti·es
  pl cal·vi·ti·es
calx
  pl calx·es
  or cal·ces
    product of calcining
calx
  pl cal·ces
    heel
ca·ly·ce·al
  or ca·li·ce·al
ca·ly·ces
  pl of calyx

ca·ly·cine
  also ca·lyc·i·nal

ca·lyc·u·lus
  pl ca·lyc·u·li

Ca·lym·ma·to·bac·
te·ri·um

ca·lyx
  also ca·lix
  pl ca·lyx·es
  or ca·ly·ces
  also ca·li·ces

cam·era lu·ci·da
cam·i·sole
cam·o·mile
  var of chamomile

cam·phor
cam·phor·ate
  cam·phor·at·ed
  cam·phor·at·ing
cam·phor·ic
cam·pim·e·ter
camp·to·cor·mia
camp·to·dac·ty·ly
  pl camp·to·dac·ty·lies

cam·py·lo·bac·ter
ca·nal
can·a·lic·u·lar
can·a·lic·u·lus
  pl can·a·lic·u·li
ca·na·lis
  pl ca·na·les

ca·na·li·za·tion
can·a·lize
  can·a·lized
  can·a·liz·ing
ca·nal of Schlemm
Can·a·va·lia

ca·na·val·in
ca·na·van·ine
can·cel·late
  or can·cel·lat·ed
can·cel·li
can·cel·lous
can·cer
can·cer·ate
  can·cer·at·ed
  can·cer·at·ing
can·cer·i·ci·dal
  or can·cer·o·ci·dal
can·cer·iza·tion
can·cer·o·gen·ic
  or can·cer·i·gen·ic
can·cer·ol·o·gist
can·cer·ol·o·gy
  pl can·cer·ol·o·gies
can·cer·o·lyt·ic
can·cer·ous
can·cer·pho·bia
  or can·cer·o·pho·bia
can·croid
can·crum oris
  pl can·cra oris
can·de·la
can·di·ci·din
can·di·da
can·di·dal
can·di·di·a·sis
  pl can·di·di·a·ses
can·dle
ca·nic·o·la fe·ver
can·id
Can·i·dae
ca·nine

ca·ni·nus
  pl ca·ni·ni

Ca·nis
ca·ni·ti·es
  pl ca·ni·ti·es

can·ker
can·na·bi·di·ol
can·na·bi·noid
can·na·bi·nol
can·na·bis
can·na·bism
can·ni·bal
can·ni·bal·ism
can·non
can·nu·la
  also can·u·la
  pl can·nu·las
  or can·nu·lae
  or can·u·las
  or can·u·lae

can·nu·lar
can·nu·late
  can·nu·lat·ed
  can·nu·lat·ing
can·nu·la·tion
can·nu·lize
  can·nu·lized
  can·nu·liz·ing
can·thar·i·dal
can·thar·i·date
  can·thar·i·dat·ed
  can·thar·i·dat·
    ing
can·thar·id·i·an
  or can·tha·rid·e·an

can·thar·i·din
can·thar·i·dism

can·tha·ris
  pl can·thar·i·des

can·thus
  pl can·thi

caou·tchouc

cap
  capped
  cap·ping

ca·pac·i·tance

ca·pac·i·ta·tion

ca·pac·i·tor

ca·pac·i·ty
  pl ca·pac·i·ties

cap·e·line

cap·il·lar·ia

ca·pil·la·ri·a·sis
  also cap·il·lar·i·o·sis
  pl ca·pil·la·ri·a·ses
  also cap·il·lar·i·o·ses

cap·il·lar·id

cap·il·lar·i·ty
  pl cap·il·lar·i·ties

cap·il·lar·o·scope

cap·il·la·ros·co·py
  also cap·il·lar·i·os·co·py
  pl cap·il·lar·i·a·ros·co·pies
  also cap·il·lar·i·os·co·pies

cap·il·lary
  pl cap·il·lar·ies

ca·pil·li·cul·ture

ca·pil·lus
  pl ca·pil·li

ca·pi·ta
  pl of caput

cap·i·tate

cap·i·ta·tum
  pl cap·i·ta·ta

cap·i·tel·lum
  pl cap·i·tel·la

ca·pit·u·lum
  pl ca·pit·u·la

ca·pon·iza·tion

ca·pon·ize
  ca·pon·ized
  ca·pon·iz·ing

cap·pit·u·lar

cap·rate

cap·re·o·my·cin

cap·ric

cap·ro·ate

ca·pro·ic

ca·pry·late

ca·pryl·ic

cap·si·cum

cap·sid

cap·sid·al

cap·so·mer
  or cap·so·mere

cap·su·la
  pl cap·su·lae

cap·su·lar

cap·su·lat·ed
  also cap·su·late

cap·su·la·tion

cap·sule

cap·su·lec·to·my
  pl cap·su·lec·to·mies

cap·su·li·tis

cap·su·lor·rha·phy
  pl cap·su·lor·rha·phies

cap·su·lot·o·my
  pl cap·su·lot·o·mies

ca·put
  pl ca·pi·ta

ca·put suc·ce·da·ne·um
  pl ca·pi·ta suc·ce·da·nea

car·a·mel

ca·ra·te

car·a·way

car·ba·chol

car·ba·mate

car·ba·maz·e·pine

car·bam·ic

carb·amide

carb·ami·no·he·mo·glo·bin

car·bar·sone

car·ba·ryl

car·ba·zole

car·ben·i·cil·lin

carb·he·mo·glo·bin
  or car·bo·he·mo·glo·bin

car·bi·nol

car·bo

car·bo·hy·drase

car·bo·hy·drate

car·bo·late

car·bo·lat·ed

car·bol·fuch·sin

car·bol·ic

car·bo·lized

car·bo·my·cin

car·bon

car·bon·ate
  car·bon·at·ed
  car·bon·at·ing
car·bon·ation
car·bon·ic
car·bon·yl·he·mo·
  glo·bin
car·boxy·he·mo·
  glo·bin
car·box·yl
car·box·yl·ase
car·box·yl·ate
  car·box·yl·at·ed
  car·box·yl·at·ing
car·box·yl·ation
car·box·yl·ic
car·boxy·meth·yl·
  cel·lu·lose
car·boxy·pep·ti·
  dase
car·bro·mal
car·bun·cle
car·bun·cu·lar
car·bun·cu·lo·sis
  pl car·bun·cu·lo·ses
car·cass
car·ce·ag
car·ci·no·em·bry·
  on·ic
car·cin·o·gen
car·ci·no·gen·e·sis
  pl car·ci·no·gen·e·ses
car·ci·no·gen·ic
car·ci·no·gen·i·cal·
  ly

car·ci·no·ge·nic·i·ty
  pl car·ci·no·ge·nic·i·
  ties
car·ci·noid
car·ci·no·lyt·ic
car·ci·no·ma
  pl car·ci·no·mas
  or car·ci·no·ma·ta
car·ci·no·ma in si·
  tu
car·ci·no·ma·toid
car·ci·no·ma·to·sis
  pl car·ci·no·ma·to·ses
car·ci·no·ma·tous
car·ci·no·sar·co·ma
  pl car·ci·no·sar·co·
  mas
  or car·ci·no·sar·co·
  ma·ta
car·ci·no·sis
  pl car·ci·no·ses
car·da·mom
car·dia
  pl car·di·ae
  or car·dias
car·di·ac
car·di·al·gia
car·di·ec·to·my
  pl car·di·ec·to·mies
car·di·nal
car·dio·ac·cel·er·a·
  tion
car·dio·ac·cel·er·a·
  tor
  also car·dio·ac·cel·er·
  a·to·ry
car·dio·ac·tive

car·dio·ac·tiv·i·ty
  pl car·dio·ac·tiv·i·ties
car·dio·cir·cu·la·to·
  ry
car·dio·dy·nam·ics
car·dio·gen·ic
car·dio·gram
car·dio·graph
car·di·og·ra·pher
car·dio·graph·ic
car·di·og·ra·phy
  pl car·di·og·ra·phies
car·dio·in·hib·i·to·
  ry
car·dio·lip·in
car·di·o·log·i·cal
car·di·ol·o·gist
car·di·ol·o·gy
  pl car·di·ol·o·gies
car·dio·meg·a·ly
  pl car·dio·meg·a·lies
car·di·om·e·ter
car·dio·met·ric
car·di·om·e·try
  pl car·di·om·e·tries
car·dio·my·op·a·
  thy
  pl car·dio·my·op·a·
  thies
car·dio·path
car·di·op·a·thy
  pl car·di·op·a·thies
car·dio·pho·bia
car·dio·plas·ty
  pl car·dio·plas·ties
car·dio·ple·gia

car·dio·pul·mo·
nary
car·dio·re·nal
car·dio·re·spi·ra·to·
ry
car·di·or·rha·phy
pl car·di·or·rha·phies
car·dio·scle·ro·sis
pl car·dio·scle·ro·ses
car·dio·scope
car·dio·spasm
car·dio·spas·tic
car·dio·ta·chom·e·
ter
car·dio·tacho·met·
ric
car·dio·ta·chom·e·
try
pl car·dio·ta·chom·e·
tries
car·dio·tho·ra·cic
car·di·ot·o·my
pl car·di·ot·o·mies
car·dio·ton·ic
car·dio·tox·ic
car·dio·tox·ic·i·ty
pl car·dio·tox·ic·i·ties
car·dio·vas·cu·lar
car·dio·ver·sion
car·dio·ver·ter
car·di·tis
Car·i·ca
car·ies
pl car·ies
ca·ri·na
pl ca·ri·nas
or ca·ri·nae

car·i·nate
car·io·gen·ic
car·io·stat·ic
car·i·ous
ca·ri·so·pro·dol
carm·al·um
car·mi·na·tive
car·mine
car·min·ic
car·mus·tine
car·ni·fi·ca·tion
car·ni·tine
Car·niv·o·ra
car·ni·vore
car·niv·o·rous
car·no·sine
car·ob
car·o·tene
car·o·ten·emia
also car·o·tin·emia
ca·rot·enoid
also ca·rot·i·noid
ca·rot·id
car·pa·ine
car·pal
car·pa·le
pl car·pa·lia
car·pec·to·my
pl car·pec·to·mies
car·phol·o·gy
pl car·phol·o·gies
car·po·meta·car·
pal
car·po·ped·al
car·pus
pl car·pi

car·ra·geen
also car·ra·gheen
car·ra·geen·an
also car·ra·geen·in
car·ri·er
Car·ri·ón's dis·ease
car·sick
car·tha·mus
car·ti·lage
car·ti·lag·i·noid
car·ti·lag·i·nous
car·un·cle
small fleshy eminence
(see carbuncle,
furuncle)
ca·run·cu·la
pl ca·run·cu·lae
car·va·crol
cas·cara
cas·cara amar·ga
cas·cara sa·gra·da
ca·se·ate
ca·se·at·ed
ca·se·at·ing
ca·se·ation
case·book
ca·sein
ca·sein·o·gen
ca·se·ous
case·work
case·work·er
cas·sette
also ca·sette
cas·sia
Cas·tel·la·ni's paint
cas·tile soap
cas·tor

cas·trate
  cas·trat·ed
  cas·trat·ing
cas·trat·er
  or cas·tra·tor
cas·tra·tion
ca·su·al·ty
  pl ca·su·al·ties
ca·su·is·tic
cat
cata·bi·o·sis
  pl cata·bi·o·ses
cat·a·bol·ic
cat·a·bol·i·cal·ly
ca·tab·o·lism
ca·tab·o·lite
ca·tab·o·lize
  ca·tab·o·lized
  ca·tab·o·liz·ing
cata·crot·ic
cat·a·lase
cat·a·lat·ic
cat·a·lep·sy
  pl cat·a·lep·sies
cat·a·lep·tic
cat·a·lep·ti·cal·ly
cat·a·lep·toid
cat·a·lo·gia
ca·tal·y·sis
  pl ca·tal·y·ses
cat·a·lyst
cat·a·lyt·ic
cat·a·lyt·i·cal·ly
cat·a·lyze
  cat·a·lyzed
  cat·a·lyz·ing
cat·a·lyz·er

cata·me·nia
cata·me·ni·al
cat·a·mite
cat·am·ne·sis
  pl cat·am·ne·ses
cat·am·nes·tic
cata·pha·sia
cat·a·pho·re·sis
  pl cat·a·pho·re·ses
cat·a·pho·ret·ic
cat·a·pla·sia
cat·a·plasm
cat·a·plas·tic
cat·a·plec·tic
cat·a·plexy
  pl cat·a·plex·ies
cat·a·ract
cat·a·ract·ous
ca·tarrh
ca·tarrh·al
Cat·ar·rhi·na
cat·ar·rhine
ca·tas·tro·phe
cat·a·stroph·ic
cata·to·nia
cata·ton·ic
cata·ton·i·cal·ly
cat·bite fe·ver
catch·ment
cat·e·chol
cat·e·chol·amine
cat·e·chol·amin·er·
  gic
cat·e·chu
cat·elec·trot·o·nus
cat·e·noid
ca·ten·u·late

cat·gut
ca·thar·sis
  pl ca·thar·ses
ca·thar·tic
ca·thect
ça·thec·tic
ca·thep·sin
cath·e·ter
cath·e·ter·iza·tion
cath·e·ter·ize
  cath·e·ter·ized
  cath·e·ter·iz·ing
ca·thex·is
  pl ca·thex·es
cath·od·al
cath·ode
cath·od·ic
cath·od·i·cal·ly
ca·thol·i·con
cat·ion
cat·ion·ic
cat·ion·i·cal·ly
cat·mint
cat·nip
  also cat·nep
ca·top·tric
cat·tery
  pl cat·ter·ies
cau·da
  pl cau·dae
cau·dad
cau·da equi·na
  pl cau·dae equi·nae
cau·da he·li·cis
  pl cau·dae he·li·cis
cau·dal
cau·date

cau·da·to·len·tic·u·
　lar
caul
cau·li·flow·er
cau·sal·gia
cau·sal·gic
caus·tic
caus·ti·cal·ly
caus·tic·i·ty
　pl caus·tic·i·ties
cau·ter
cau·ter·ant
cau·ter·iza·tion
cau·ter·ize
　cau·ter·ized
　cau·ter·iz·ing
cau·tery
　pl cau·ter·ies
ca·va
　pl ca·vae
ca·val
cav·al·ry bone
cav·ern
cav·er·no·ma
　pl cav·er·no·mas
　or cav·er·no·ma·ta
cav·er·nos·to·my
　pl cav·er·nos·to·mies
cav·ern·ous
cav·i·tary
cav·i·tate
　cav·i·tat·ed
　cav·i·tat·ing
cav·i·ta·tion
cav·i·ty
　pl cav·i·ties

cav·og·ra·phy
　pl cav·og·ra·phies
ca·vo·sur·face
ca·vum
　pl ca·va
ca·vy
　pl ca·vies
ce·cal
ce·cec·to·my
　pl ce·cec·to·mies
ce·ci·tis
ce·co·pexy
　pl ce·co·pex·ies
ce·cos·to·my
　pl ce·cos·to·mies
ce·cot·o·my
　pl ce·cot·o·mies
ce·cum
　pl ce·ca
ce·dar·wood
ce·la·tion
ce·li·ac
ce·li·os·co·py
　pl ce·li·os·co·pies
ce·li·ot·o·my
　pl ce·li·ot·o·mies
cel·lif·u·gal
　or cel·lu·lif·u·gal
cel·lip·e·tal
　or cel·lu·lip·e·tal
cell-me·di·at·ed
cel·lo·bi·ose
cell of Clau·di·us
cell of Cor·ti
cell of Dei·ters
cell of Hen·sen
cel·loi·din

cel·lose
cel·lu·la
　pl cel·lu·lae
cel·lu·lar
cel·lu·lar·i·ty
　pl cel·lu·lar·i·ties
cel·lu·lase
cel·lule
cel·lu·lif·u·gal
　var of cellifugal
cel·lu·lin
cel·lu·lip·e·tal
　var of cellipetal
cel·lu·lite
cel·lu·li·tis
cel·lu·lo·lyt·ic
cel·lu·lose
cel·lu·los·ic
Cel·sius
ce·ment
ce·men·ta·tion
ce·ment·i·cle
ce·ment·i·fi·ca·
　tion
ce·ment·o·blast
ce·mento·enam·
　el
ce·men·to·ma
　pl ce·men·to·mas
　or ce·men·to·ma·ta
ce·men·tum
cen·es·the·sia
cen·es·thet·ic
ce·no·ge·net·ic
　or coe·no·ge·net·ic
cen·sor
cen·so·ri·al

cen·te·sis
  pl cen·te·ses
cen·ti·grade
cen·ti·gram
cen·ti·li·ter
cen·ti·me·ter
cen·ti·nor·mal
cen·ti·pede
cen·ti·poise
cen·ti·stoke
cen·tra
  pl of centrum
cen·trad
cen·tral
cen·tric
cen·trif·u·gal
cen·trif·u·gal·iza·
  tion
cen·trif·u·gal·
  ize
  cen·trif·u·gal·
    ized
  cen·trif·u·gal·iz·
    ing
cen·trif·u·ga·tion
cen·tri·fuge
  cen·tri·fuged
  cen·tri·fug·
    ing
cen·tri·lob·u·lar
cen·tri·ole
cen·trip·e·tal
cen·tro·lec·i·thal
cen·tro·mere
cen·tro·mer·ic
cen·tro·some
cen·tro·so·mic

cen·tro·sphere
cen·trum
  pl cen·trums
  or cen·tra
Cen·tru·roi·des
Cepha·elis
ceph·a·lad
ceph·a·lal·gia
ceph·a·lex·in
ceph·al·he·ma·to·
  ma
  pl ce·phal·he·ma·to·
    mas
  or ce·phal·he·ma·to·
    ma·ta
ce·phal·ic
ce·phal·i·cal·ly
ceph·a·lin
ceph·a·li·za·tion
ceph·a·lo·cau·dal
ceph·a·lo·gram
ceph·a·lom·e·ter
ceph·a·lo·met·ric
ceph·a·lom·e·try
  pl ceph·a·lom·e·tries
ceph·a·lo·pel·vic
ceph·a·lo·pod
Ceph·a·lop·o·da
ceph·a·lop·o·dan
ceph·a·lor·i·dine
ceph·a·lo·spo·rin
Ceph·a·lo·spo·ri·um
ceph·a·lo·thin
ceph·a·lo·tho·ra·
  cop·a·gus
  pl ceph·a·lo·tho·ra·
    cop·a·gi

ce·ra al·ba

ce·ra·ceous
ce·ra fla·va
cer·amide
cer·amide·tri·hexo·
  si·dase
cer·amide·tri·hexo·
  side
ce·rate
cer·a·to·hy·al
  or cer·a·to·hy·oid
cer·car·ia
  pl cer·car·i·ae
cer·car·i·al
cer·clage
Cer·co·pi·the·ci·
  dae
cer·co·pith·e·coid
Cer·co·pi·the·cus
cer·cus
  pl cer·ci
cere
  cered
  cer·ing
ce·rea flex·i·bil·i·
  tas
ce·re·al
cer·e·bel·lar
cer·e·bel·li·tis
cer·e·bel·lo·pon·
  tine
cer·e·bel·lo·ru·bral
cer·e·bel·lum
  pl cer·e·bel·lums
  or cer·e·bel·la
ce·re·bral

cer·e·brate
  cer·e·brat·ed
  cer·e·brat·ing
cer·e·bra·tion
cere·bri·form
cer·e·brip·e·tal
cer·e·broid
cer·e·bron·ic
cer·e·brose
ce·re·bro·side
ce·re·bro·spi·nal
ce·re·bro·to·nia
ce·re·bro·vas·cu·lar
ce·re·brum
  pl ce·re·brums
  or ce·re·bra

cere·cloth
cere·ment
Ce·ren·kov ra·di·a·tion
  also Che·ren·kov ra·di·a·tion

cer·e·sin
ce·ri·um
ce·roid
cer·ti·fi·able
cer·ti·fi·ably
cer·ti·fi·ca·tion
cer·ti·fy
  cer·ti·fied
  cer·ti·fy·ing
ce·ru·lo·plas·min
ce·ru·men
ce·ru·mi·nous
cer·vi·cal
cer·vi·cec·to·my
  pl cer·vi·cec·to·mies

cer·vi·ci·tis
cer·vi·co·fa·cial
cer·vi·co·tho·rac·ic
cer·vi·co·vag·i·nal
cer·vix
  pl cer·vi·ces
  or cer·vix·es
cer·vix cor·nu
cer·vix ute·ri
ce·sar·e·an
  or cae·sar·e·an
  also ce·sar·i·an
  or cae·sar·i·an

ce·si·um
Ces·to·da
ces·tode
ces·to·di·a·sis
  pl ces·to·di·a·ses
ces·toid
Ces·toi·dea
cet·ri·mide
ce·tyl·py·ri·din·i·um
cev·a·dil·la
cev·a·dine
ce·vi·tam·ic
cgs
Cha·ber·tia
chafe
  chafed
  chaf·ing
Cha·gas' dis·ease
cha·go·ma
  pl cha·go·mas
  or cha·go·ma·ta
chain
chair·side

cha·la·sia
cha·la·za
  pl cha·la·zae
  or cha·la·zas
cha·la·zi·on
  pl cha·la·zia
chal·i·co·sis
  pl chal·i·co·ses
chalk
chalk·stone
chalky
chal·lenge
  chal·lenged
  chal·leng·ing
cha·lone
cha·ly·be·ate
cham·ber
Cham·ber·land fil·ter
cham·o·mile
  or cam·o·mile
chan·cre
chan·cri·form
chan·croid
chan·croi·dal
chan·crous
chan·nel
chao·tro·pic
chap
  chapped
  chap·ping
char·ac·ter
char·ac·ter·is·tic
char·ac·ter·is·ti·cal·ly
char·ac·ter·olog·i·cal

char·ac·ter·ol·o·gist

char·ac·ter·ol·o·gy
pl char·ac·ter·ol·o·gies

cha·ras

char·bon

char·coal

Char·cot-Ley·den crys·tals

Char·cot-Ma·rie-Tooth dis·ease

Char·cot's joint
or Char·cot joint

charge
charged
charg·ing

char·la·tan

Charles' law
also Charles's law

char·ley horse

char·ta
pl char·tae

char·tu·la
pl char·tu·lae

Chas·tek pa·ral·y·sis

chaul·moo·gra

chaul·moo·grate

chaul·moo·gric

check·bite

check·up

Che·diak-Hi·ga·shi syn·drome

cheek·bone

cheil·ec·tro·pi·on
also chil·ec·tro·pi·on

chei·li·tis
or chi·li·tis

chei·lo·plas·tic

chei·lo·plas·ty
pl chei·lo·plas·ties

chei·los·chi·sis
pl chei·los·chi·ses

chei·lo·sis
pl chei·lo·ses

chei·ro·kin·es·thet·ic

chei·rol·o·gy
or chi·rol·o·gy
pl chei·rol·o·gies
or chi·rol·o·gies

chei·ro·pom·pho·lyx

chei·ro·scope

che·late
che·lat·ed
che·lat·ing

che·la·tion

che·la·tor

che·lic·era
pl che·lic·er·ae

chel·i·do·ni·um

che·loid
var of keloid

chem·i·cal

che·mi·lu·mi·nes·cence

che·mi·lu·mi·nes·cent

chemi·os·mot·ic

che·mi·sorb

che·mi·sorp·tion

chem·ist

chem·is·try
pl chem·is·tries

che·mo·au·to·troph

che·mo·au·to·tro·phic

che·mo·au·tot·ro·phy
pl che·mo·au·tot·ro·phies

che·mo·cep·tor

che·mo·dec·to·ma
pl che·mo·dec·to·mas
or che·mo·dec·to·ma·ta

che·mo·dif·fer·en·ti·a·tion

che·mo·ki·ne·sis
pl che·mo·ki·ne·ses

chemo·ki·net·ic

che·mo·nu·cle·ol·y·sis
pl che·mo·nu·cle·ol·y·ses

che·mo·pal·li·dec·to·my
pl che·mo·pal·li·dec·to·mies

che·mo·pro·phy·lac·tic

che·mo·pro·phy·lax·is
pl che·mo·pro·phy·lax·es

che·mo·re·cep·tion

che·mo·re·cep·tive

che·mo·re·cep·tor

che·mo·re·flex

che·mo·re·sis·tance

che·mo·re·sis·tant

che·mo·sen·si·tive

chemo·sen·si·tiv·i·ty
pl chemo·sen·si·tiv·i·ties

che·mo·sen·so·ry

che·mo·sis
pl che·mo·ses

chem·os·mo·sis
pl chem·os·mo·ses

chem·os·mot·ic

che·mo·stat

che·mo·ster·il·ant

che·mo·ster·il·iza·tion

che·mo·ster·il·ize
che·mo·ster·il·ized
che·mo·ster·il·iz·ing

che·mo·sur·gery
pl che·mo·sur·ger·ies

che·mo·sur·gi·cal

che·mo·syn·the·sis
pl che·mo·syn·the·ses

che·mo·syn·thet·ic

che·mo·tac·tic

che·mo·tac·ti·cal·ly

che·mo·tax·is
pl che·mo·tax·es

che·mo·ther·a·peu·sis
pl che·mo·ther·a·peu·ses

che·mo·ther·a·peu·tant

che·mo·ther·a·peu·tic

che·mo·ther·a·peu·ti·cal

che·mo·ther·a·peu·ti·cal·ly

che·mo·ther·a·peu·tics

che·mo·ther·a·pist

che·mo·ther·a·py
pl che·mo·ther·a·pies

che·mot·ic

che·mo·tro·pic

che·mo·tro·pi·cal·ly

che·mot·ro·pism

che·no·de·ox·y·cho·lic
or che·no·des·ox·y·cho·lic

Che·no·po·di·um

che·no·po·di·um oil

Che·ren·kov ra·di·a·tion
var of Cerenkov radiation

cher·ry
pl cher·ries

cher·ub·ism

Cheyne-Stokes res·pi·ra·tion

chi·asm

chi·as·ma
pl chi·as·ma·ta

chi·as·mat·ic

chig·ger

chi·goe

chil·blain

child
pl chil·dren

child·bear·ing

child·bed

child·birth

child·hood

chil·ec·tro·pi·on
var of cheilectropion

chi·li·tis
var of cheilitis

Chi·lo·mas·tix

Chi·lop·o·da

chi·lop·o·dan

chi·me·ra
or chi·mae·ra

chi·me·ric

chi·me·rism

chim·pan·zee

chin·bone

chinch

chi·ni·o·fon

chi·on·ablep·sia

chip-blow·er

chi·ral

chi·ral·i·ty
pl chi·ral·i·ties

chi·rol·o·gy
var of cheirology

chi·ro·po·di·al

chi·rop·o·dist

chi·rop·o·dy
pl chi·rop·o·dies

chi·ro·prac·tic

chi·ro·prac·tor
chi·ro·prax·is
   pl chi·ro·prax·es
chi·rur·geon
chi·rur·gi·cal
chi·tin
chi·tin·ous
chla·myd·ia
   pl chla·myd·iae
Chla·myd·i·a·ce·ae
chla·myd·ial
chla·mydo·spore
chlo·as·ma
   pl chlo·as·ma·ta
chlor·ace·to·phe·
  none
   var of chloroaceto-
    phenone
chlor·ac·ne
chlo·ral
chlo·ral·form·
  amide
chlo·ral·ose
chlo·ral·osed
chlo·ram·bu·cil
chlo·ra·mine
chlor·am·phen·i·
  col
chlor·ane·mia
chlor·ane·mic
chlo·rate
chlor·cy·cli·zine
chlor·dan
chlor·dane
chlor·di·az·epox·
  ide
chlo·rel·la

chlo·rel·lin
chlor·e·mia
chlor·gua·nide
   var of chloroguanide
chlor·hex·i·dine
chlo·ride
chlo·ri·nate
  chlo·ri·nat·ed
  chlo·ri·nat·ing
chlo·ri·na·tion
chlo·rine
chlo·rite
chlor·mer·o·drin
chlo·ro·ace·tic
chlo·ro·ace·to·phe·
  none
   or chlor·ace·to·phe·
    none
chlo·ro·ane·mia
chlo·ro·az·o·din
chlo·ro·bu·ta·nol
chlo·ro·cre·sol
chlo·ro·form
chlo·ro·gua·nide
   or chlor·gua·nide
chlo·ro·leu·ke·mia
chlo·ro·ma
   pl chlo·ro·mas
   or chlo·ro·ma·ta
chlo·rom·a·tous
chlo·ro·per·cha
chlo·ro·phe·nol
   also chlor·phe·nol
chlo·ro·phen·o·
  thane
chlo·ro·phyll
chlo·ro·phyl·lase

chlo·ro·phyl·lide
chlo·ro·phyl·lose
chlo·ro·phyl·lous
chlo·ro·pia
chlo·ro·pic·rin
Chlo·rop·i·dae
chlo·ro·plast
chlo·ro·plas·tic
chlo·ro·pro·caine
chlo·rop·sia
chlo·ro·quine
chlo·ro·sis
   pl chlo·ro·ses
chlo·ro·then
chlo·ro·thi·a·zide
chlo·ro·thy·mol
chlo·rot·ic
chlo·ro·tri·an·i·
  sene
chlo·rous
chlo·ro·xy·le·nol
chlor·phen·e·sin
chlor·phe·nol
   var of chlorophenol
chlor·prom·a·zine
chlor·prop·amide
chlor·tet·ra·cy·
  cline
chlor·thal·i·done
cho·a·na
   pl cho·a·nae
cho·a·nal
choke
  choked
  chok·ing
cho·la·gog·ic
cho·la·gogue

cho·lane
chol·an·gio·gram
chol·an·gio·graph·
ic
chol·an·gi·og·ra·
phy
  pl chol·an·gi·og·ra·
  phies

chol·an·gi·ole
chol·an·gi·o·lit·ic
chol·an·gi·o·li·tis
  pl chol·an·gi·o·lit·i·
  des

chol·an·gi·o·ma
  pl chol·an·gi·o·mas
  or chol·an·gi·o·ma·ta

chol·an·gi·tis
  pl chol·an·git·i·des

cho·lan·ic
chol·ano·poi·e·sis
  pl chol·ano·poi·e·ses

chol·an·threne
cho·late
cho·le·cal·cif·er·ol
cho·le·chro·mo·
poi·e·sis
  pl cho·le·chro·mo·
  poi·e·ses

cho·le·cyst
cho·le·cys·ta·gogue
cho·le·cys·tec·to·
mized
cho·le·cys·tec·to·
my
  pl cho·le·cys·tec·to·
  mies

cho·le·cys·ten·ter·
os·to·my
  or cho·le·cys·to·en·
  ter·os·to·my
  pl cho·le·cys·ten·ter·
  os·to·mies
  or cho·le·cys·to·en·
  ter·os·to·mies

cho·le·cys·tic
cho·le·cys·ti·tis
  pl cho·le·cys·tit·i·des

cho·le·cys·to·gram
cho·le·cys·to·
graph·ic
cho·le·cys·tog·ra·
phy
  pl cho·le·cys·tog·ra·
  phies

cho·le·cys·to·ki·
net·ic
cho·le·cys·to·ki·nin
cho·le·cys·tor·rha·
phy
  pl cho·le·cys·tor·rha·
  phies

cho·le·cys·tos·to·
my
  pl cho·le·cys·tos·to·
  mies

cho·le·cys·tot·o·my
  pl cho·le·cys·tot·o·
  mies

cho·le·doch·al
cho·le·do·chi·tis
cho·led·o·cho·du·o·
de·nos·to·my
  pl cho·led·o·cho·du·o·
  de·nos·to·mies

cho·led·o·cho·je·ju·
nos·to·my
  pl cho·led·o·cho·je·ju·
  nos·to·mies

cho·led·o·cho·li·
thi·a·sis
  pl cho·led·o·cho·li·
  thi·a·ses

cho·led·o·cho·li·
thot·o·my
  pl cho·led·o·cho·li·
  thot·o·mies

cho·led·o·chor·ra·
phy
  pl cho·led·o·chor·ra·
  phies

cho·led·o·chos·to·
my
  pl cho·led·o·chos·to·
  mies

cho·led·o·chot·o·
my
  pl cho·led·o·chot·o·
  mies

cho·led·o·chus
  pl cho·led·o·chi

cho·le·glo·bin
cho·le·ic
cho·le·lith
cho·le·li·thi·a·sis
  pl cho·le·li·thi·a·ses

cho·le·mia
cho·le·mic
cho·le·poi·e·sis
  pl cho·le·poi·e·ses

cho·le·poi·et·ic
chol·era
chol·e·ra·ic

chol·era in·fan·
  tum
cho·le·re·sis
  pl cho·le·re·ses
cho·le·ret·ic
cho·ler·ic
chol·er·i·form
chol·er·oid
cho·le·sta·sis
  pl cho·le·sta·ses
cho·le·stat·ic
cho·les·te·a·to·ma
  pl cho·les·te·a·to·mas
  or cho·les·te·a·to·ma·
  ta
cho·les·te·a·to·ma·
  tous
cho·les·ter·ic
cho·les·ter·ol
cho·les·ter·ol·emia
  or cho·les·ter·emia
cho·les·ter·ol·osis
  pl cho·les·ter·ol·oses
cho·les·ter·o·sis
  pl cho·les·ter·o·ses
cho·le·styr·amine
cho·lic
cho·line
cho·lin·er·gic
cho·lin·er·gi·cal·ly
cho·lin·es·ter·ase
cho·li·no·lyt·ic
cho·li·no·mi·met·ic
cho·li·no·re·cep·tor
cho·lor·rhea
chol·uria
chon·dral

chon·dri
  pl of chondrus
chon·dri·fi·ca·tion
chon·dri·fy
  chon·dri·fied
  chon·dri·fy·ing
chon·drio·som·al
chon·drio·some
chon·dro·blast
chon·dro·blas·tic
chon·dro·clast
chon·dro·cra·ni·
  um
  pl chon·dro·cra·nia
chon·dro·cyte
chon·dro·dys·pla·
  sia
chon·dro·dys·tro·
  phia
chon·dro·dys·tro·
  phic
chon·dro·dys·tro·
  phy
  pl chon·dro·dys·tro·
  phies
chon·dro·gen·e·sis
  pl chon·dro·gen·e·ses
chon·dro·ge·net·ic
chon·dro·gen·ic
chon·dro·glos·sus
  pl chon·dro·glos·si
chon·droid
chon·droi·tin
chon·droi·tin·sul·
  fu·ric

chon·dro·ma
  pl chon·dro·mas
  also chon·dro·ma·ta
chon·dro·ma·la·cia
chon·dro·ma·tous
chon·dro·mu·coid
chon·dro-os·teo·
  dys·tro·phy
  pl chon·dro-os·teo·
  dys·tro·phies
chon·dro·pha·ryn·
  ge·us
  pl chon·dro·pha·ryn·
  gei
chon·dro·phyte
chon·dro·pro·tein
chon·dro·sar·co·
  ma
  pl chon·dro·sar·co·
  mas
  or chon·dro·sar·co·
  ma·ta
chon·dro·ster·nal
chon·drot·o·my
  pl chon·drot·o·mies
chon·dro·xi·phoid
Cho·part's joint
chor·da
  pl chor·dae
chord·al
chor·da·meso·
  derm
chor·da·meso·der·
  mal
Chor·da·ta
chor·date

chor·da ten·din·ea
pl chor·dae ten·din·e·ae

chor·da tym·pa·ni
chor·dee
chor·di·tis
chor·do·ma
pl chor·do·mas
or chor·do·ma·ta

chor·dot·o·my
var of cordotomy

cho·rea
cho·re·at·ic
cho·re·ic
cho·re·i·form
cho·reo·ath·e·toid
or cho·reo·ath·e·tot·ic

cho·reo·ath·e·to·sis
pl cho·reo·ath·e·to·ses

cho·re·oid
cho·rio·al·lan·to·ic
cho·rio·al·lan·to·is
pl cho·rio·al·lan·to·ides

cho·rio·an·gi·o·ma
pl cho·rio·an·gi·o·mas
or cho·rio·an·gi·o·ma·ta

cho·rio·cap·il·lar·is
cho·rio·car·ci·no·ma
pl cho·rio·car·ci·no·mas
or cho·rio·car·ci·no·ma·ta

cho·rio·ep·i·the·li·o·ma
pl cho·rio·ep·i·the·li·o·mas
or cho·rio·ep·i·the·li·o·ma·ta

cho·rio·ep·i·the·li·o·ma·tous
cho·ri·oid
var of choroid

cho·ri·o·ma
pl cho·ri·o·mas
or cho·ri·o·ma·ta

cho·rio·men·in·gi·tis
pl cho·rio·men·in·git·i·des

cho·ri·on
cho·ri·on·ep·i·the·li·o·ma
pl cho·ri·on·ep·i·the·li·o·mas
or cho·ri·on·ep·i·the·li·o·ma·ta

cho·ri·on fron·do·sum
cho·ri·on·ic
Cho·ri·op·tes
cho·ri·op·tic
cho·rio·ret·i·nal
cho·rio·ret·i·ni·tis
also cho·roi·do·ret·i·ni·tis
pl cho·rio·ret·i·nit·i·des
also cho·roi·do·ret·i·nit·i·des

cho·roid
also cho·ri·oid
noun

cho·roid
or cho·roi·dal
adjective

cho·roi·de·re·mia
cho·roid·itis
or cho·ri·oid·itis

cho·roi·do·iri·tis
cho·roid·op·a·thy
pl cho·roid·op·a·thies

chro·maf·fin
chro·maf·fi·no·ma
pl chro·maf·fi·no·mas
or chro·maf·fi·no·ma·ta

chro·mate
chro·mat·ic
chro·ma·tic·i·ty
pl chro·ma·tic·i·ties

chro·ma·tid
chro·ma·tin
chro·ma·tin·ic
chro·ma·tism
chro·mato·gram
chro·mato·graph
chro·mato·graph·er
chro·mato·graph·ic
chro·mato·graph·i·cal·ly
chro·ma·tog·ra·phy
pl chro·ma·tog·ra·phies

chro·ma·toid
chro·ma·tol·y·sis
pl chro·ma·tol·y·ses

chro·mato·lyt·ic
chro·ma·tom·e·ter

chro·mato·phore
chro·mato·phor·ic
chro·ma·top·sia
chro·ma·to·sis
  pl chro·ma·to·ses

chrome
chrom·es·the·sia
chro·mic
chro·mi·dro·sis
  pl chro·mi·dro·ses

chro·mi·um
chro·mo·bac·te·ri·um
  pl chro·mo·bac·te·ria

chro·mo·blast
chro·mo·blas·to·
  my·co·sis
  pl chro·mo·blas·to·
  my·co·ses

chro·mo·cen·ter
chro·mo·cyte
chro·mo·gen
chro·mo·gen·ic
chro·mo·mere
chro·mone
chro·mo·ne·ma
  pl chro·mo·ne·ma·ta

chro·mo·ne·mal
chro·mo·ne·ma·tal
chro·mo·ne·mat·ic
chro·mo·phil
chro·mo·phobe
chro·mo·phy·to·sis
  pl chro·mo·phy·to·ses

chro·mo·plast
chro·mo·pro·tein

chro·mos·co·py
  pl chro·mos·co·pies

chro·mo·som·al
chro·mo·some
chron·ax·ie
  also chron·axy
  or chron·ax·ia
  pl chron·ax·ies
  also chron·ax·ias

chro·nax·im·e·ter
chro·nax·i·met·ric
chro·nax·im·e·try
  pl chro·nax·im·e·tries

chron·ic
  also chron·i·cal

chro·nic·i·ty
  pl chro·nic·i·ties

chro·no·graph
chro·no·graph·ic
chro·nog·ra·phy
  pl chro·nog·ra·phies

chro·nom·e·ter
chro·nom·e·try
  pl chro·nom·e·tries

chro·no·trop·ic
chro·not·ro·pism
chrys·a·ro·bin
chry·si·a·sis
  pl chry·si·a·ses

Chrys·o·mya
Chrys·ops
chryso·ther·a·py
  pl chryso·ther·a·pies

Chvos·tek's sign
  or Chvos·tek sign

chyl·an·gi·o·ma
  pl chyl·an·gi·o·mas
  or chyl·an·gi·o·ma·ta

chyle
chy·lif·er·ous
chy·li·fi·ca·tion
chy·li·form
chy·lo·cele
chy·lo·mi·cron
chy·lo·mi·cro·ne·
  mia
chy·lo·peri·to·ne·
  um
  pl chy·lo·peri·to·ne·
   um
  or chy·lo·peri·to·nea

chy·lo·pneu·mo·
  tho·rax
  pl chy·lo·pneu·mo·
   tho·rax·es
  or chy·lo·pneu·mo·
   tho·ra·ces

chy·lo·poi·e·sis
  pl chy·lo·poi·e·ses

chy·lo·poi·et·ic
chy·lo·tho·rax
  pl chy·lo·tho·rax·es
  or chy·lo·tho·ra·ces

chy·lous
chy·lu·ria
chyme
chy·mi·fi·ca·tion
chy·mo·pa·pa·in
chy·mo·sin
chy·mo·tryp·sin
chy·mo·tryp·sin·o·
  gen
chy·mo·tryp·tic
chy·mous
cic·a·tri·cial

ci·ca·trix
  pl ci·ca·tri·ces

cic·a·tri·zant

cic·a·tri·za·tion

cic·a·trize
  cic·a·trized
  ci·ca·triz·ing

cic·u·tox·in

ci·gua·tera

ci·gua·tox·in

cil·i·ary

Cil·i·a·ta

cil·i·ate

cil·i·at·ed

cil·i·ate·ly

cil·i·a·tion

Cil·i·oph·o·ra

cil·i·oph·o·ran

cil·io·ret·i·nal

cil·i·um
  pl cil·ia

ci·met·i·dine

ci·mex
  pl ci·mi·ces

Ci·mic·i·dae

cim·i·cif·u·ga

cin·cho·na

cin·chon·amine

cin·chon·ic

cin·cho·ni·dine

cin·cho·nine

cin·cho·nism

cin·cho·nize
  cin·cho·nized
  cin·cho·niz·ing

cin·cho·phen

cine·an·gio·car·dio·
  graph·ic

cine·an·gio·car·di·
  og·ra·phy
  pl cine·an·gio·car·di·
    og·ra·phies

cine·an·gio·graph·
  ic

cine·an·gi·og·ra·
  phy
  pl cine·an·gi·og·ra·
    phies

cine·flu·o·ro·graph·
  ic

cine·flu·o·rog·ra·
  phy
  pl cine·flu·o·rog·ra·
    phies

cin·e·mat·o·graph

cin·e·mat·o·graph·
  ic

cin·e·mat·o·graph·
  i·cal·ly

cin·e·ma·tog·ra·
  phy
  pl cin·e·ma·tog·ra·
    phies

cin·e·ole

cine·pho·to·mi·cro·
  graph

cin·e·plas·tic
  also ki·ne·plas·tic

cin·e·plas·ty
  also ki·ne·plas·ty
  pl cin·e·plas·ties
  also ki·ne·plas·ties

cine·ra·dio·graph·
  ic

cine·ra·di·og·ra·
  phy
  pl cine·ra·di·og·ra·
    phies

ci·ne·rea

cine·roent·gen·og·
  ra·phy
  pl cine·roent·gen·og·
    ra·phies

cin·gu·late

cin·gu·lec·to·my
  pl cin·gu·lec·to·mies

cin·gu·lot·o·my
  pl cin·gu·lot·o·mies

cin·gu·lum
  pl cin·gu·la

cin·na·bar

cin·na·mate

cin·nam·ic

cin·na·mon

cir·ca·di·an

circ·an·nu·al

cir·ci·nate

cir·cle

cir·cle of Wil·lis

cir·cu·late
  cir·cu·lat·ed
  cir·cu·lat·ing

cir·cu·la·tion

cir·cu·la·to·ry

cir·cu·lin

cir·cu·lus
  pl cir·cu·li

cir·cum·cise
  cir·cum·cised
  cir·cum·cis·ing

cir·cum·cis·er

cleanser

cir·cum·ci·sion

cir·cum·cor·ne·al

cir·cum·duct

cir·cum·duc·tion

cir·cum·flex

cir·cum·len·tal

cir·cum·nu·cle·ar

cir·cum·oral

cir·cum·scribed

cir·cum·stan·ti·al·i·ty
  pl cir·cum·stan·ti·al·i·ties

cir·cum·val·late

cir·rho·sis
  pl cir·rho·ses

cir·rhot·ic

cir·rus
  pl cir·ri

cir·soid

cis·plat·in
  or cis-plat·i·num

cis·tern

cis·ter·na
  pl cis·ter·nae

cis·ter·na chy·li
  pl cis·ter·nae chy·li

cis·ter·nal

cis·ter·nal·ly

cis·ter·na mag·na
  pl cis·ter·nae mag·nae

cis·ter·nog·ra·phy
  pl cis·ter·nog·ra·phies

cis·tron

Ci·tel·lus

cit·ral

cit·rate

cit·rat·ed

cit·ric

cit·rin

ci·tri·nin

cit·ro·nel·la

ci·trov·o·rum fac·tor

cit·rul·lin

cit·rul·line

cit·rul·lin·emia

cit·rus
  pl cit·rus·es
  or cit·rus

clair·voy·ance

clair·voy·ant

clam·my
  clam·mi·er
  clam·mi·est

clamp

clap

cla·rif·i·cant

clar·i·fi·ca·tion

clar·i·fi·er

clar·i·fy
  clar·i·fied
  clar·i·fy·ing

Clarke's col·umn

clas·ma·to·sis
  pl clas·ma·to·ses

clasp

class

clas·sic

clas·si·cal

clas·si·fi·ca·tion

clas·si·fy
  clas·si·fied
  clas·si·fy·ing

clas·tic

clath·rate

clau·di·ca·tion

claus·tro·phil·ia

claus·tro·pho·bia

claus·tro·pho·bic

claus·tro·pho·bi·cal·ly

claus·trum
  pl claus·tra

cla·va
  pl cla·vae

clav·a·cin

cla·val

cla·vate

clav·i·cle

cla·vic·u·la
  pl cla·vic·u·lae

cla·vic·u·lar

cla·vic·u·lec·to·my
  pl cla·vic·u·lec·to·mies

clav·i·form

clav·i·for·min

cla·vus
  pl cla·vi

claw

clawed

Clay·ton gas

clean

cleanse
  cleansed
  cleans·ing

cleans·er

clear
clear·ance
cleav·age
cleft
clei·do·ic
clei·dot·o·my
  pl clei·dot·o·mies
cle·oid
cli·mac·ter·ic
cli·mac·te·ri·um
  pl cli·mac·te·ria
cli·mac·tic
cli·ma·to·ther·a·py
  pl cli·ma·to·ther·a·
    pies
cli·max
clin·da·my·cin
clin·ic
clin·i·cal
cli·ni·cian
clin·i·co·path·o·log·
  ic
  or clin·i·co·path·o·
    log·i·cal
clin·i·co·path·o·log·
  i·cal·ly
cli·no·dac·ty·ly
  pl cli·no·dac·ty·lies
cli·noid
clip
clit·i·on
  pl clit·ia
cli·to·ral
  also cli·tor·ic
clit·o·ri·dec·to·my
  pl clit·o·ri·dec·to·
    mies

cli·to·ris
  pl cli·to·ri·des
cli·vus
  pl cli·vi
clo·aca
  pl clo·acae
clo·acal
clo·a·ci·tis
clo·fi·brate
clo·mi·phene
clon·al
clone
  cloned
  clon·ing
clon·ic
clo·nic·i·ty
  pl clo·nic·i·ties
clon·i·co·ton·ic
clo·ni·dine
clo·nism
clo·nor·chi·a·sis
  also clo·nor·chi·o·sis
  pl clo·nor·chi·a·ses
  also clo·nor·chi·o·ses
Clo·nor·chis
clo·nus
clos·trid·i·al
clos·trid·i·um
  pl clos·trid·ia
clo·sure
clot
  clot·ted
  clot·ting
clove
clo·ven foot
clo·ven-foot·ed
clo·ven-hoofed

clox·a·cil·lin
clubbed
club·bing
club·foot
  pl club·feet
club·foot·ed
club·hand
clump
Clut·ton's joints
cly·sis
  pl cly·ses
clys·ma
  pl clys·ma·ta
clys·ter
cne·mi·al
cne·mis
  pl cnem·i·des
cni·do·blast
co·ac·er·vate
co·ac·er·va·tion
co·ad·ap·ta·tion
co·adapt·ed
coag time
co·ag·u·la·bil·i·ty
co·ag·u·la·ble
co·ag·u·lant
co·ag·u·lase
co·ag·u·late
  co·ag·u·lat·ed
  co·ag·u·lat·ing
co·ag·u·la·tion
co·ag·u·la·tor
co·ag·u·la·to·ry
co·ag·u·lin
co·ag·u·lom·e·ter
co·ag·u·lop·a·thy
  pl co·ag·u·lop·a·thies

co·ag·u·lum
 pl co·ag·u·la
 or co·ag·u·lums

co·apt

co·ap·ta·tion

co·arct

co·arc·ta·tion

coarse

coat

coat·ed

Coats's dis·ease

co·bal·a·min
 also co·bal·a·mine

co·balt

co·bal·tic

co·bal·tous

co·bra

co·ca

co·caine

co·cain·ism

co·cain·iza·tion

co·cain·ize
 co·cain·ized
 co·cain·iz·ing

co·car·box·yl·ase

co·car·cin·o·gen

co·car·cin·o·gen·ic

coc·cal

coc·ci
 pl of coccus

coc·cid·ia
 pl of coccidium

Coc·cid·ia

coc·cid·i·al

coc·cid·i·an

coc·cid·i·oi·dal

coc·cid·i·oi·des

coc·cid·i·oi·din

coc·cid·i·oi·do·my·
 co·sis
 pl coc·cid·i·oi·do·my·
  co·ses

coc·cid·io·my·co·
 sis
 pl coc·cid·io·my·co·
  ses

coc·cid·i·o·sis
 pl coc·cid·i·o·ses

coc·cid·io·stat

coc·cid·i·um
 pl coc·cid·ia

coc·co·ba·cil·la·ry

coc·co·ba·cil·lus
 pl coc·co·ba·cil·li

coc·co·gen·ic
 also coc·ci·gen·ic

coc·coid

coc·cu·lus
 pl coc·cu·lus

coc·cus
 pl coc·ci

coc·cy·dyn·ia

coc·cy·geal

coc·cy·gec·to·my
 pl coc·cy·gec·to·mies

coc·cyg·eus
 pl coc·cyg·ei

coc·cy·go·dyn·ia

coc·cyx
 pl coc·cy·ges
 also coc·cyx·es

co·chi·neal

co·chle·a
 pl co·chle·as
 or co·chle·ae

co·chle·ar

co·chle·ar·i·form

co·chle·ate

co·chleo·ves·tib·u·
 lar

Coch·lio·my·ia

co·chro·mato·
 graph

co·chro·ma·tog·ra·
 phy
 pl co·chro·ma·tog·ra·
  phies

co·cil·la·na

cock·eye

cock·eyed

cock·roach

co·coa

co·con·scious

co·co·nut

coc·to·sta·ble

co·cul·ti·vate
 co·cul·ti·vat·ed
 co·cul·ti·vat·ing

co·cul·ti·va·tion

cod
 pl cod
 also cods

co·da·mine

code
 cod·ed
 cod·ing

co·de·car·box·yl·
 ase

co·deine

co·dex
 pl co·di·ces

cod-liv·er oil

co·dom·i·nant

co·don

co·ef·fi·cient

co·elec·tro·pho·re·sis

Coe·len·ter·a·ta

coe·len·ter·ate

coe·lom
pl coe·loms
or coe·lo·ma·ta

coe·lo·mate

coe·lo·mic

coe·no·cyte

coe·no·cyt·ic

coe·no·ge·net·ic
var of cenogenetic

coe·nu·ro·sis
or coe·nu·ri·a·sis
pl coe·nu·ro·ses
or coe·nu·ri·a·ses

coe·nu·rus
pl coe·nu·ri

co·en·zy·mat·ic

co·en·zy·mat·i·cal·ly

co·en·zyme

co·en·zyme A

co·en·zyme Q

co·fac·tor

cog·ni·tion

cog·ni·tive

co·he·sion

co·he·sive

Cohn·heim's ar·ea

co·ho·ba

co·ho·ba·tion

co·hosh

co·ital

co·ition

co·ition·al

co·itus

co·itus in·ter·rup·tus

co·itus res·er·va·tus

co·la
pl of colon

co·la·mine

col·chi·cine

col·chi·cum

cold

cold-blood·ed

col·ec·to·my
pl col·ec·to·mies

co·le·op·te·ra

co·le·op·te·ran

co·le·op·te·rist

co·le·op·te·rous

co·li

co·li·ba·cil·la·ry

co·li·ba·cil·lo·sis
pl co·li·ba·cil·lo·ses

col·ic
noun
paroxysmal abdominal pain

col·ic
adjective
relating to colic

co·lic
adjective
relating to the colon

co·li·cin
also co·li·cine

co·li·ci·no·ge·nic

co·li·ci·no·ge·nic·i·ty
pl co·li·ci·no·ge·nic·i·ties

co·li·ci·nog·e·ny
pl co·li·ci·nog·e·nies

col·icky

co·li·form

co·lin·ear

co·lin·ear·i·ty
pl co·lin·ear·i·ties

co·li·phage

co·lis·tin

co·li·tis

col·la
pl of collum

col·la·gen

col·la·ge·nase

col·la·gen·ic

col·la·gen·o·lyt·ic

col·la·ge·no·sis
pl col·la·ge·no·ses

col·lag·e·nous

col·lapse

col·lapsed

col·laps·ing

col·laps·ibil·i·ty

col·laps·ible

col·lar

col·lar·bone

col·lat·er·al

Col·les' frac·ture

col·lic·u·lus
pl col·lic·u·li

col·li·mate
  col·li·mat·ed
  col·li·mat·ing
col·li·ma·tion
col·li·ma·tor
col·li·qua·tion
col·liq·ua·tive
col·lo·di·on
col·loid
col·loi·dal
col·loi·do·cla·sia
col·loi·do·clas·tic
col·lum
  pl col·la
col·lu·nar·i·um
  pl col·lu·nar·ia
col·lu·to·ri·um
  pl col·lu·to·ria
col·lyr·i·um
  pl col·lyr·ia
  or col·lyr·i·ums
col·o·bo·ma
  pl col·o·bo·ma·ta
col·o·bo·ma·tous
co·lo·co·lic
co·lom·bo
  var of calumba
co·lon
  pl co·lons
  or co·la
co·lon·ic
col·o·ni·za·tion
col·o·nize
  col·o·nized
  col·o·niz·ing
co·lon·o·scope
co·lon·o·scop·ic

co·lo·nos·co·py
  pl co·lo·nos·co·pies
col·o·ny
  pl col·o·nies
col·o·pexy
  pl col·o·pex·ies
co·lo·proc·tos·to·my
  pl co·lo·proc·tos·to·mies
col·or-blind
col·or blind·ness
co·lo·rec·tal
col·or·im·e·ter
col·or·i·met·ric
col·or·i·met·ri·cal·ly
col·or·im·e·try
  pl col·or·im·e·tries
co·los·to·mize
  co·los·to·mized
  co·los·to·miz·ing
co·los·to·my
  pl co·los·to·mies
co·los·tral
co·los·trum
co·lot·o·my
  pl co·lot·o·mies
col·pec·to·my
  pl col·pec·to·mies
col·peu·ryn·ter
col·peu·ry·sis
col·pi·tis
col·po·cen·te·sis
  pl col·po·cen·te·ses
col·po·clei·sis
  pl col·po·clei·ses

col·po·per·i·ne·or·rha·phy
  pl col·po·per·i·ne·or·rha·phies
col·po·pexy
  pl col·po·pex·ies
col·po·plas·ty
  pl col·po·plas·ties
col·por·rha·phy
  pl col·por·rha·phies
col·po·scope
col·po·scop·ic
col·po·scop·i·cal·ly
col·pos·co·py
  pl col·pos·co·pies
col·po·stat
col·pot·o·my
  pl col·pot·o·mies
col·u·brid
Co·lu·bri·dae
co·lum·bin
co·lum·bi·um
col·u·mel·la
  pl col·u·mel·lae
col·u·mel·lar
col·u·mel·late
co·lum·na
  pl co·lum·nae
  also co·lum·nas
co·lum·nar
co·ma
co·ma·tose
com·bat fa·tigue
com·e·do
  pl com·e·do·nes

com·e·do·car·ci·no·ma
   pl com·e·do·car·ci·no·mas
   or com·e·do·car·ci·no·ma·ta

com·men·sal
com·men·sal·ism
com·mi·nute
   com·mi·nut·ed
   com·mi·nut·ing
com·mi·nu·tion
com·mis·su·ra
   pl com·mis·su·rae

com·mis·sur·al
com·mis·sure
com·mis·sur·ot·o·my
   pl com·mis·sur·ot·o·mies

com·mo·tio
com·mu·ni·ca·bil·i·ty
   pl com·mu·ni·ca·bil·i·ties

com·mu·ni·ca·ble
com·mu·ni·cate
   com·mu·ni·cat·ed
   com·mu·ni·cat·ing
com·mu·ni·ca·tion
com·pac·ta
com·par·a·tive
com·part·men·tal·iza·tion

com·part·men·tal·ize
   com·part·men·tal·ized
   com·part·men·tal·iz·ing
com·part·men·ta·tion
com·pat·i·bil·i·ty
   pl com·pat·i·bil·i·ties
com·pat·i·ble
com·pen·sate
   com·pen·sat·ed
   com·pen·sat·ing
com·pen·sa·tion
com·pen·sa·to·ry
com·pe·tence
com·pe·ten·cy
   pl com·pe·ten·cies
com·pe·tent
com·pet·i·tive
com·plain
com·plaint
com·ple·ment
com·ple·men·tar·i·ty
   pl com·ple·men·tar·i·ties
com·ple·men·ta·ry
com·ple·men·ta·tion
com·plete
com·plex
com·plex·ion
com·plex·ioned
com·plex·us
com·pli·ance

com·pli·cate
   com·pli·cat·ed
   com·pli·cat·ing
com·pli·ca·tion
com·pos men·tis
com·pound
com·press
com·pres·sion
com·pres·sor
com·pro·mise
   com·pro·mised
   com·pro·mis·ing
Comp·ton ef·fect
com·pul·sion
com·pul·sive
com·pul·siv·i·ty
   pl com·pul·siv·i·ties
con·al·bu·min
co·nar·i·um
   pl co·nar·ia
co·na·tion
co·na·tive
con·ca·nav·a·lin
Con·ca·to's dis·ease
con·cave
con·cav·i·ty
   pl con·cav·i·ties
con·ca·vo-con·cave
con·ceive
   con·ceived
   con·ceiv·ing
con·cen·trate
   con·cen·trat·ed
   con·cen·trat·ing
con·cen·tra·tion
con·cen·tra·tor

con·cen·tric
con·cen·tri·cal·ly
con·cept
con·cep·tion
con·cep·tive
con·cep·tu·al
con·cep·tus
conch
  pl conchs
  or conch·es
con·cha
  pl con·chae
con·chal
con·cor·dance
con·cor·dant
con·cres·cence
con·cre·tio cor·dis
con·cre·tion
con·cuss
con·cus·sion
con·cus·sive
con·dens·able
con·den·sa·tion
con·dense
  con·densed
  con·dens·ing
con·dens·er
con·di·ment
con·di·men·tal
con·di·tion
  con·di·tioned
  con·di·tion·ing
con·di·tion·able
con·di·tion·al
con·dom
con·duct
con·duc·tance

con·duc·tion
con·duc·tive
con·duc·tiv·i·ty
  pl con·duc·tiv·i·ties
con·duc·tor
con·duc·to·ri·al
con·du·ran·go
con·dy·lar
con·dy·lar·thro·sis
  pl con·dy·lar·thro·ses
con·dyle
con·dy·lec·to·my
  pl con·dy·lec·to·mies
con·dyl·i·on
con·dy·loid
con·dy·lo·ma
  pl con·dy·lo·ma·ta
  also con·dy·lo·mas
con·dy·lo·ma acu·
  mi·na·tum
  pl con·dy·lo·ma·ta
  acu·mi·na·ta
con·dy·lo·ma·tous
cone·nose
con·fab·u·late
  con·fab·u·lat·ed
  con·fab·u·lat·ing
con·fab·u·la·tion
con·fab·u·la·to·ry
con·fec·tio
  pl con·fec·ti·o·nes
con·fec·tion
con·fig·u·ra·tion
con·fig·u·ra·tion·al
con·fig·u·ra·tive

con·fine
  con·fined
  con·fin·ing
con·fine·ment
con·flict
con·flic·tu·al
con·flu·ence of si·
  nus·es
con·flu·ens si·nu·
  um
con·flu·ent
con·fo·cal
con·for·ma·tion
con·form·er
con·fused
con·fu·sion
con·geal
con·ge·la·tion
con·ge·ner
con·ge·ner·ic
con·gen·i·tal
con·gest·ed
con·ges·tion
con·ges·tive
con·gi·us
  pl con·gii
con·glo·bate
  con·glo·bat·ed
  con·glo·bat·ing
con·glom·er·ate
  con·glom·er·at·
  ed
  con·glom·er·at·
  ing
con·glom·er·a·tion

con·glu·ti·nate
  con·glu·ti·nat·ed
  con·glu·ti·nat·
    ing
con·glu·ti·na·tion
con·glu·ti·nin
Con·go red
con·gress
con·hy·drine
co·ni
  pl of conus
con·i·cal
  or con·ic
co·nid·i·al
co·nid·i·al
co·nid·io·phore
co·nid·i·oph·o·rous
co·nid·io·spore
co·nid·i·um
  pl co·nid·ia
co·ni·ine
co·ni·um
con·iza·tion
con·ju·gal
con·ju·gant
con·ju·gase
con·ju·ga·ta
  pl con·ju·ga·tae
con·ju·gate
  con·ju·gat·ed
  con·ju·gat·ing
con·ju·ga·tion
con·ju·ga·tion·al
con·junc·ti·va
  pl con·junc·ti·vas
  or con·junc·ti·vae
con·junc·ti·val

con·junc·ti·vi·tis
con·junc·tivo·plas·
  ty
  pl con·junc·tivo·plas·
    ties
con·junc·tivo·rhi·
  nos·to·my
  pl con·junc·tivo·rhi·
    nos·to·mies
con·nec·tor
Conn's syn·drome
co·noid
  or co·noi·dal
con·san·guine
con·san·guin·e·ous
con·san·guin·i·ty
  pl con·san·guin·i·ties
con·science
con·scious
con·sen·su·al
con·ser·va·tion
con·ser·va·tive
con·serve
  con·served
  con·serv·ing
con·sol·i·da·tion
con·so·lute
con·spe·cif·ic
con·stant
con·stel·la·tion
con·sti·pate
  con·sti·pat·ed
  con·sti·pat·ing
con·sti·pa·tion
con·sti·tu·tion
con·sti·tu·tive
con·strict

con·stric·tion
con·stric·tive
con·stric·tor
con·sult
con·sul·tant
con·sul·ta·tion
con·sum·ma·to·ry
con·sump·tion
con·sump·tive
con·tact
con·ta·gion
con·ta·gious
con·ta·gium
  pl con·ta·gia
con·tam·i·nant
con·tam·i·nate
  con·tam·i·nat·ed
  con·tam·i·nat·
    ing
con·tam·i·na·tion
con·tam·i·na·tive
con·tam·i·na·tor
con·tent
con·ti·gu·ity
  pl con·ti·gu·ities
con·tig·u·ous
con·ti·nence
con·ti·nent
con·ti·nu·ity
  pl con·ti·nu·it·ies
con·tin·u·ous
con·tour
con·tra·cep·tion
con·tra·cep·tive
con·tract
con·tract·ibil·i·ty
  pl con·tract·ibil·i·ties

con·tract·ible
con·trac·tile
con·trac·til·i·ty
  pl con·trac·til·i·ties
con·trac·tion
con·trac·tor
con·trac·ture
con·tra·in·di·cate
  con·tra·in·di·cat·ed
  con·tra·in·di·cat·ing
con·tra·in·di·ca·tion
con·tra·lat·er·al
con·tre·coup
con·trec·ta·tion
con·trol
  con·trolled
  con·trol·ling
con·tuse
  con·tused
  con·tus·ing
con·tu·sion
co·nus
  pl co·ni
co·nus ar·te·ri·o·sus
  pl co·ni ar·te·ri·o·si
co·nus med·ul·lar·is
con·va·lesce
  con·va·lesced
  con·va·lesc·ing
con·va·les·cence
con·va·les·cent
con·val·la·tox·in

con·vec·tion
con·vec·tive
con·verge
  con·verged
  con·verg·ing
con·ver·gence
con·ver·gent
con·ver·sion
con·vex
con·vex·i·ty
  pl con·vex·i·ties
con·vexo-con·cave
con·vexo-con·vex
con·vo·lute
  con·vo·lut·ed
con·vo·lu·tion
con·vo·lu·tion of Bro·ca
con·vol·vu·lus
  pl con·vol·vu·lus·es
  or con·vol·vu·li
con·vul·sant
con·vulse
  con·vulsed
  con·vuls·ing
con·vul·sion
con·vul·sive
Coo·ley's ane·mia
Coo·lidge tube
Coombs test
Coo·pe·ria
coop·er·id
Coo·per's lig·a·ment
co·or·di·nate
  co·or·di·nat·ed
  co·or·di·nat·ing

co·or·di·na·tion
co·os·si·fi·ca·tion
co·os·si·fy
  co·os·si·fied
  co·os·si·fy·ing
coo·tie
co·pai·ba
cope
  coped
  cop·ing
co·pe·pod
Co·pep·o·da
co·pol·y·mer
co·po·ly·mer·iza·tion
co·po·ly·mer·ize
  co·po·ly·mer·ized
  co·po·ly·mer·iz·ing
cop·per
cop·per·head
cop·pery
cop·ro·an·ti·body
  pl cop·ro·an·ti·bod·ies
cop·ro·lag·nia
cop·ro·lag·nist
cop·ro·la·lia
cop·ro·lith
cop·ro·pha·gia
co·proph·a·gist
co·proph·a·gous
  or cop·ro·phag·ic
co·proph·a·gy
  pl co·proph·a·gies
cop·ro·phil·ia
cop·ro·phil·i·ac

cop·ro·phil·ic
cop·roph·i·lous
cop·ro·por·phy·rin
co·pros·ta·nol
co·pros·ter·ol
cop·u·la
 pl cop·u·las
 also cop·u·lae

cop·u·late
 cop·u·lat·ed
 cop·u·lat·ing
cop·u·la·tion
cop·u·la·to·ry
co·quille
cor·a·cid·i·um
 pl cor·a·cid·ia

cor·a·co·acro·mi·al
cor·a·co·bra·chi·a·lis
 pl cor·a·co·bra·chi·a·les

cor·a·co·cla·vic·u·lar
cor·a·co·hu·mer·al
cor·a·coid
cor bo·vi·num
cord
cor·date
cor·dec·to·my
 pl cor·dec·to·mies

cor·dial
cor·dia pul·mo·na·lia
 pl of cor pulmonale

cor·di·form

cor·dot·o·my
 or chor·dot·o·my
 pl cor·dot·o·mies
 or chor·dot·o·mies
core
co·re·pres·sor
co·ri·an·der
Co·ri cy·cle
Co·ri es·ter
co·ri·um
 pl co·ria

corm
cor·nea
cor·ne·al
cor·ne·itis
cor·neo·scler·al
cor·ne·ous
cor·ner
cor·ne·um
 pl cor·nea

cor·nic·u·late
cor·nic·u·lum
 pl cor·nic·u·la

cor·ni·fi·ca·tion
cor·ni·fy
 cor·ni·fied
 cor·ni·fy·ing
cor·nu
 pl cor·nua

cor·nu·al
corny
corn·i·er
corn·i·est
co·ro·na
co·ro·nal
co·ro·nale

co·ro·na ra·di·a·ta
 pl co·ro·nae ra·di·a·tae

cor·o·nary
 pl cor·o·nar·ies

co·ro·na·vi·rus
cor·o·ner
cor·o·net
co·ro·ni·on
 pl co·ro·nia

cor·o·ni·tis
cor·o·noid
cor·o·noid·ec·to·my
 pl cor·o·noid·ec·to·mies

cor·po·ra
 pl of corpus

cor·po·ral
cor·po·ra quad·ri·gem·i·na
cor·po·re·al
corpse
corps·man
 pl corps·men

cor·pu·lence
cor·pu·len·cy
 pl cor·pu·len·cies

cor·pu·lent
cor pul·mo·na·le
 pl cor·dia pul·mo·na·lia

cor·pus
 pl cor·po·ra

cor·pus al·bi·cans
 pl cor·po·ra al·bi·can·tia

cor·pus cal·lo·sum
pl cor·po·ra cal·lo·sa

cor·pus ca·ver·no·sum
pl cor·po·ra ca·ver·no·sa

cor·pus·cle

cor·pus·cle of Herbst

cor·pus·cle of Krause

cor·pus·cu·lar

cor·pus de·lic·ti
pl cor·po·ra de·lic·ti

cor·pus he·mor·rhag·i·cum

cor·pus lu·te·um
pl cor·po·ra lu·tea

cor·pus spon·gi·o·sum

cor·pus stri·a·tum
pl cor·po·ra stri·a·ta

cor·pus uteri

cor·rect

cor·rect·able

cor·rec·tion

cor·rec·tive

Cor·ri·gan's pulse
or Cor·ri·gan pulse

cor·ri·gent

cor·rode

cor·rod·ed

cor·rod·ing

cor·ro·sion

cor·ro·sive

cor·ru·ga·tor

cor·tex
pl cor·ti·ces
or cor·tex·es

cor·ti·cal

cor·ti·cate

cor·ti·cif·u·gal

cor·ti·cip·e·tal

cor·ti·co·af·fer·ent

cor·ti·co·bul·bar

cor·ti·co·ef·fer·ent

cor·ti·coid

cor·ti·co·pon·tine

cor·ti·co·pon·to·cer·e·bel·lar

cor·ti·co·ru·bral

cor·ti·co·spi·nal

cor·ti·co·ste·roid

cor·ti·co·ste·rone

cor·ti·co·tha·lam·ic

cor·ti·co·tro·pic
also cor·ti·co·tro·phic

cor·ti·co·tro·pin
or cor·ti·co·tro·phin

cor·tin

Cor·ti's gan·gli·on

cor·ti·sol

cor·ti·sone

co·ryd·a·lis

Cor·y·ne·bac·te·ri·a·ce·ae

Cor·y·ne·bac·te·ri·um
pl cor·y·ne·bac·te·ria

co·ryne·form

co·ry·za

co·ry·zal

cos·met·ic

cos·ta
pl cos·tae

cos·tal

cos·tec·to·my
pl cos·tec·to·mies

cos·tive

cos·to·cen·tral

cos·to·cer·vi·cal

cos·to·chon·dral

cos·to·cla·vic·u·lar

cos·to·cor·a·coid

cos·to·di·a·phrag·mat·ic

cos·to·phren·ic

cos·to·tome

cos·to·trans·verse

cos·to·trans·ver·sec·to·my
pl cos·to·trans·ver·sec·to·mies

cos·to·ver·te·bral

cos·to·xi·phoid

cot

co·tar·nine

co·throm·bo·plas·tin

co·trans·duc·tion

cot·ton

cot·ton·mouth

cot·ton·seed

cot·y·le·don

cot·y·le·don·ary

cot·y·loid

couch

cough

cou·lomb

cou·ma·phos

cou·ma·rin

coun·sel
  coun·seled
    or coun·selled
  coun·sel·ing
    or coun·sel·ling
coun·sel·ee
coun·sel·or
  or coun·sel·lor

count
count·er
coun·ter·act
coun·ter·ac·tion
coun·ter·con·di·
  tion·ing
coun·ter·cur·rent
coun·ter·ir·ri·tant
coun·ter·ir·ri·tate
  coun·ter·ir·ri·tat·
    ed
  coun·ter·ir·ri·tat·
    ing
coun·ter·ir·ri·ta·
  tion
coun·ter·open·ing
coun·ter·pho·bic
coun·ter·pul·sa·
  tion
coun·ter·punc·ture
coun·ter·shock
coun·ter·stain
coun·ter·trac·tion
coun·ter·trans·fer·
  ence
cou·pling
course
  pl cours·es

cou·vade
Cou·ve·laire uter·
  us
  pl Cou·ve·laire uteri
co·va·lence
co·va·len·cy
  pl co·va·len·cies
co·va·lent
cov·er glass
cov·er·slip
cow·age
  or cow·hage
Cow·dria
Cow·per's gland
cow·pox
coxa
  pl cox·ae
Cox·i·el·la
cox·i·tis
  pl cox·it·i·des
coxo·fem·o·ral
Cox·sack·ie vi·rus
crab
cra·dle
cramp
cra·ni·acro·mi·al
cra·ni·ad
cra·ni·al
cra·ni·al·gia
cra·ni·ate
cra·ni·ec·to·my
  pl cra·ni·ec·to·mies
cra·nio·ce·re·bral
cra·nio·cla·sis
  pl cra·nio·cla·ses
cra·nio·fa·cial
cra·nio·fe·nes·tria

cra·nio·graph
cra·ni·ol·o·gy
  pl cra·ni·ol·o·gies
cra·ni·om·e·ter
cra·nio·met·ric
  or cra·nio·met·ri·cal
cra·ni·om·e·try
  pl cra·ni·om·e·tries
cra·ni·op·a·gus
  pl cra·ni·op·a·gi
cra·ni·op·a·thy
  pl cra·ni·op·a·thies
cra·nio·pha·ryn·
  geal
cra·nio·pha·ryn·gi·
  o·ma
  pl cra·nio·pha·ryn·gi·
    o·mas
  or cra·nio·pha·ryn·gi·
    o·ma·ta
cra·nio·phore
cra·nio·plas·ty
  pl cra·nio·plas·ties
cra·nio·ra·chis·chi·
  sis
  pl cra·nio·ra·chis·chi·
    ses
cra·nio·sa·cral
cra·ni·os·chi·sis
  pl cra·ni·os·chi·ses
cra·nio·scop·ic
cra·ni·os·co·pist
cra·ni·os·co·py
  pl cra·ni·os·co·pies
cra·nio·ste·no·sis
  pl cra·nio·ste·no·ses

cra·nio·syn·os·to·
sis
   pl cra·nio·syn·os·to·
   ses
   or cra·nio·syn·os·to·
   sis·es

cra·nio·ta·bes
   pl cra·nio·ta·bes

cra·nio·tome
cra·ni·ot·o·my
   pl cra·ni·ot·o·mies

cra·ni·um
   pl cra·ni·ums
   or cra·nia

crap·u·lous
cra·ter
cra·ter·iza·tion
craw-craw
C-re·ac·tive pro·
tein
crease
   creased
   creas·ing
cre·atine
cre·at·i·nine
cre·atin·uria
cre·mains
cre·mas·ter
cre·mas·ter·ic
cre·mate
   cre·mat·ed
   cre·mat·ing
cre·ma·tion
cre·ma·to·ri·um
   pl cre·ma·to·ri·ums
   or cre·ma·to·ria

cre·ma·to·ry
   pl cre·ma·to·ries

crème
   pl crèmes

cre·nat·ed
   also cre·nate

cre·na·tion
cren·o·cyte
cre·o·sote
crep·i·tant
crep·i·tate
   crep·i·tat·ed
   crep·i·tat·ing
crep·i·ta·tion
crep·i·tus
   pl crep·i·tus

cres·cent
cre·sol
crest
cre·ta
cre·tin
cre·tin·ism
cre·tin·oid
cre·tin·ous
Creutz·feldt-Ja·kob
dis·ease
   also Creutz·feld-Ja·
   cob dis·ease

crev·ice
cre·vic·u·lar
cri·bra·tion
crib·ri·form
cri·ce·tid
Cri·ce·ti·dae
cri·co·ar·y·te·noid
cri·coid

cri·coid·ec·to·my
   pl cri·coid·ec·to·mies

cri·co·pha·ryn·geal
cri·co·thy·roid
cri·co·thy·roi·de·us
   pl cri·co·thy·roi·dei

cri du chat syn·
drome
crim·i·no·log·i·cal
crim·i·nol·o·gist
crim·i·nol·o·gy
   pl crim·i·nol·o·gies

crip·ple
   crip·pled
   crip·pling
crip·pler
cri·sis
   pl cri·ses

cris·ta
   pl cris·tae

cris·ta acus·ti·ca
   pl cris·tae acus·ti·cae

cris·ta gal·li
cri·thid·ia
cri·thid·i·al
cri·thid·i·form
crit·i·cal
crock
cro·cus
   pl cro·cus·es
   also cro·cus
   or cro·ci

Crohn's dis·ease
cross·abil·i·ty
   pl cross·abil·i·ties

cross·able
cross·bred

cross·breed
  cross·bred
  cross·breed·ing
cross·bridge
cross-eye
  pl cross-eyes
cross-eyed
cross-fer·tile
cross-fer·til·iza·
  tion
cross-fer·til·ize
  cross-fer·til·ized
  cross-fer·til·iz·
    ing
cross-fir·ing
cross·ing-over
cross-link
cross·match
cross·match·ing
cross·over
cross-re·act
cross-re·ac·tion
cross-re·ac·tive
cross-re·ac·tiv·i·ty
  pl cross-re·ac·tiv·i·ties
cross sec·tion
cross-sec·tion·al
cross-ster·ile
cross-ste·ril·i·ty
  pl cross-ste·ril·i·ties
cross-tol·er·ance
cro·ta·lid
Cro·tal·i·dae
cro·ta·lin
cro·ta·line
cro·ta·lism
Cro·ta·lus

cro·taph·i·on
crotch
cro·tin
cro·ton
Cro·ton bug
croup
croup·ous
croupy
  croup·i·er
  croup·i·est
crow's-foot
  pl crow's-feet
cru·ci·ate
cru·ci·ble
cru·ra ce·re·bri
cru·ra for·ni·cis
cru·ral
crus
  pl cru·ra
crust
crus·ta
  pl crus·tae
crus·ta·cea
crus·ta·cean
crutch
cry·mo·ther·a·py
  pl cry·mo·ther·a·pies
cryo·bi·o·log·i·cal
cryo·bi·ol·o·gist
cryo·bi·ol·o·gy
  pl cryo·bi·ol·o·gies
cryo·cau·tery
  pl cryo·cau·ter·ies
cryo·ex·trac·tion
cryo·ex·trac·tor
cryo·fi·brin·o·gen
cryo·gen

cryo·gen·ic
cryo·gen·i·cal·ly
cryo·gen·ics
cryo·glob·u·lin
cryo·glob·u·lin·
  emia
cry·on·ics
cryo·phil·ic
cryo·pre·cip·i·tate
cryo·pre·cip·i·ta·
  tion
cryo·pres·er·va·
  tion
cryo·pre·serve
  cryo·pre·served
  cryo·pre·serv·ing
cryo·probe
cryo·pro·tec·tant
cryo·pro·tec·tive
cryo·pro·tein
cryo·scope
cry·os·co·py
  pl cry·os·co·pies
cryo·stat
cryo·stat·ic
cryo·sur·geon
cryo·sur·gery
  pl cryo·sur·ger·ies
cryo·sur·gi·cal
cryo·ther·a·py
  pl cryo·ther·a·pies
crypt
crypt·ec·to·my
  pl crypt·ec·to·mies
cryp·tic
cryp·ti·cal·ly
cryp·ti·tis

cryp·to·bi·o·sis
 pl cryp·to·bi·o·ses

cryp·to·coc·cal

cryp·to·coc·co·sis
 pl cryp·to·coc·co·ses

cryp·to·coc·cus
 pl cryp·to·coc·ci

cryp·to·crys·tal·line

crypt of Lie·ber·kühn

crypt of Mor·ga·gni

cryp·to·gam

Cryp·to·ga·mia

cryp·to·gam·ic

cryp·tog·a·mous

cryp·to·ge·net·ic

cryp·to·gen·ic

cryp·tom·ne·sia

cryp·tom·ne·sic

crypt·or·chid

crypt·or·chi·dism
 also crypt·or·chism

cryp·to·spo·rid·i·o·sis
 pl cryp·to·spo·rid·i·o·ses

Cryp·to·spo·rid·i·um

cryp·to·xan·thin

cryp·to·xan·thol

cryp·to·zo·ite

crys·tal

crys·tal·line

crys·tal·liz·able

crys·tal·li·za·tion

crys·tal·lize
 also crys·tal·ize

crys·tal·lized
 also crys·tal·ized

crys·tal·liz·ing
 also crys·tal·iz·ing

crys·tal·lo·gram

crys·tal·log·ra·pher

crys·tal·lo·graph·ic
 or crys·tal·lo·graph·i·cal

crys·tal·log·ra·phy
 pl crys·tal·log·ra·phies

crys·tal·lu·ria

Cteno·ce·phal·i·des

cu·beb

cu·bi·tal

cu·bi·tus
 pl cu·bi·ti

cu·boid

cu·boi·dal

cu·cum·ber

cud·bear

cui·rass

cul-de-sac
 pl culs-de-sac
 also cul-de-sacs

cul-de-sac of Doug·las

cul·do·cen·te·sis
 pl cul·do·cen·te·ses

cul·do·scop·ic

cul·dos·co·py
 pl cul·dos·co·pies

cul·dot·o·my
 pl cul·dot·o·mies

cu·lex

Cu·lic·i·dae

cu·li·cide

cu·li·cine

Cu·li·coi·des

cul·men

cul·ti·vate
  cul·ti·vat·ed
  cul·ti·vat·ing

cul·ti·va·tion

cul·tur·al

cul·ture
  cul·tured
  cul·tur·ing

cu·mu·la·tive

cu·mu·lus
 pl cu·mu·li

cu·mu·lus ooph·o·rus

cu·ne·ate

cu·ne·i·form

cu·ne·us
 pl cu·nei

cu·nic·u·lus
 pl cu·nic·u·li

cun·ni·lin·guism

cun·ni·lin·gus
 also cun·ni·linc·tus

cun·nus
 pl cun·ni

cu·pre·ine

cu·pric

cu·pu·la
 pl cu·pu·lae

cur·able

cu·ra·re
 also cu·ra·ri

cu·ra·ri·form

cu·ra·rine
cu·ra·ri·za·tion
cu·ra·rize
  cu·ra·rized
  cu·ra·riz·ing
cu·ra·tive
cur·er
cu·ret·tage
cu·rette
  also cu·ret
  cu·rett·ed
  cu·rett·ing
cu·rette·ment
cu·rie
cu·ri·um
Cur·ling's ul·cer
cur·rent
cur·va·ture
cush·ing·oid
Cush·ing's dis·ease
cush·ion
cusp
cus·pid
cus·pi·date
cus·to·di·al
cu·ta·ne·ous
cut·down
Cu·te·re·bra
Cu·te·reb·ri·dae
cu·ti·cle
cu·tic·u·lar
cu·tic·u·lar·iza·tion
cu·tic·u·lar·ized
cu·ti·re·ac·tion
cu·tis
  pl cu·tes
  or cu·tis·es

cu·tis an·se·ri·na
  pl cu·tes an·se·ri·nae
cu·tis ve·ra
  pl cu·tes ve·rae
cu·vette
Cu·vie·ri·an vein
cy·an·ic
cy·a·nide
cy·a·no·ac·ry·late
cy·a·no·co·bal·a·min
  also cy·a·no·co·bal·a·mine
cy·ano·gen
cy·a·no·gen·e·sis
  pl cy·a·no·gen·e·ses
cy·a·no·ge·net·ic
  or cy·a·no·gen·ic
cy·a·no·met·he·mo·glo·bin
  or cy·an·met·he·mo·glo·bin
cy·ano·phile
  also cy·ano·phil
cy·a·noph·i·lous
  also cy·a·no·phil·ic
cy·a·nosed
cy·a·no·sis
  pl cy·a·no·ses
cy·a·not·ic
cy·an·urate
cy·an·uric
cy·ber·nat·ed
cy·ber·na·tion
cy·ber·net·ic
cy·ber·net·i·cal
cy·ber·ne·ti·cian

cy·ber·net·ics
cy·borg
cy·ca·sin
cy·cla·mate
cy·clan·de·late
cy·clase
cy·claz·o·cine
cy·cle
cy·clec·to·my
  pl cy·clec·to·mies
cy·clic
cy·cli·cal
cy·clic AMP
cy·clic GMP
cy·clic·i·ty
  pl cy·clic·i·ties
cy·cli·tis
cy·cli·zine
cy·clo·bar·bi·tal
cy·clo·di·al·y·sis
  pl cy·clo·di·al·y·ses
cy·clo·dia·ther·my
  pl cy·clo·dia·ther·mies
cy·clo·di·ene
cy·clo·hex·i·mide
cy·clo·hex·yl·a·mine
cy·cloid
cy·clo·ox·y·gen·ase
cy·clo·pho·ria
cy·clo·phor·ic
cy·clo·phos·pha·mide
cy·clo·phre·nia
Cy·clo·phyl·lid·ea
cy·clo·phyl·lid·e·an

cy·clo·pia
cy·clo·ple·gia
cy·clo·ple·gic
cy·clo·pro·pane
cy·clops
 pl cy·clo·pes
   individual with one eye

cy·clops
 pl cy·clops
   water flea

cy·clo·ser·ine
cy·clo·sis
 pl cy·clo·ses

cy·clo·spor·in A
cy·clo·spor·ine
cy·clo·stome
Cy·clos·to·mi
cy·clo·thyme
cy·clo·thy·mia
cy·clo·thy·mic
cy·clot·o·my
 pl cy·clot·o·mies

cy·clo·tro·pia
cy·e·sis
 pl cy·e·ses

cyl·in·droid
cyl·in·dro·ma
 pl cyl·in·dro·mas
 or cyl·in·dro·ma·ta

cyl·in·dru·ria
cy·ma·rin
cy·ma·rose
cym·ba
 pl cym·bae

cy·no·mol·gus
cy·no·pho·bia

cy·pro·hep·ta·dine
cy·prot·er·one
cyr·tom·e·ter
cyst
cyst·ad·e·no·ma
 pl cyst·ad·e·no·mas
 or cyst·ad·e·no·ma·ta

cyst·ad·e·no·ma·tous
cys·ta·mine
cys·ta·thi·o·nine
cys·te·amine
cys·tec·to·my
 pl cys·tec·to·mies

cys·teine
cys·tic
cys·ti·cer·cal
cys·ti·cer·ci·a·sis
 pl cys·ti·cer·ci·a·ses

cys·ti·cer·coid
cys·ti·cer·co·sis
 pl cys·ti·cer·co·ses

cys·ti·cer·cus
 pl cys·ti·cer·ci

cys·ti·cid·al
cys·tig·er·ous
cys·tine
cys·ti·no·sis
 pl cys·ti·no·ses

cys·ti·not·ic
cys·tin·uria
cys·tin·uric
cys·tit·ic
cys·ti·tis
 pl cys·tit·i·des

cys·to·cele
cys·to·cer·cous

cys·to·gas·tros·to·my
 pl cys·to·gas·tros·to·mies

cys·to·gram
cys·to·graph·ic
cys·tog·ra·phy
 pl cys·tog·ra·phies

cys·toid
cy·sto·je·ju·nos·to·my
 pl cy·sto·je·ju·nos·to·mies

cys·to·lith
cys·to·li·thi·a·sis
 pl cys·to·li·thi·a·ses

cys·to·lith·ic
cys·to·li·thot·o·my
 pl cys·to·li·thot·o·mies

cys·to·ma
 pl cys·to·mas
 or cys·to·ma·ta

cys·to·ma·tous
cys·tom·e·ter
cys·to·met·ric
cys·to·met·ro·gram
cys·to·me·trog·ra·phy
 pl cys·to·me·trog·ra·phies

cys·tom·e·try
 pl cys·tom·e·tries

cys·to·plas·ty
 pl cys·to·plas·ties

cys·to·py·eli·tis

cys·to·py·elog·ra·
phy
pl cys·to·py·elog·ra·
phies

cys·to·py·elo·ne·
phri·tis
pl cys·to·py·elo·ne·
phrit·i·des
also cys·to·py·elo·ne·
phri·tis·es

cys·tor·rha·phy
pl cys·tor·rha·phies

cys·to·sar·co·ma
pl cys·to·sar·co·mas
or cys·to·sar·co·ma·ta

cys·to·scope
cys·to·scoped
cys·to·scop·ing

cys·to·scop·ic

cys·tos·co·pist

cys·tos·co·py
pl cys·tos·co·pies

cys·tos·to·my
pl cys·tos·to·mies

cys·to·tome

cys·tot·o·my
pl cys·tot·o·mies

cys·to·ure·ter·itis

cys·to·ure·thro·cele

cys·to·ure·thro·
gram

cys·to·ure·thro·
graph·ic

cys·to·ure·throg·ra·
phy
pl cys·to·ure·throg·ra·
phies

cys·to·ure·thro·
scope

cys·to·ure·thros·co·
py
pl cys·to·ure·thros·co·
pies

cyst·ous

cyt·ar·a·bine

cy·ti·dine

cy·ti·dyl·ic

cyt·i·sine

cy·to·ar·chi·tec·ton·
ics

cy·to·ar·chi·tec·tur·
al

cy·to·ar·chi·tec·
ture

cy·to·cha·la·sin

cy·to·chem·i·cal

cy·to·chem·ist

cy·to·chem·is·try
pl cy·to·chem·is·tries

cy·to·chrome

cytochrome

cy·toc·i·dal

cy·to·di·ag·no·sis
pl cy·to·di·ag·no·ses

cy·to·di·ag·nos·tic

cy·to·dif·fer·en·ti·a·
tion

cy·to·gen·e·sis
pl cy·to·gen·e·ses

cy·to·ge·net·i·cal

cy·to·ge·net·i·cist

cy·to·ge·net·ics

cy·toid

cy·to·ki·ne·sis
pl cy·to·ki·ne·ses

cy·to·ki·net·ic

cy·to·log·i·cal
or cy·to·log·ic

cy·tol·o·gist

cy·tol·o·gy
pl cy·tol·o·gies

cy·to·ly·sin

cy·tol·y·sis
pl cy·tol·y·ses

cy·to·lyt·ic

cy·to·me·gal·ic

cy·to·meg·a·lo·vi·
rus

cy·to·mem·brane

cy·tom·e·ter

cy·to·met·ric

cy·tom·e·try
pl cy·tom·e·tries

cy·to·mor·pho·log·
i·cal

cy·to·mor·phol·o·
gy
pl cy·to·mor·phol·o·
gies

cy·to·mor·pho·sis
pl cy·to·mor·pho·ses

cy·ton

cy·to·path·ic

cy·to·patho·gen·ic

cy·to·patho·ge·nic·
i·ty
pl cy·to·patho·ge·nic·
i·ties

cy·to·patho·log·ic
also cy·to·patho·log·i·cal

cy·to·pa·thol·o·gist

cy·to·pa·thol·o·gy
pl cy·to·pa·thol·o·gies

cy·to·pem·phis

cy·to·pemp·sis

cy·to·pe·nia

cy·to·pe·nic

cy·to·phag·ic

cy·to·phar·ynx

cy·to·phil·ic

cy·to·pho·tom·e·ter

cy·to·pho·to·met·ric

cy·to·pho·to·met·ri·cal·ly

cy·to·pho·tom·e·try
pl cy·to·pho·tom·e·tries

cy·to·phys·i·o·log·i·cal

cy·to·phys·i·ol·o·gy
pl cy·to·phys·i·ol·o·gies

cy·to·plasm

cy·to·plas·mic

cy·to·plas·mi·cal·ly

cy·to·poi·e·sis
pl cy·to·poi·e·ses

cy·to·ryc·tes
pl cy·to·ryc·tes

cy·to·sine

cy·to·skel·e·tal

cy·to·skel·e·ton

cy·to·sol

cy·to·sol·ic

cy·to·some

cy·to·spec·tro·pho·tom·e·try
pl cy·to·spec·tro·pho·tom·e·tries

cy·to·stat·ic

cy·to·stat·i·cal·ly

cy·to·stome

cy·to·tax·o·nom·ic

cy·to·tax·on·o·my
pl cy·to·tax·on·o·mies

cy·to·tech

cy·to·tech·ni·cian

cy·to·tech·nol·o·gist

cy·to·tech·nol·o·gy
pl cy·to·tech·nol·o·gies

cy·to·tox·ic

cy·to·tox·ic·i·ty
pl cy·to·tox·ic·i·ties

cy·to·tox·in

cy·to·tro·pho·blast

cy·to·tro·pho·blas·tic

cy·to·tro·pic

D

dac·rya
pl of dacryon

dac·ryo·ad·e·nec·to·my
pl dac·ryo·ad·e·nec·to·mies

dac·ry·o·cyst

dac·ryo·cys·tec·to·my
pl dac·ryo·cys·tec·to·mies

dac·ryo·cys·ti·tis

dac·ryo·cys·to·rhi·nos·to·my
pl dac·ryo·cys·to·rhi·nos·to·mies

dac·ryo·cys·tos·to·my
pl dac·ryo·cys·tos·to·mies

dac·ryo·cys·tot·o·my
pl dac·ryo·cys·tot·o·mies

dac·ryo·lith

dac·ry·on
pl dac·rya

dac·ryo·ste·no·sis
pl dac·ryo·ste·no·ses

dac·ti·no·my·cin

dac·tyl

dac·tyl·i·on

dac·ty·log·ra·pher

dac·ty·log·ra·phy
pl dac·ty·log·ra·phies

dac·tyl·o·scop·ic

dac·ty·los·co·py
pl dac·ty·los·co·pies

dac·ty·lo·sym·phy·sis
pl dac·ty·lo·sym·phy·ses

dal·ton

Dal·ton·ism

Dal·ton's law

dam·mar
or dam·ar

damp

dan·de·li·on

dan·der

dan·druff

dan·druffy

Da·nysz phe·nom·e·non

daph·ne

dap·pen

dap·sone

Da·rier's dis·ease

D'Ar·son·val cur·rent

dar·tos

Dar·win·ian

Dar·win·ian

Dar·win·ism

Dar·win·ist

Dar·win's tu·ber·cle

da·ta

da·tu·ra

Dau·ben·ton's plane

daugh·ter

dau·no·my·cin

dau·no·ru·bi·cin

day·dream

day·dream·er

de·acid·i·fi·ca·tion

de·acid·i·fy
de·acid·i·fied
de·acid·i·fy·ing

de·ac·ti·vate
de·ac·ti·vat·ed
de·ac·ti·vat·ing

de·ac·ti·va·tion

dead
pl dead

dead·li·ness

dead·ly
dead·li·er
dead·li·est

dead·ly night·shade

deaf

deaf·en
deaf·ened
deaf·en·ing

deaf·en·ing·ly

de·af·fer·en·ta·tion

deaf-mute

deaf-mute·ness

deaf-mut·ism

deaf·ness

de·am·i·dase

de·am·i·nase
also des·am·i·nase

de·am·i·nate
de·am·i·nat·ed
de·am·i·nat·ing

de·am·i·na·tion

de·am·i·ni·za·tion

de·am·i·nize
de·am·i·nized
de·am·i·niz·ing

death·bed

de·bil·i·tate
de·bil·i·tat·ed
de·bil·i·tat·ing

de·bil·i·ta·tion

de·bil·i·ty
pl de·bil·i·ties

de·bride

de·brid·ed

de·brid·ing

de·bride·ment

de·bris
pl de·bris

deca·gram
var of dekagram

de·cal·ci·fi·ca·tion

de·cal·ci·fy
de·cal·ci·fied
de·cal·ci·fy·ing

deca·li·ter
var of dekaliter

deca·me·ter
var of dekameter

deca·me·tho·ni·um

dec·a·no·ic

de·cant

de·can·ta·tion

deca·pep·tide

de·cap·i·tate
de·cap·i·tat·ed
de·cap·i·tat·ing

de·cap·i·ta·tion

de·cap·su·late
de·cap·su·lat·ed
de·cap·su·lat·ing

de·cap·su·la·tion

de·car·box·yl·ase

de·car·box·yl·ate
  de·car·box·y·lat·ed
  de·car·box·y·lat·ing
de·car·box·yl·ation
de·cay
de·cease
  de·ceased
  de·ceas·ing
de·ceased
  pl de·ceased
de·ce·dent
de·cel·er·ate
  de·cel·er·at·ed
  de·cel·er·at·ing
de·cel·er·a·tion
de·cer·e·brate
  de·cer·e·brat·ed
  de·cer·e·brat·ing
de·cer·e·bra·tion
de·chlo·ri·nate
  de·chlo·ri·nat·ed
  de·chlo·ri·nat·ing
de·chlo·ri·na·tion
deci·bel
de·cid·ua
  pl de·cid·uae
de·cid·ua ba·sa·lis
de·cid·ua cap·su·lar·is
de·cid·u·al
de·cid·ua pa·ri·etal·is
de·cid·u·ate
de·cid·u·itis

de·cid·u·o·sis
  pl de·cid·u·o·ses
de·cid·u·ous
deci·gram
deci·li·ter
deci·me·ter
de·cline
  de·clined
  de·clin·ing
de·clive
de·clot
  de·clot·ted
  de·clot·ting
de·coct
de·coc·tion
de·coc·tum
  pl de·coc·ta
de·col·or·ant
de·col·or·ation
de·col·or·iza·tion
de·col·or·ize
  de·col·or·ized
  de·col·or·iz·ing
de·col·or·iz·er
de·com·pen·sate
  de·com·pen·sat·ed
  de·com·pen·sat·ing
de·com·pen·sa·tion
de·com·pen·sa·to·ry
de·com·pos·abil·i·ty
  pl de·com·pos·abil·i·ties
de·com·pos·able

de·com·pose
de·com·posed
de·com·pos·ing
de·com·pos·er
de·com·po·si·tion
de·com·press
de·com·pres·sion
de·com·pres·sive
de·con·di·tion
de·con·gest
de·con·ges·tant
de·con·ges·tion
de·con·ges·tive
de·con·tam·i·nate
  de·con·tam·i·nat·ed
  de·con·tam·i·nat·ing
de·con·tam·i·na·tion
de·cor·ti·cate
  de·cor·ti·cat·ed
  de·cor·ti·cat·ing
de·cor·ti·ca·tion
de·crep·i·ta·tion
de·cu·bi·tal
de·cu·bi·tus
  pl de·cu·bi·ti
de·cus·sate
  de·cus·sat·ed
  de·cus·sat·ing
de·cus·sa·tio
  pl de·cus·sa·ti·o·nes
de·cus·sa·tion

de·dif·fer·en·ti·ate
  de·dif·fer·en·ti·
    at·ed
  de·dif·fer·en·ti·
    at·ing
de·dif·fer·en·ti·a·
  tion
deep
deep·ly
deer·fly
de·fat
  de·fat·ted
  de·fat·ting
def·e·cate
  def·e·cat·ed
  def·e·cat·ing
def·e·ca·tion
de·fect
de·fec·tive
de·fem·i·ni·za·tion
de·fem·i·nize
  de·fem·i·nized
  de·fem·i·niz·ing
de·fense
de·fen·sive
def·er·ent
def·er·en·tial
de·fer·ves·cence
de·fi·bril·late
  de·fi·bril·lat·ed
  de·fi·bril·lat·ing
de·fi·bril·la·tion
de·fi·bril·la·tor
de·fi·brin·ate
  de·fi·brin·at·ed
  de·fi·brin·at·ing
de·fi·brin·ation

de·fi·cien·cy
  pl de·fi·cien·cies
de·fi·cient
def·i·ni·tion
de·fin·i·tive
de·flect
de·flec·tion
de·flo·rate
  de·flo·rat·ed
  de·flo·rat·ing
de·flo·ra·tion
de·flo·res·cence
de·flu·vi·um
de·fo·cus
  de·fo·cused
  de·fo·cus·ing
de·formed
de·for·mi·ty
  pl de·for·mi·ties
de·gen·er·a·cy
  pl de·gen·er·a·cies
de·gen·er·ate
  de·gen·er·at·ed
  de·gen·er·at·ing
de·gen·er·a·tion
de·gen·er·a·tive
de·germ·ation
de·glu·ti·tion
deg·ra·da·tion
deg·ra·da·tive
de·grade
de·gran·u·late
  de·gran·u·lat·ed
  de·gran·u·lat·ing
de·gran·u·la·tion
de·gree
de·greed

de·gust
de·gus·ta·tion
de·hisce
  de·hisced
  de·hisc·ing
de·his·cence
de·hu·mid·i·fi·ca·
  tion
de·hu·mid·i·fi·er
de·hu·mid·i·fy
  de·hu·mid·i·fied
  de·hu·mid·i·fy·
    ing
de·hy·drase
de·hy·dra·tase
de·hy·drate
  de·hy·drat·ed
  de·hy·drat·ing
de·hy·dra·tion
de·hy·dra·tor
de·hy·dro·ace·tic
de·hy·dro·ascor·bic
de·hy·dro·cho·late
7-de·hy·dro·cho·
  les·ter·ol
de·hy·dro·cho·lic
11-de·hy·dro·cor·ti·
  co·ste·rone
de·hy·dro·epi·an·
  dros·ter·one
de·hy·dro·ge·nase
de·hy·dro·ge·nate
  de·hy·dro·ge·nat·
    ed
  de·hy·dro·ge·nat·
    ing

de·hy·dro·ge·na·
tion
de·hy·dro·ge·nize
de·hy·dro·ge·
nized
de·hy·dro·ge·niz·
ing
de·hy·dro·iso·an·
dros·ter·one
de·hyp·no·tize
de·hyp·no·tized
de·hyp·no·tiz·ing
de·in·sti·tu·tion·al·
iza·tion
de·in·sti·tu·tion·al·
ize
de·in·sti·tu·tion·
al·ized
de·in·sti·tu·tion·
al·iz·ing
de·ion·iza·tion
de·ion·ize
de·ion·ized
de·ion·iz·ing
de·ion·iz·er
Dei·ters' cell
dé·jà vu
de·jec·ta
de·ject·ed
de·jec·tion
deka·gram
or deca·gram
deka·li·ter
or deca·li·ter
deka·me·ter
or deca·me·ter

de·lam·i·nate
de·lam·i·nat·ed
de·lam·i·nat·ing
de·lam·i·na·tion
de·lead
del·e·te·ri·ous
de·le·tion
de·lin·quen·cy
pl de·lin·quen·cies
de·lin·quent
del·i·ques·cence
del·i·ques·cent
de·lir·i·ant
de·lir·i·ous
de·lir·i·um
de·lir·i·um tre·
mens
de·liv·er
de·liv·ered
de·liv·er·ing
de·liv·ery
pl de·liv·er·ies
de·lo·mor·phous
or de·lo·mor·phic
de·louse
de·loused
de·lous·ing
del·phin·i·um
del·ta
del·toid
del·toi·de·us
pl del·toi·dei
de·lude
de·lud·ed
de·lud·ing
de·lu·sion
de·lu·sion·al

de·mar·cate
de·mar·cat·ed
de·mar·cat·ing
de·mar·ca·tion
also de·mar·ka·tion
de·mas·cu·lin·iza·
tion
de·mas·cu·lin·ize
de·mas·cu·lin·
ized
de·mas·cu·lin·iz·
ing
dem·e·car·i·um
de·ment·ed
de·men·tia
de·men·tial
de·men·tia par·a·
lyt·i·ca
pl de·men·ti·ae par·a·
lyt·i·cae
de·men·tia prae·
cox
demi·lune
demi·lune of Gian·
nuz·zi
demi·lune of Hei·
den·hain
de·min·er·al·iza·
tion
de·min·er·al·ize
de·min·er·al·ized
de·min·er·al·iz·
ing
dem·o·dec·tic
de·mo·dex
de·mog·ra·pher
de·mo·graph·ic

de·mo·graph·i·cal·
ly
de·mog·ra·phy
pl de·mog·ra·phies
de·mon·o·ma·nia
dem·on·strate
dem·on·strat·ed
dem·on·strat·ing
dem·on·stra·tion
dem·on·stra·tor
de·mul·cent
de·my·elin·at·ing
de·my·eli·na·tion
de·my·elin·isa·tion
de·my·elin·iza·tion
de·na·tur·ant
de·na·tur·ation
de·na·ture
de·na·tured
de·na·tur·ing
den·drite
den·drit·ic
den·dro·den·drit·ic
den·droid
den·dron
pl den·drons
also den·dra
de·ner·vate
de·ner·vat·ed
de·ner·vat·ing
de·ner·va·tion
den·gue
de·ni·al
dcn·i·da·tion
de·ni·tri·fi·ca·tion
de·ni·tri·fi·er

de·ni·tri·fy
de·ni·tri·fied
de·ni·tri·fy·ing
de·ni·trog·e·nate
de·ni·trog·e·nat·
ed
de·ni·trog·e·nat·
ing
de·ni·trog·e·na·tion
dens
pl den·tes
den·sim·e·ter
den·si·met·ric
den·si·tom·e·ter
den·si·to·met·ric
den·si·tom·e·try
pl den·si·tom·e·tries
den·si·ty
pl den·si·ties
dent
den·tal
den·tal·ly
den·tate
den·tes
pl of dens
den·ti·cle
den·tic·u·late
or den·tic·u·lat·ed
den·ti·frice
den·tig·er·ous
den·tin
or den·tine
den·tin·al
den·tin·o·blast
den·tino·enam·el
den·tino·gen·e·sis
pl den·tino·gen·e·ses

den·tino·gen·ic
den·ti·noid
den·ti·no·ma
pl den·ti·no·mas
also den·ti·no·ma·ta
den·tist
den·tist·ry
pl den·tist·ries
den·ti·tion
den·to·fa·cial
den·toid
den·tu·lous
den·ture
den·tur·ist
de·nu·da·tion
de·nude
de·nud·ed
de·nud·ing
de·odor·ant
de·odor·iza·tion
de·odor·ize
de·odor·ized
de·odor·iz·ing
de·odor·iz·er
de·ox·i·da·tion
de·ox·i·dize
de·ox·i·dized
de·ox·i·diz·ing
de·ox·i·diz·er
de·oxy·cho·late
also des·oxy·cho·late
de·oxy·cho·lic
or des·oxy·cho·lic
de·oxy·cor·ti·co·ste·
rone
var of des·oxy·cor·ti·
co·ste·rone

de·oxy·cy·ti·dine
de·ox·y·gen·ate
  de·ox·y·gen·at·ed
  de·ox·y·gen·at·
    ing
de·ox·y·gen·at·ed
de·ox·y·gen·ation
de·oxy·ri·bo·nu·
  cle·ase
  also des·oxy·ri·bo·nu·
    cle·ase

de·oxy·ri·bo·nu·
  cle·ic
  also des·oxy·ri·bo·nu·
    cle·ic

de·oxy·ri·bo·nu·
  cleo·pro·tein
  also des·oxy·ri·bo·nu·
    cleo·pro·tein

de·oxy·ri·bo·nu·
  cle·o·tide
  also des·oxy·ri·bo·nu·
    cle·o·tide

de·oxy·ri·bose
  also des·oxy·ri·bose

de·pan·cre·atize
  de·pan·cre·
    atized
  de·pan·cre·atiz·
    ing
de·pen·dence
de·pen·dent
de·pen·dent·ly
de·per·son·al·iza·
  tion

de·per·son·al·ize
  de·per·son·al·
    ized
  de·per·son·al·iz·
    ing
de·phos·phor·y·late
  de·phos·phor·y·
    lat·ed
  de·phos·phor·y·
    lat·ing
de·phos·phor·y·la·
  tion
de·pig·ment
de·pig·men·ta·tion
dep·i·late
  dep·i·lat·ed
  dep·i·lat·ing
dep·i·la·tion
de·pil·a·to·ry
de·plete
  de·plet·ed
  de·plet·ing
de·ple·tion
de·po·lar·iza·tion
de·po·lar·ize
  de·po·lar·ized
  de·po·lar·iz·ing
  de·po·lar·iz·er
de·po·lym·er·ase
de·po·ly·mer·iza·
  tion
de·po·ly·mer·ize
  de·po·ly·mer·
    ized
  de·po·ly·mer·iz·
    ing

de·pos·it
  de·pos·it·ed
  de·pos·it·ing
de·pot
de·press
de·pres·sant
de·pres·sion
de·pres·sive
de·pres·sor
de·pres·sor sep·ti
de·pri·va·tion
de·prive
  de·prived
  de·priv·ing
de·pro·tein·ate
  de·pro·tein·at·ed
  de·pro·tein·at·
    ing
de·pro·tein·ation
de·pro·tein·iza·tion
de·pro·tein·ize
  de·pro·tein·ized
  de·pro·tein·iz·
    ing
dep·u·rate
  dep·u·rat·ed
  dep·u·rat·ing
dep·u·ra·tion
de·Quer·vain's dis·
  ease
de·range
  de·ranged
  de·rang·ing
de·range·ment
de·re·al·iza·tion
de·re·ism
de·re·is·tic

de·re·press
de·re·pres·sion
der·i·va·tion
de·riv·a·tive
de·rive
  de·rived
  de·riv·ing
der·ma
derm·abra·sion
Der·ma·cen·tor
der·mal
der·ma·nys·sid
Der·ma·nys·si·dae
Der·ma·nys·sus
der·ma·tit·ic
der·ma·ti·tis
  pl der·ma·tit·is·es
  or der·ma·tit·i·des
Der·ma·to·bia
der·ma·to·fi·bro·
  ma
  pl der·ma·to·fi·bro·
    mas
  also der·ma·to·fi·bro·
    ma·ta
der·ma·to·fi·bro·
  sar·co·ma
  pl der·ma·to·fi·bro·
    sar·co·mas
  or der·ma·to·fi·bro·
    sar·co·ma·ta
der·ma·to·fi·bro·
  sar·co·ma pro·tu·
  ber·ans
der·ma·to·glyph·ic
der·ma·to·glyph·
  ics
der·ma·to·graph·ia

der·ma·to·graph·
  ism
der·ma·tog·ra·phy
  pl der·ma·tog·ra·
    phies
der·ma·to·his·to·
  log·ic
der·ma·to·his·tol·o·
  gy
  pl der·ma·to·his·tol·o·
    gies
der·ma·toid
der·ma·to·log·ic
  or der·ma·to·log·i·cal
  adjective
der·ma·to·log·i·cal
  noun
der·ma·tol·o·gist
der·ma·tol·o·gy
  pl der·ma·tol·o·gies
der·ma·to·mal
der·ma·tome
der·ma·to·mic
der·ma·to·my·co·
  sis
  pl der·ma·to·my·co·
    ses
der·ma·to·my·o·si·
  tis
  pl der·ma·to·my·o·si·
    tis·es
  or der·ma·to·my·o·sit·
    i·des
der·ma·to·path·ia
der·ma·to·path·ic
der·ma·to·pa·thol·
  o·gist

der·ma·to·pa·thol·
  o·gy
  pl der·ma·to·pa·thol·
    o·gies
der·ma·top·a·thy
  pl der·ma·top·a·thies
der·ma·to·phyte
der·ma·to·phyt·ic
der·ma·to·phy·tid
der·ma·to·phy·to·
  sis
  pl der·ma·to·phy·to·
    ses
der·ma·to·plas·ty
  pl der·ma·to·plas·ties
der·ma·to·scle·ro·
  sis
  pl der·ma·to·scle·ro·
    ses
der·ma·to·sis
  pl der·ma·to·ses
der·ma·to·ther·a·py
  pl der·ma·to·ther·a·
    pies
der·ma·to·zoo·no·
  sis
  pl der·ma·to·zoo·no·
    ses
der·mic
der·mis
der·mi·tis
der·mo·graph·ia
der·mo·graph·ic
der·mog·ra·phism
der·moid
  also der·moi·dal
der·mom·e·ter
der·mo·ne·crot·ic

der·mop·a·thy
 pl der·mop·a·thies

der·mo·tro·pic
der·ren·ga·de·ra
de·sat·u·rate
 de·sat·u·rat·ed
 de·sat·u·rat·ing
de·sat·u·ra·tion
des·ce·met·o·cele
Des·ce·met's mem·
 brane
de·scen·sus
de·scent
de·sen·si·ti·za·tion
de·sen·si·tize
 de·sen·si·tized
 de·sen·si·tiz·ing
de·sen·si·tiz·er
de·sex
de·sex·u·al·iza·tion
de·sex·u·al·ize
 de·sex·u·al·ized
 de·sex·u·al·iz·ing
des·ic·cant
des·ic·cate
 des·ic·cat·ed
 des·ic·cat·ing
des·ic·ca·tion
de·sic·ca·tive
des·ic·ca·tor
de·sign
de·si·pra·mine
des·meth·yl·imip·
 ra·mine
des·mo·cra·ni·um
 pl des·mo·cra·ni·ums
 or des·mo·cra·nia

des·mo·cyte
des·moid
des·mo·lase
des·mo·some
des·mos·ter·ol
deso·mor·phine
de·sorb
de·sorp·tion
des·oxy·cho·late
 var of deoxycholate
des·oxy·cho·lic
 var of deoxycholic
des·oxy·cor·ti·co·
 ste·rone
 or de·oxy·cor·ti·co·
 ste·rone
des·oxy·cor·tone
des·oxy·ri·bo·nu·
 cle·ase
 var of deoxyribonu-
 clease
des·oxy·ri·bo·nu·
 cle·ic
 var of deoxyribonu-
 cleic
des·oxy·ri·bo·nu·
 cleo·pro·tein
 var of deoxyribonu-
 cleoprotein
des·oxy·ri·bo·nu·
 cle·o·tide
 var of deoxyribonu-
 cleotide
des·oxy·ri·bose
 var of deoxyribose
de·spe·ci·ate
 de·spe·ci·at·ed
 de·spe·ci·at·ing

de·spe·ci·a·tion
des·qua·mate
 des·qua·mat·ed
 des·qua·mat·ing
des·qua·ma·tion
des·qua·ma·tive
des·qua·ma·to·ry
des·thio·bi·o·tin
de·stru·do
de·syn·chro·ni·za·
 tion
de·syn·chro·nize
 de·syn·chro·
 nized
 de·syn·chro·niz·
 ing
de·tec·tor
de·ter·gent
de·te·ri·o·rate
 de·te·ri·o·rat·ed
 de·te·ri·o·rat·ing
de·te·ri·o·ra·tion
de·ter·mi·nant
de·ter·mi·nate
de·ter·mi·na·tion
de·ter·mine
 de·ter·mined
 de·ter·min·ing
de·ter·min·er
de·ter·min·ism
de·ter·min·ist
de·ter·min·is·tic
de·ter·min·is·ti·cal·
 ly
de·ter·sive
de·tick
de·tor·sion

de·tox
de·tox·i·cant
de·tox·i·cate
  de·tox·i·cat·ed
  de·tox·i·cat·ing
de·tox·i·ca·tion
de·tox·i·fi·ca·tion
de·tox·i·fi·er
de·tox·i·fy
  de·tox·i·fied
  de·tox·i·fy·ing
de·tri·tion
de·tri·tus
  pl de·tri·tus
de·tru·sor
de·tru·sor uri·nae
de·tu·ba·tion
de·tu·mes·cence
de·tu·mes·cent
deu·ter·anom·a·lous
deu·ter·anom·a·ly
  pl deu·ter·anom·a·lies
deu·ter·an·ope
deu·ter·an·opia
deu·ter·an·opic
deu·te·ri·um
deu·to·plasm
deu·to·plas·mic
deu·to·plas·mol·y·sis
  pl deu·to·plas·mol·y·ses
de·vas·cu·lar·iza·tion
de·vas·cu·lar·ized
de·vel·op

de·vel·op·ment
de·vel·op·men·tal
de·vi·ance
de·vi·ant
de·vi·ate
de·vi·a·tion
de·vice
de·vi·tal·iza·tion
de·vi·tal·ize
  de·vi·tal·ized
  de·vi·tal·iz·ing
dew·claw
dew·lap
dew·lapped
de·worm
dex
dexa·meth·a·sone
dex·ter
dex·ter·i·ty
  pl dex·ter·i·ties
dex·ter·ous
  or dex·trous
dex·trad
dex·tral
dex·tral·i·ty
  pl dex·tral·i·ties
dex·tran
dex·tran·ase
dex·trin
  also dex·trine
dex·trino·gen·ic
dex·tro
dex·tro·am·phet·amine
dex·tro·car·dia
dex·tro·car·di·al

dex·tro·car·dio·gram
dex·troc·u·lar
dex·troc·u·lar·i·ty
  pl dex·troc·u·lar·i·ties
dex·tro·po·si·tion
dex·tro·pro·poxy·phene
dex·tro·ro·ta·tion
dex·tro·ro·ta·to·ry
  also dex·tro·ro·ta·ry
dex·trose
dex·trous
  var of dexterous
dex·tro·ver·sion
di·a·be·tes
di·a·be·tes in·sip·i·dus
di·a·be·tes mel·li·tus
di·a·bet·ic
di·a·be·to·gen·ic
di·ac·e·tin
di·ace·tyl·mor·phine
dia·der·mal
  or dia·der·mat·ic
  or dia·der·mic
di·a·do·cho·ki·ne·sia
  or di·a·do·ko·ki·ne·sia
di·a·do·cho·ki·ne·sis
  pl di·a·do·cho·ki·ne·ses

di·a·do·cho·ki·net·
  ic
  or di·a·do·ko·ki·net·ic

di·ag·nos·able
  also di·ag·nose·able

di·ag·nose
  di·ag·nosed
  di·ag·nos·ing

di·ag·no·sis
  pl di·ag·no·ses

di·ag·nos·tic
  also di·ag·nos·ti·cal

di·ag·nos·ti·cian

dia·ki·ne·sis
  pl dia·ki·ne·ses

dia·ki·net·ic

Dia·lis·ter

di·al·lel

di·al·lyl

di·al·lyl·bar·bi·tu·
  ric

di·al·y·sance

di·al·y·sate
  or di·al·y·zate

di·al·y·sis
  pl di·al·y·ses

di·a·lyt·ic

di·a·lyz·abil·i·ty
  pl di·a·lyz·abil·i·ties

di·a·lyz·able

di·a·lyze
  di·a·lyzed
  di·a·lyz·ing

di·a·lyz·er

di·am·e·ter

di·amide

di·amine

di·ami·no·di·phe·
  nyl

dia·mor·phine

dia·pause

di·a·paus·ing

di·a·pe·de·sis
  pl di·a·pe·de·ses

di·a·pe·det·ic

di·a·per
  di·a·pered
  di·a·per·ing

di·aph·a·nom·e·ter

di·aph·a·no·met·ric

di·aph·a·no·scope

di·aph·a·nos·co·py
  pl di·aph·a·nos·co·
  pies

di·aph·o·rase

di·a·pho·re·sis
  pl di·a·pho·re·ses

di·a·pho·ret·ic

di·a·phragm

di·a·phrag·ma sel·
  lae

di·a·phrag·mat·ic

di·aph·y·se·al
  or di·a·phys·i·al

di·a·phy·sec·to·my
  pl di·a·phy·sec·to·
  mies

di·aph·y·sis
  pl di·aph·y·ses

di·apoph·y·sis
  pl di·apoph·y·ses

di·ap·to·mid

Di·ap·to·mus

di·ar·rhea
  also di·ar·rhoea

di·ar·rhe·al

di·ar·rhe·ic

di·ar·rhet·ic

di·ar·thro·di·al

di·ar·thro·sis
  pl di·ar·thro·ses

di·ar·tic·u·lar

di·as·chi·sis
  pl di·as·chi·ses

di·a·scope

di·a·scop·ic

di·as·co·py
  pl di·as·co·pies

di·a·stase

di·as·ta·sis
  pl di·as·ta·ses

di·a·stat·ic

di·a·ste·ma
  pl di·a·ste·ma·ta

di·a·ste·mat·ic

di·a·ste·ma·to·my·
  e·lia
  or di·a·ste·reo·mer

di·a·ste·reo·iso·
  mer·ic

di·as·to·le

di·a·stol·ic

dia·ther·mic

dia·ther·mo·co·ag·
  u·la·tion

dia·ther·my
  pl dia·ther·mies

di·ath·e·sis
  pl di·ath·e·ses

di·a·thet·ic

di·a·tom
di·a·to·ma·ceous
di·atom·ic
di·at·o·mite
dia·tri·zo·ate
di·az·e·pam
di·a·zine
di·azo
di·azo·ben·zene·
sul·fon·ic
di·a·zo·ni·um
di·azo re·ac·tion
di·az·o·ti·za·tion
di·az·o·tize
    di·az·o·tized
    di·az·o·tiz·ing
di·az·ox·ide
di·ba·sic
di·benz·an·thra·
cene
    or 1,2:5,6-di·benz·an·
    thra·cene

*Di·both·rio·ceph·a·
lus*
di·bu·caine
di·bu·tyl
di·car·box·yl·ic
di·cary·on
    var of dikaryon
di·cary·o·tic
    var of dikaryotic
di·cen·tric
di·ceph·a·lus
    pl di·ceph·a·li
di·chlo·ra·mine-T

di·chlor·eth·yl sul·
fide
    also di·chlo·ro·eth·yl
    sul·fide
di·chlo·ro·ben·
zene
di·chlo·ro·di·flu·o·
ro·meth·ane
di·chlo·ro·meth·
ane
2,4-di·chlo·ro·
phen·oxy·ace·tic
ac·id
    also di·chlo·ro·phen·
    oxy·ace·tic ac·id
di·chlor·vos
di·cho·ri·al
di·cho·ri·on·ic
dich·otic
dich·oti·cal·ly
di·chot·o·mous
di·chot·o·my
    pl di·chot·o·mies
di·chro·ic
di·chro·ism
di·chro·mat
di·chro·mate
di·chro·mat·ic
di·chro·ma·tism
di·chro·ma·top·sia
Dick test
di·clox·a·cil·lin
di·cou·ma·rin
Di·cro·coe·li·i·dae
Di·cro·coe·li·um
di·crot·ic
di·cro·tism

Dic·ty·o·cau·lus
dic·tyo·ki·ne·sis
    pl dic·tyo·ki·ne·ses
dic·tyo·some
di·cu·ma·rol
    also di·cou·ma·rol
di·cy·clo·mine
di·dac·tic
di·del·phia
di·del·phic
Di·del·phis
diel·drin
di·en·ce·phal·ic
di·en·ceph·a·lon
die·ner
di·en·es·trol
Di·ent·amoe·ba
di·es·ter
di·es·trous
    also di·es·tru·al
di·es·trus
    also di·es·trum
di·et
di·etari·ly
di·etary
    pl di·etar·ies
di·et·er
di·etet·ic
di·etet·i·cal·ly
di·eth·yl
di·eth·yl·car·bam·
azine
di·eth·yl·pro·pi·on
di·eth·yl·stil·bes·
trol
di·eti·tian
    or di·eti·cian

Die·tl's cri·sis
di·e·to·ther·a·py
pl di·e·to·ther·a·pies
dif·fer·en·tia
pl dif·fer·en·ti·ae
dif·fer·en·tial
dif·fer·en·ti·ate
dif·fer·en·ti·at·ed
dif·fer·en·ti·at·
ing
dif·fer·en·ti·a·tion
dif·flu·ent
dif·fract
dif·frac·tion
dif·fu·sate
dif·fuse
dif·fused
dif·fus·ing
dif·fus·ibil·i·ty
pl dif·fus·ibil·i·ties
dif·fus·ible
dif·fu·sion
dif·fu·sion·al
di·ga·met·ic
di·gas·tric
di·gas·tri·cus
Di·ge·nea
di·ge·ne·an
di·gen·e·sis
pl di·gen·e·ses
di·ge·net·ic
di·gest
di·ges·ta
di·ges·tant
di·gest·er
also di·ges·tor

di·gest·ibil·i·ty
pl di·gest·ibil·i·ties
di·gest·ible
di·ges·tion
di·ges·tive
dig·i·lan·id
or dig·i·lan·ide
dig·it
dig·i·tal
dig·i·tal·in
dig·i·tal·is
dig·i·ta·li·za·tion
dig·i·ta·lize
dig·i·ta·lized
dig·i·ta·liz·ing
dig·i·tal·ose
dig·i·tate
dig·i·ta·tion
dig·i·ti·grade
dig·i·to·nin
dig·i·to·plan·tar
digi·toxi·gen·in
digi·tox·in
dig·i·tox·ose
di·glos·sia
di·glyc·er·ide
di·gox·in
di·hy·brid
di·hy·drate
di·hy·drat·ed
di·hy·dro·chlo·ride
di·hy·dro·co·de·
inone
di·hy·dro·er·go·cor·
nine
di·hy·dro·er·got·a·
mine

di·hy·dro·mor·phi·
none
di·hy·dro·strep·to·
my·cin
di·hy·dro·tachy·ste·
rol
di·hy·dro·tes·tos·
ter·one
di·hy·dro·the·elin
di·hy·droxy
di·hy·droxy·ac·e·
tone
1,25-di·hy·droxy·
cho·le·cal·cif·er·
ol
di·hy·droxy·phe·
nyl·al·a·nine·
di·hy·droxy·phe·
nyl·al·a·nine
or 3,4-di·hy·droxy·
phe·nyl·al·a·nine
dopa

di·hy·droxy·phe·
nyl·al·a·nine
or L-3,4-di·hy·droxy·
phe·nyl·al·a·nine
or L-di·hy·droxy·phe·
nyl·al·a·nine
L-dopa

di·io·do·hy·droxy·
quin
di·io·do·hy·droxy·
quin·o·line
di·io·do·ty·ro·sine
di·iso·pro·pyl
di·kary·on
also di·cary·on

di·kary·o·tic
  also di·cary·o·tic
di·lac·er·ate
  di·lac·er·at·ed
  di·lac·er·at·ing
di·lac·er·a·tion
di·la·ta·tion
di·la·ta·tor
di·late
  di·lat·ed
  di·lat·ing
di·la·tion
di·la·tor
dil·do
  pl dil·dos
dil·u·ent
di·lute
  di·lut·ed
  di·lut·ing
di·lu·tion
di·lut·or
  also di·lut·er
di·men·hy·dri·nate
di·mer
di·mer·cap·rol
di·mer·ic
di·mer·iza·tion
di·mer·ize
  di·mer·ized
  di·mer·iz·ing
di·meth·yl·ni·tros·
  amine
di·meth·yl·poly·si·
  lox·ane
di·meth·yl·tryp·ta·
  mine

di·meth·yl·tu·bo·
  cu·ra·rine
di·mor·phic
di·mor·phism
di·mor·phous
dim·ple
  dim·pled
  dim·pling
di·ni·tro-*o*-cre·sol
  also di·ni·tro-or·tho-
  cre·sol
di·ni·tro·phe·nol
Di·no·fla·gel·la·ta
di·no·fla·gel·late
di·nu·cle·o·tide
Di·oc·to·phy·me
di·o·done
di·op·ter
di·op·tom·e·ter
di·op·tom·e·try
  pl di·op·tom·e·tries
di·op·tric
  also di·op·tri·cal
di·ose
di·os·gen·in
di·otic
di·ovu·lar
di·ox·ane
  also di·ox·an
di·ox·ide
di·ox·in
di·oxy·ben·zone
di·pen·tene
di·pep·ti·dase
di·pep·tide
Di·pet·a·lo·ne·ma

Di·pet·a·lo·ne·mat·
  i·dae
di·pha·sic
di·phen·an
di·phen·hy·dra·
  mine
di·phe·nol
di·phen·oxy·late
di·phe·nyl·amine
di·phe·nyl·amine·
  chlor·ar·sine
di·phe·nyl·chlo·ro·
  ar·sine
  also di·phe·nyl·chlor·
  ar·sine

di·phe·nyl·hy·dan·
  to·in
di·phos·gene
di·phos·phate
2,3-di·phos·pho·
  glyc·er·ate
  also di·phos·pho·glyc·
  er·ate

di·phos·pho·gly·
  cer·ic ac·id
  or 1,3-di·phos·pho·
  glyc·er·ic ac·id

di·phos·pho·pyr·i·
  dine
diph·the·ria
diph·the·ri·al
diph·the·ric
diph·the·rit·ic
diph·the·rit·ic
diph·the·roid

di·phyl·lo·both·ri·
a·sis
pl di·phyl·lo·both·ri·
a·ses

Di·phyl·lo·both·ri·
i·dae

*Di·phyl·lo·both·ri·
um*

di·phy·odont

dip·la·cu·sis
pl dip·la·cu·ses

di·ple·gia

di·plo·ba·cil·lary

dip·lo·ba·cil·lus
pl dip·lo·ba·cil·li

dip·lo·blas·tic

dip·lo·car·dia

dip·lo·car·di·ac

di·plo·coc·cal

dip·lo·coc·cin

dip·lo·coc·coid

dip·lo·coc·cus
pl dip·lo·coc·ci

dip·loe

dip·lo·et·ic

di·plo·ic

dip·loid

dip·loi·dy
pl dip·loi·dies

dip·lo·kar·y·ot·ic

dip·lo·mate

dip·lo·my·elia

dip·lo·ne·ma

dip·lo·neu·ral

dip·lont

dip·lon·tic

dip·lo·phase

dip·lo·pia

dip·lo·pic

dip·lo·some

dip·lo·tene

di·po·lar

di·pole

di·pro·so·pus

dip·so·ma·nia

dip·so·ma·ni·ac

dip·so·ma·ni·a·cal

Dip·tera

dip·ter·an

di·py·gus
pl di·py·gi

di·py·li·di·a·sis
pl di·py·li·di·a·ses

Di·py·lid·i·um

di·pyr·i·dam·ole

di·rec·tive

di·rec·tor

di·rhin·ic

Di·ro·fi·lar·ia

di·ro·fi·lar·i·al

di·ro·fil·a·ri·a·sis
pl di·ro·fil·a·ri·a·ses

dirty
dirt·i·er
dirt·i·est

dis·abil·i·ty
pl dis·abil·i·ties

dis·able
dis·abled
dis·abling

dis·able·ment

di·sac·cha·ri·dase

di·sac·cha·ride

dis·ag·gre·gate
dis·ag·gre·gat·ed
dis·ag·gre·gat·ing
dis·ag·gre·ga·tion

dis·ar·tic·u·late
dis·ar·tic·u·lat·ed
dis·ar·tic·u·lat·
ing
dis·ar·tic·u·la·tion

dis·as·sim·i·late
dis·as·sim·i·lat·
ed
dis·as·sim·i·lat·
ing
dis·as·sim·i·la·tion
dis·as·sim·i·la·tive

dis·charge
dis·charged
dis·charg·ing

dis·ci
pl of discus

dis·ci·form

dis·cis·sion

dis·clos·ing

dis·co·blas·tic

dis·co·blas·tu·la
pl dis·co·blas·tu·las
or dis·co·blas·tu·lae

dis·co·gas·tru·la
pl dis·co·gas·tru·las
or dis·co·gas·tru·lae

dis·co·gram
var of diskogram

dis·cog·ra·phy
var of diskography

dis·coid

dis·coi·dal

dis·co·pla·cen·ta
dis·cor·dance
dis·cor·dant
dis·crete
dis·crim·i·nate
  dis·crim·i·nat·ed
  dis·crim·i·nat·
    ing
dis·crim·i·na·tion
dis·cus
  pl dis·ci
dis·cus pro·lig·er·
  us
dis·ease
dis·eased
dis·equi·lib·ri·um
  pl dis·equi·lib·ri·ums
  or dis·equi·lib·ria
dis·func·tion
  var of dysfunction
dis·ha·bit·u·ate
  dis·ha·bit·u·at·ed
  dis·ha·bit·u·at·
    ing
dis·ha·bit·u·a·tion
dis·har·mo·ny
  pl dis·har·mo·nies
dis·in·fect
dis·in·fec·tant
dis·in·fec·tion
dis·in·fest
dis·in·fes·tant
dis·in·fes·ta·tion
dis·in·hi·bi·tion
dis·in·hib·i·to·ry
dis·in·sec·tion
dis·in·sect·iza·tion

dis·in·ser·tion
dis·in·te·grate
  dis·in·te·grat·ed
  dis·in·te·grat·ing
dis·in·te·gra·tion
dis·in·te·gra·tor
dis·in·ter
dis·in·tox·i·cate
  dis·in·tox·i·cat·
    ed
  dis·in·tox·i·cat·
    ing
dis·in·tox·i·ca·tion
dis·junc·tion
disk·ec·to·my
  pl disk·ec·to·mies
disk·o·gram
  also disc·o·gram
dis·kog·ra·phy
  also dis·cog·ra·phy
  pl dis·kog·ra·phies
  also dis·cog·ra·phies
dis·lo·cate
  dis·lo·cat·ed
  dis·lo·cat·ing
dis·lo·ca·tion
dis·mem·ber
  dis·mem·bered
  dis·mem·ber·ing
dis·mem·ber·ment
di·so·di·um
di·so·di·um ed·e·
  tate
di·so·mic
di·so·mus
  pl di·so·mi
  or di·so·mus·es

dis·or·der
dis·or·dered
dis·or·der·ing
dis·or·ga·ni·za·tion
dis·or·ga·nize
dis·or·ga·nized
dis·or·ga·niz·ing
dis·ori·ent
dis·ori·en·tate
dis·ori·en·tat·ed
dis·ori·en·tat·ing
dis·ori·en·ta·tion
dis·pa·rate
dis·par·i·ty
  pl dis·par·i·ties
dis·pen·sa·ry
  pl dis·pen·sa·ries
dis·pen·sa·tion
dis·pen·sa·to·ry
  pl dis·pen·sa·to·ries
dis·pense
dis·pensed
dis·pens·ing
di·sper·my
  pl di·sper·mies
dis·pers·al
dis·perse
dis·persed
dis·pers·ing
dis·per·sion
dis·per·sive
dis·place
dis·placed
dis·plac·ing
dis·place·ment
dis·pro·por·tion
dis·rupt

docimasy

dis·rup·tion
dis·rup·tive
dis·sect
dis·sec·tion
dis·sec·tor
dis·sem·i·nat·ed
dis·sem·i·na·tion
dis·sep·i·ment
dis·sim·i·late
  dis·sim·i·lat·ed
  dis·sim·i·lat·ing
dis·sim·i·la·tion
dis·so·ciant
dis·so·ci·ate
  dis·so·ci·at·ed
  dis·so·ci·at·ing
dis·so·ci·a·tion
dis·so·cia·tive
dis·so·lu·tion
dis·solv·able
dis·solve
  dis·solved
  dis·solv·ing
dis·solv·er
dis·so·nance
dis·tad
dis·tal
dis·tal·ly
dis·tem·per
dis·tem·per·oid
dis·tend
dis·ten·si·bil·i·ty
  pl dis·ten·si·bil·i·ties
dis·ten·si·ble
dis·ten·sile
dis·ten·sion
  or dis·ten·tion

dis·till
  also dis·til
  dis·tilled
  dis·till·ing
dis·til·late
dis·til·la·tion
dis·to·buc·cal
dis·to·buc·cal·ly
dis·to·clu·sion
dis·to·lin·gual
Dis·to·ma·ta
di·sto·mate
di·sto·ma·to·sis
  pl di·sto·ma·to·ses
di·stome
di·sto·mi·a·sis
  pl di·sto·mi·a·ses
dis·tor·tion
dis·tract
dis·trac·tion
dis·tress
dis·tri·bu·tion
dis·tur·bance
dis·turbed
di·sul·fide
di·sul·fi·ram
di·ure·sis
  pl di·ure·ses
di·uret·ic
di·uret·i·cal·ly
di·ur·nal
di·va·lent
di·verge
  di·verged
  di·verg·ing
di·ver·gence
di·ver·gent

di·ver·tic·u·lar
di·ver·tic·u·lec·to·
  my
  pl di·ver·tic·u·lec·to·
    mies
di·ver·tic·u·li·tis
di·ver·ti·cu·lop·exy
  pl di·ver·ti·cu·lop·ex·
    ies
di·ver·tic·u·lo·sis
  pl di·ver·tic·u·lo·ses
di·ver·tic·u·lum
  pl di·ver·tic·u·la
di·vide
  di·vid·ed
  di·vid·ing
di·vi·sion
di·vi·sion·al
di·vulse
  di·vulsed
  di·vuls·ing
di·vul·sion
di·vul·sor
di·zy·got·ic
di·zy·gous
diz·zi·ly
diz·zi·ness
diz·zy
  diz·zi·er
  diz·zi·est
DNA poly·mer·ase
DN·ase
  also DNA·ase
Do·bell's so·lu·tion
doc·i·ma·sia
doc·i·ma·sy
  pl doc·i·ma·sies

doc·tor
  doc·tored
  doc·tor·ing
do·dec·a·no·ic
dol
dol·i·cho·ce·phal·ic
dol·i·cho·ceph·a·ly
  pl dol·i·cho·ceph·a·lies
dol·i·cho·cra·ni·al
dol·i·cho·hi·er·ic
dol·i·cho·pel·lic
Dol·i·cho·psyl·li·dae
dol·i·chu·ran·ic
do·lor
do·lo·rif·ic
do·lo·ri·met·ric
do·lo·ri·met·ri·cal·ly
do·lo·rim·e·try
  pl do·lo·rim·e·tries
do·lo·rol·o·gy
  pl do·lo·rol·o·gies
do·lor·ous
do·mi·cil·i·ary
dom·i·nance
dom·i·nant
dom·i·na·tor
do·nee
Don Juan·ism
  pl Don Juan·isms
Don·nan equi·lib·ri·um
do·nor
Don·o·van body
do·pa

do·pa·mine
do·pa·mi·ner·gic
Dopp·ler ef·fect
do·ra·pho·bia
dor·sa
  pl of dorsum
dor·sad
dor·sal
dor·sa·lis
  pl dor·sa·les
dor·sa·lis pe·dis
dor·si·duct
dor·si·flex
dor·si·flex·ion
dor·si·flex·or
dor·si·spi·nal
dor·so·lat·er·al
dor·so·lum·bar
dor·so·me·di·al
dor·so·ven·tral
dor·so·ven·tral·i·ty
  pl dor·so·ven·tral·i·ties
dor·sum
  pl dor·sa
dos·age
dose
  dosed
  dos·ing
do·sim·e·ter
  also dose·me·ter
do·si·met·ric
do·sim·e·try
  pl do·sim·e·tries
dot·age
dou·blet

douche
  douched
  douch·ing
Doug·las bag
Doug·las's cul-de-sac
Doug·las's pouch
dou·rine
Do·ver's pow·der
down·growth
Down's syn·drome
  or Down syn·drome
dox·e·pin
doxo·ru·bi·cin
doxy·cy·cline
dox·yl·amine
drachm
  var of dram
drac·on·ti·a·sis
  pl drac·on·ti·a·ses
dra·cun·cu·li·a·sis
  pl dra·cun·cu·li·a·ses
dra·cun·cu·lo·sis
  pl dra·cun·cu·lo·ses
Dra·cun·cu·lus
draft
drafty
dra·gée
drain·age
dram
  also drachm
dra·ma·ti·za·tion
dras·tic
dras·ti·cal·ly

draw
  drew
  drawn
  draw·ing
draw·sheet
dream
  dreamed
  dreamt
  dream·ing
dream·er
dream·work
drep·a·no·cyte
drep·a·no·cyt·ic
drep·a·no·cy·to·sis
  pl drep·a·no·cy·to·ses
drink
  drank
  drunk
  drink·ing
Drink·er res·pi·ra·tor
dro·mo·ma·nia
dro·mo·trop·ic
drop·let
drop·per
drop·per·ful
drop·si·cal
drop·sy
  pl drop·sies
dro·soph·i·la
drows·i·ly
drows·i·ness
drowsy
  drows·i·er
  drows·i·est
drug·fast
drug·gist

drug·mak·er
drug·store
drum·head
drum·stick
drunk
drunk·ard
drunk·en
drunk·o·me·ter
druse
  pl dru·sen
dry
  adjective
  dri·er
  dri·est
dry
  verb
  dried
  dry·ing
dry-nurse
  verb
  dry-nursed
  dry-nurs·ing
dry nurse
  noun
du·al·ism
du·al·ist
du·al·is·tic
Du·boi·sia
Du Bois-Rey·mond's law
  or Du Bois-Rey·mond prin·ci·ple
Du·chenne
Du·crey's ba·cil·lus
duc·tal
duc·tile

duc·til·i·ty
  pl duc·til·i·ties
duc·tion
duct of Bar·tho·lin
duct of Bel·li·ni
duct of Cu·vier
duct of Ri·vi·nus
duct of San·to·ri·ni
duct of Wir·sung
duct·ule
duc·tu·lief·fe·ren·tes
duc·tu·lus
  pl duc·tu·li
duc·tu·lus ab·er·rans
  pl duc·tu·li ab·er·ran·tes
duc·tus
  pl duc·tus
duc·tus ar·te·ri·o·sus
duc·tus cho·le·do·chus
duc·tus co·chle·ar·is
duc·tus de·fer·ens
  pl duc·tus de·fer·en·tes
duc·tus ejac·u·la·to·ri·us
duc·tus re·uni·ens
duc·tus ve·no·sus
Duf·fy
Dührs·sen's in·ci·sions
dul·ci·tol

Du·long and Pe·
tit's law
dum·dum fe·ver
dump·ing syn·
drome
du·o·de·nal
du·o·de·nal
du·o·de·nec·to·my
pl du·o·de·nec·to·
mies
du·o·de·ni·tis
du·o·de·no·cho·led·
o·chot·o·my
pl du·o·de·no·cho·led·
o·chot·o·mies
du·o·de·nog·ra·phy
pl du·o·de·nog·ra·
phies
du·o·de·no·je·ju·nal
du·o·de·no·je·ju·
nos·to·my
pl du·o·de·no·je·ju·
nos·to·mies
du·o·de·not·o·my
pl du·o·de·not·o·mies
du·o·de·num
pl du·o·de·na
or du·o·de·nums
du·plex
du·pli·cate
du·pli·cat·ed
du·pli·cat·ing
du·pli·ca·tion
du·pli·ca·ture
Du·puy·tren's con·
trac·ture
du·ral
du·ra ma·ter

dwarf
pl dwarfs
or dwarves
dwarf·ism
dy·ad
dy·ad·ic
dy·ad·i·cal·ly
dy·dro·ges·ter·one
dye
dyed
dye·ing
dy·nam·ic
also dy·nam·i·cal
dy·nam·ics
dy·na·mo·gen·e·sis
pl dy·na·mo·gen·e·ses
dy·na·mo·gen·ic
dy·na·mog·e·ny
pl dy·na·mog·e·nies
dy·na·mom·e·ter
dy·na·mo·met·ric
dyne
dy·phyl·line
dys·acou·sia
dys·acou·sis
pl dys·acou·ses
dys·ad·ap·ta·tion
dys·ar·thria
dys·ar·thric
dys·ar·thro·sis
pl dys·ar·thro·ses
dys·au·to·no·mia
dys·au·to·nom·ic
dys·ba·rism
dys·cal·cu·lia
dys·che·zia
dys·che·zic

dys·chon·dro·pla·
sia
dys·chro·mia
dys·cra·sia
dys·di·ad·o·cho·ki·
ne·sia
or dys·di·ad·o·ko·ki·
ne·sia
dys·en·do·crin·ism
dys·en·ter·ic
dys·en·ter·i·form
dys·en·tery
pl dys·en·ter·ies
dys·er·gia
dys·er·gy
pl dys·er·gies
dys·es·the·sia
dys·es·thet·ic
dys·func·tion
also dis·func·tion
dys·func·tion·al
dys·func·tion·ing
dys·gam·ma·glob·
u·li·ne·mia
dys·gen·e·sis
pl dys·gen·e·ses
dys·gen·ic
dys·ger·mi·no·ma
pl dys·ger·mi·no·mas
or dys·ger·mi·no·ma·
ta
dys·geu·sia
dys·gon·ic
dys·graph·ia
dys·hi·dro·sis
or dys·idro·sis
pl dys·hi·dro·ses
or dys·idro·ses

dys·kary·o·sis
  pl dys·kary·o·ses
  or dys·kary·o·sis·es

dys·ker·a·to·sis
  pl dys·ker·a·to·ses

dys·ker·a·tot·ic

dys·ki·ne·sia

dys·ki·net·ic

dys·la·lia

dys·lec·tic

dys·lex·ia

dys·lex·ic

dys·lo·gia

dys·men·or·rhea

dys·men·or·rhe·ic

dys·met·ria

dys·mor·phism

dys·on·to·ge·net·ic

dys·os·mia

dys·os·to·sis
  pl dys·os·to·ses

dys·os·tot·ic

dys·pa·reu·nia

dys·pep·sia

dys·pep·tic

dys·pep·ti·cal·ly

dys·pha·gia

dys·phag·ic

dys·pha·sia

dys·pha·sic

dys·phe·mia

dys·pho·nia

dys·phon·ic

dys·pho·ria

dys·phor·ic

dys·pi·tu·itar·ism

dys·pla·sia

dys·plas·tic

dys·pnea

dys·pne·ic

dys·prax·ia

dys·pro·si·um

dys·pro·tein·emia

dys·pro·tein·emic

dys·reg·u·la·tion

dys·rhyth·mia

dys·rhyth·mic

dys·se·ba·cia

dys·syn·er·gy
  pl dys·syn·er·gies

dys·syn·er·gia

dys·syn·er·gic

dys·thy·mia

dys·thy·mic

dys·to·cia
  or dys·to·kia

dys·to·nia

dys·to·nia mus·cu·lo·rum de·for·mans

dys·ton·ic

dys·to·pia

dys·to·pic

dys·tro·phic

dys·tro·phy
  pl dys·tro·phies

dys·uria

dys·uric

E

ear·ache

ear·drum

eared

ear·lobe

ear·piece

ear·plug

ear·wax

Eb·er·thel·la

ebri·e·ty
  pl ebri·e·ties

eb·ul·lism

eb·ur·nat·ed

eb·ur·na·tion

ec·bol·ic

ec·cen·tric

ec·cen·tri·cal·ly

ec·chon·dro·ma
  pl ec·chon·dro·ma·ta
  or ec·chon·dro·mas

ec·chy·mosed

ec·chy·mo·sis
  pl ec·chy·mo·ses

ec·chy·mot·ic

ec·co·pro·ti·co·phor·ic

ec·crine

ec·cri·nol·o·gy
  pl ec·cri·nol·o·gies

ec·dys·ial

ec·dy·sis
  pl ec·dy·ses

ec·dy·sone
  also ec·dy·son

ec·go·nine

echi·no·coc·co·sis
  pl echi·no·coc·co·ses

echi·no·coc·cus
  pl echi·no·coc·ci

echi·no·derm

Echi·no·der·ma·ta
echi·no·der·ma·
　tous
echi·nu·late
echi·nu·la·tion
echo
　pl ech·oes
echo·car·dio·gram
echo·car·dio·
　graph·ic
echo·car·di·og·ra·
　phy
　pl echo·car·di·og·ra·
　phies
echo·en·ceph·a·lo·
　gram
echo·en·ceph·a·lo·
　graph·ic
echo·en·ceph·a·
　log·ra·phy
　pl echo·en·ceph·a·
　log·ra·phies
echo·gram
echo·graph
echo·graph·ic
echo·graph·i·cal·
　ly
echog·ra·phy
　pl echog·ra·phies
echo·ki·ne·sis
　pl echo·ki·ne·ses
echo·la·lia
echo·lal·ic
echo·mim·ia
echo·prac·tic
echo·prax·ia
echo·thi·o·phate

echo·vi·rus
Eck fis·tu·la
ec·lamp·sia
ec·lamp·tic
eclec·tic
eclec·ti·cal·ly
eclec·ti·cism
eco·log·i·cal
　also eco·log·ic
ecol·o·gist
ecol·o·gy
　pl ecol·o·gies
écor·ché
ec·pho·ria
　pl ec·pho·rias
　or ec·pho·ri·ae
ec·pho·rize
　ec·pho·rized
　ec·pho·riz·ing
écra·seur
ec·sta·sy
　pl ec·sta·sies
ec·stat·ic
ec·tad
ec·ta·sia
ec·ta·sis
　pl ec·ta·ses
ec·tat·ic
ect·eth·moid
ec·thy·ma
ec·thy·ma·tous
ec·to·blast
ec·to·blas·tic
ec·to·car·dia
ec·to·chon·dral
ec·to·com·men·
　sal

ec·to·crine
ec·to·cyst
ec·to·derm
ec·to·der·mal
ec·to·en·zyme
ec·to·gen·ic
ec·tog·e·nous
ec·to·mere
ec·to·mer·ic
ec·to·morph
ec·to·mor·phic
ec·to·mor·phy
　pl ec·to·mor·phies
ec·to·par·a·site
ec·to·par·a·sit·ic
ec·to·phyte
ec·to·phyt·ic
ec·to·pia
ec·top·ic
ec·top·i·cal·ly
ec·to·pla·cen·ta
ec·to·pla·cen·tal
ec·to·plasm
ec·to·plas·mic
ec·to·py
　pl ec·to·pies
ec·to·sarc
ect·os·te·al
ec·to·thrix
ec·tro·dac·ty·lous
ec·tro·dac·ty·ly
　pl ec·tro·dac·ty·lies
ec·tro·me·lia
ec·tro·me·lic
ec·tro·pi·on
ec·tro·pi·um
ec·ze·ma

ec·ze·ma·ti·za·tion
ec·ze·ma·toid
ec·zem·a·tous
ede·ma
edem·a·tous
Eden·ta·ta
eden·tate
eden·tu·lous
Ed·ing·er-West·phal nu·cle·us
ed·ro·pho·ni·um
ef·face
  ef·faced
  ef·fac·ing
ef·face·ment
ef·fect
ef·fec·tive
ef·fec·tive·ness
ef·fec·tor
ef·fer·ent
  conducting outward
  from a center (see
  afferent)
ef·fer·ent·ly
ef·fer·vesce
  ef·fer·vesced
  ef·fer·vesc·ing
ef·fer·ves·cence
  the process of giving off
  gas bubbles
  (see efflorescence*)*
ef·fer·ves·cent
ef·fleu·rage
ef·flo·resce
  ef·flo·resced
  ef·flo·resc·ing

ef·flo·res·cence
  a rash, also the process
  of forming a pow-
  dery chemical crust
  (see effervescence*)*
ef·flo·res·cent
ef·flu·vi·um
  pl ef·flu·via
  or ef·flu·vi·ums
ef·flux
ef·fuse
ef·fu·sion
egest
eges·ta
eges·tion
eges·tive
ego
  pl egos
ego·cen·tric
ego·cen·tri·cal·ly
ego·cen·tric·i·ty
  pl ego·cen·tric·i·ties
ego·cen·trism
ego-de·fense
  also ego-de·fence
ego-dys·ton·ic
ego-in·volve
  ego-in·volved
  ego-in·volv·ing
ego-in·volve·ment
ego·ism
ego·ist
ego·is·tic
  or ego·is·ti·cal
ego·ma·nia
ego·ma·ni·ac
ego·ma·ni·a·cal

egoph·o·ny
  pl egoph·o·nies
ego-syn·ton·ic
ego·tism
ego·tist
ego·tis·tic
  or ego·tis·ti·cal
ei·det·ic
ei·det·i·cal·ly
Eijk·man test
ei·ko·nom·e·ter
Ei·me·ria
ei·me·ri·an
Ei·me·ri·idae
ein·stei·ni·um
ejac·u·late
  ejac·u·lat·ed
  ejac·u·lat·ing
ejac·u·la·tion
ejac·u·la·tio prae·cox
ejac·u·la·tor
ejac·u·la·to·ry
ejac·u·lum
  pl ejac·u·la
ejec·ta
elab·o·rate
  elab·o·rat·ed
  elab·o·rat·ing
elab·o·ra·tion
elap·id
Elap·i·dae
elas·mo·branch
  pl elas·mo·branchs
Elas·mo·bran·chii
elas·tase
elas·ti·ca

elas·tic·i·ty
pl elas·tic·i·ties

elas·tin

elas·to·lyt·ic

elas·tom·e·ter

elas·tom·e·try
pl elas·tom·e·tries

elas·to·plast

elas·to·sis
pl elas·to·ses

elat·ed

ela·tion

el·bow

el·der

el·der·ber·ry
pl el·der·ber·ries

ele·cam·pane

elec·tive

Elec·tra com·plex

elec·tro·anal·y·sis
pl elec·tro·anal·y·ses

elec·tro·an·a·lyt·ic
or elec·tro·an·a·lyt·i·cal

elec·tro·an·es·the·sia

elec·tro·car·dio·gram

elec·tro·car·dio·graph

elec·tro·car·dio·graph·ic

elec·tro·car·dio·graph·i·cal·ly

elec·tro·car·di·og·ra·phy
pl elec·tro·car·di·og·ra·phies

elec·tro·cau·ter·iza·tion

elec·tro·cau·tery
pl elec·tro·cau·ter·ies

elec·tro·chem·i·cal

elec·tro·chem·is·try
pl elec·tro·chem·is·tries

elec·tro·chro·ma·tog·ra·phy
pl elec·tro·chro·ma·tog·ra·phies

elec·tro·co·ag·u·late

elec·tro·co·ag·u·lat·ed

elec·tro·co·ag·u·lat·ing

elec·tro·co·ag·u·la·tion

elec·tro·co·ag·u·la·tive

elec·tro·co·ma

elec·tro·con·trac·til·i·ty
pl elec·tro·con·trac·til·i·ties

elec·tro·con·vul·sive

elec·tro·cor·ti·cal

elec·tro·cor·ti·co·gram

elec·tro·cor·ti·co·graph·ic

elec·tro·cor·ti·co·graph·i·cal·ly

elec·tro·cor·ti·cog·ra·phy
pl elec·tro·cor·ti·cog·ra·phies

elec·tro·cor·tin

elec·tro·cute

elec·tro·cut·ed

elec·tro·cut·ing

elec·tro·cu·tion

elec·trode

elec·tro·der·mal

elec·tro·des·ic·ca·tion

elec·tro·di·ag·nos·tic

elec·tro·di·al·y·sis
pl elec·tro·di·al·y·ses

elec·tro·di·a·lyt·ic

elec·tro·di·a·lyze

elec·tro·di·a·lyzed

elec·tro·di·a·lyz·ing

elec·tro·di·a·lyz·er

elec·tro·en·ceph·a·lo·gram

elec·tro·en·ceph·a·lo·graph

electrophorus

elec·tro·en·ceph·a·log·ra·pher

elec·tro·en·ceph·a·lo·graph·ic

elec·tro·en·ceph·a·lo·graph·i·cal·ly

elec·tro·en·ceph·a·log·ra·phy
pl elec·tro·en·ceph·a·log·ra·phies

elec·tro·en·ceph·a·log·ra·pher

elec·tro·en·dos·mo·sis
pl elec·tro·en·dos·mo·ses

elec·tro·gen·e·sis
pl elec·tro·gen·e·ses

elec·tro·gen·ic

elec·tro·gram

elec·tro·graph·ic

elec·tro·graph·i·cal·ly

elec·trog·ra·phy
pl elec·trog·ra·phies

elec·tro·hys·tero·graph

elec·tro·hys·ter·og·ra·phy
pl elec·tro·hys·ter·og·ra·phies

elec·tro·ky·mo·graph

elec·tro·ky·mo·graph·ic

elec·tro·ky·mog·ra·phy
pl elec·tro·ky·mog·ra·phies

elec·trol·o·gist

elec·trol·y·sis
pl elec·trol·y·ses

elec·tro·lyte

elec·tro·lyt·ic

elec·tro·lyze
elec·tro·lyzed
elec·tro·lyz·ing

elec·tro·mag·net

elec·tro·mag·net·ic

elec·tro·mag·net·i·cal·ly

elec·tro·myo·gram

elec·tro·myo·graph

elec·tro·myo·graph·ic

elec·tro·myo·graph·i·cal·ly

elec·tro·my·og·ra·phy
pl elec·tro·my·og·ra·phies

elec·tron

elec·tro·nar·co·sis
pl elec·tro·nar·co·ses

elec·tron-dense

elec·tro·neg·a·tive

elec·tro·neg·a·tiv·i·ty
pl elec·tro·neg·a·tiv·i·ties

elec·tro·nys·tag·mo·graph·ic

elec·tro·nys·tag·mog·ra·phy
pl elec·tro·nys·tag·mog·ra·phies

elec·tro·oc·u·lo·gram

elec·tro·oc·u·lo·graph·ic

elec·tro·oc·u·log·ra·phy
pl elec·tro·oc·u·log·ra·phies

elec·tro·os·mo·sis
pl elec·tro·os·mo·ses

elec·tro·os·mot·ic

elec·tro·phe·ro·gram

elec·tro·phil·ic

elec·tro·phi·lic·ity
pl elec·tro·phi·lic·ities

elec·tro·pho·rese
elec·tro·pho·resed
elec·tro·pho·res·ing

elec·tro·pho·re·sis
pl elec·tro·pho·re·ses

elec·tro·pho·ret·ic

elec·tro·pho·ret·i·cal·ly

elec·tro·pho·reto·gram

elec·troph·o·rus
pl elec·troph·o·ri

elec·tro·phren·ic

elec·tro·phys·i·o·log·i·cal
  also elec·tro·phys·i·o·log·ic

elec·tro·phys·i·ol·o·gist

elec·tro·phys·i·ol·o·gy
  pl elec·tro·phys·i·ol·o·gies

elec·tro·pos·i·tive

elec·tro·py·rex·ia

elec·tro·re·sec·tion

elec·tro·ret·i·no·gram

elec·tro·ret·i·no·graph

elec·tro·ret·i·no·graph·ic

elec·tro·ret·i·nog·ra·phy
  pl elec·tro·ret·i·nog·ra·phies

elec·tro·scope

elec·tro·shock

elec·tro·sleep

elec·tro·stim·u·la·tion

elec·tro·sur·gery
  pl elec·tro·sur·ger·ies

elec·tro·sur·gi·cal

elec·tro·tax·is
  pl elec·tro·tax·es

elec·tro·ther·a·py
  pl elec·tro·ther·a·pies

elec·tro·tome

elec·tro·ton·ic

elec·trot·o·nus

elec·trot·ro·pism

elec·tu·ary
  pl elec·tu·ar·ies

el·e·doi·sin

el·e·phan·ti·as·ic

el·e·phan·ti·a·sis
  pl el·e·phan·ti·a·ses

el·e·phan·toid

el·e·vat·ed

el·e·va·tion

el·e·va·tor

elim·i·nant

elim·i·nate
  elim·i·nat·ed
  elim·i·nat·ing

elim·i·na·tion

elim·i·na·tive

elix·ir

el·lag·ic

el·lip·to·cyte

el·lip·to·cy·to·sis
  pl el·lip·to·cy·to·ses

elon·gate
  elon·gat·ed
  elon·gat·ing

elon·ga·tion

el·u·ant
  or el·u·ent

el·u·ate

elute
  elut·ed
  elut·ing

elu·tion

elu·tri·a·tion

ema·ci·ate
  ema·ci·at·ed
  ema·ci·at·ing

ema·ci·a·tion

em·a·nate
  em·a·nat·ed
  em·a·nat·ing

em·a·na·tion

eman·ci·pa·tion

emas·cu·late
  emas·cu·lat·ed
  emas·cu·lat·ing

emas·cu·la·tion

emas·cu·la·tome

emas·cu·la·tor

Em·ba·dom·o·nas

em·balm

em·balm·er

em·balm·ment

em·bar·rass

em·bar·rass·ment

em·bed
  em·bed·ded
  em·bed·ding

em·bed·ment

em·bo·lec·to·my
  pl em·bo·lec·to·mies

em·bo·le·mia

em·bol·ic

em·bo·lism

em·bo·li·za·tion

emulsoidal

em·bo·lize
  em·bo·lized
  em·bo·liz·ing
em·bo·lo·la·lia
em·bo·lus
  pl em·bo·li
em·bo·ly
  pl em·bo·lies
em·bra·sure
em·bro·cate
  em·bro·cat·ed
  em·bro·cat·ing
em·bro·ca·tion
em·bryo
  pl em·bry·os
em·bryo·car·dia
em·bryo·gen·e·sis
  pl em·bryo·gen·e·ses
em·bryo·ge·net·ic
em·bryo·gen·ic
em·bry·og·e·ny
  pl em·bry·og·e·nies
em·bry·oid
em·bry·o·log·i·cal
  also em·bry·o·log·ic
em·bry·ol·o·gist
em·bry·ol·o·gy
  pl em·bry·ol·o·gies
em·bry·o·ma
  pl em·bry·o·mas
  or em·bry·o·ma·ta
em·bry·o·nal
em·bry·o·nate
  em·bry·o·nat·ed
  em·bry·o·nat·ing
em·bry·on·ic

em·bry·on·i·cal·ly
em·bry·op·a·thy
  pl em·bry·op·a·thies
em·bryo·phore
em·bryo·tome
em·bry·ot·o·my
  pl em·bry·ot·o·mies
em·bryo·tox·i·ci·ty
  pl em·bryo·tox·i·ci·ties
em·bryo·tox·on
em·bry·o·trophe
  or em·bry·o·troph
em·ery
  pl em·er·ies
eme·sis
  pl eme·ses
emet·ic
emet·i·cal·ly
em·e·tine
em·i·nence
em·i·nen·tia
em·is·sary
emis·sion
emis·siv·i·ty
  pl emis·siv·i·ties
em·men·a·gog·ic
em·men·a·gogue
em·me·trope
em·me·tro·pia
em·me·trop·ic
em·o·din
emol·lient
emo·tion
emo·tion·al

emo·tion·al·i·ty
  pl emo·tion·al·i·ties
em·path·ic
em·path·i·cal·ly
em·pa·thize
  em·pa·thized
  em·pa·thiz·ing
em·pa·thy
  pl em·pa·thies
em·phy·se·ma
em·phy·se·ma·tous
em·phy·se·mic
em·pir·ic
  noun
em·pir·i·cal
  or em·pir·ic
  adjective
em·pir·i·cism
em·pros·thot·o·nos
em·py·ema
  pl em·py·ema·ta
  or em·py·emas
em·py·emic
em·py·reu·ma
  pl em·py·reu·ma·ta
em·py·reu·mat·ic
emul·si·fi·ca·tion
emul·si·fi·er
emul·si·fy
  emul·si·fied
  emul·si·fy·ing
emul·sion
emul·sive
emul·soid
emul·soi·dal

emunc·to·ry
  pl emunc·to·ries

enam·el

enam·e·lo·ma
  pl enam·e·lo·mas
  or enam·e·lo·ma·ta

en·an·them
  or en·an·the·ma
  pl en·an·thems
  or en·an·the·ma·ta

en·an·the·ma·tous

en·an·tio·mer

en·an·tio·mer·ic

en·an·tio·morph

en·an·tio·mor·
  phic
  or en·an·tio·mor·
  phous

en·an·tio·mor·
  phism

en·ar·thro·di·al

en·ar·thro·sis
  pl en·ar·thro·ses

en·cap·su·late

en·cap·su·lat·ed

en·cap·su·lat·
  ing

en·cap·su·la·tion

en·ceinte

en·ce·phal·ic

en·ceph·a·lit·ic

en·ceph·a·li·tis
  pl en·ceph·a·lit·i·
  des

en·ceph·a·lit·o·
  gen

en·ceph·a·lit·o·
  gen·ic

en·ceph·a·li·to·zo·
  on
  pl en·ceph·a·li·
  to·zoa

en·ceph·a·lo·cele

en·ceph·a·lo·gram

en·ceph·a·lo·
  graph

en·ceph·a·lo·
  graph·ic

en·ceph·a·lo·
  graph·i·cal·ly

en·ceph·a·log·ra·
  phy
  pl en·ceph·a·log·ra·
  phies

en·ceph·a·loid

en·ceph·a·lo·ma·
  la·cia

en·ceph·a·lo·ma·
  lac·ic

en·ceph·a·lo·men·
  in·gi·tis
  pl en·ceph·a·lo·men·
  in·git·i·des

en·ceph·a·lo·me·
  nin·go·cele

en·ceph·a·lo·mere

en·ceph·a·lo·mer·
  ic

en·ceph·a·lo·my·
  elit·ic

en·ceph·a·lo·my·
  eli·tis
  pl en·ceph·a·lo·my·
  elit·i·des

en·ceph·a·lo·my·
  elop·a·thy
  pl en·ceph·a·lo·my·
  elop·a·thies

en·ceph·a·lo·myo·
  car·di·tis

en·ceph·a·lon
  pl en·ceph·a·la

en·ceph·a·lo·path·
  ic

en·ceph·a·lop·a·
  thy
  pl en·ceph·a·lop·a·
  thies

en·ceph·a·lo·sis
  pl en·ceph·a·lo·ses

en·chon·dral

en·chon·dro·ma
  pl en·chon·dro·mas
  or en·chon·dro·ma·
  ta

en·chon·dro·ma·
  tous

en·clave

en·cop·re·sis

en·crust

en·crus·ta·tion

en·cyst

en·cys·ta·tion

en·cyst·ment

end·ame·ba
  also end·amoe·ba
  pl end·ame·bas
  or end·ame·bae
  also end·amoe·bas
  or end·amoe·bae

end·am·e·bi·a·sis
  also end·am·oe·bi·a·sis
  pl end·am·e·bi·a·ses
  also end·am·oe·bi·a·ses

end·ame·bic
  also end·amoe·bic

End·amoe·ba
End·amoe·bi·dae
end·ar·ter·ec·to·my
  pl end·ar·ter·ec·to·mies

end·ar·te·ri·al
end·ar·te·ri·tis
  also en·do·ar·te·ri·tis

end·ar·te·ri·tis ob·lit·er·ans
end·ar·te·ri·um
  pl end·ar·te·ria

end·ar·tery
end·au·ral
end·brain
end-di·a·stol·ic
en·dem·ic
en·dem·i·cal·ly
en·de·mic·i·ty
  pl en·de·mic·i·ties

en·de·mism
end·er·gon·ic
en·der·mat·ic
en·der·mic
en·do·ab·dom·i·nal

en·do·an·eu·rys·mor·rha·phy
  pl en·do·an·eu·rys·mor·rha·phies

en·do·bi·ot·ic
en·do·blast
en·do·blas·tic
en·do·bron·chi·al
en·do·car·di·al
en·do·car·di·tis
en·do·car·di·um
  pl en·do·car·dia

en·do·cer·vi·cal
en·do·cer·vi·ci·tis
en·do·cer·vix
  pl en·do·cer·vi·ces

en·do·chon·dral
en·do·cra·ni·al
en·do·crine
en·do·cri·no·log·ic
  or en·do·cri·no·log·i·cal

en·do·cri·nol·o·gist
en·do·cri·nol·o·gy
  pl en·do·cri·nol·o·gies

en·do·crin·o·path·ic
en·do·cri·nop·a·thy
  pl en·do·cri·nop·a·thies

en·do·cyst

en·do·cyt·ic
en·do·cy·tose
  en·do·cy·tosed
  en·do·cy·tos·ing
en·do·cy·to·sis
  pl en·do·cy·to·ses

en·do·cy·tot·ic
en·do·derm
en·do·der·mal
end·odon·tia
end·odon·tic
end·odon·ti·cal·ly
end·odon·tics
end·odon·tist
en·do·en·zyme
en·do·eryth·ro·cyt·ic
en·dog·a·mous
en·dog·a·my
  pl en·dog·a·mies

en·do·gas·tric
en·do·gas·tri·cal·ly
en·dog·e·nous
  also en·do·gen·ic

en·do·gna·thi·on
En·do·li·max
en·do·lymph
en·do·lym·phat·ic
en·do·me·so·derm
en·do·me·so·der·mal
en·do·me·tri·al

en·do·me·tri·o·ma
    pl en·do·me·tri·o·mas
    or en·do·me·tri·o·ma·ta

en·do·me·tri·o·sis
    pl en·do·me·tri·o·ses

en·do·me·tri·tis

en·do·me·tri·um
    pl en·do·me·tria

en·do·mi·to·sis
    pl en·do·mi·to·ses

en·do·mi·tot·ic

en·do·mix·is

en·do·morph

en·do·mor·phic

en·do·mor·phy
    pl en·do·mor·phies

en·do·myo·car·di·al

en·do·myo·car·di·um
    pl en·do·myo·car·dia

en·do·my·si·um
    pl en·do·my·sia

en·do·neu·ri·al

en·do·neu·ri·um
    pl en·do·neu·ria

en·do·nu·cle·ase

en·do·nu·cleo·lyt·ic

en·do·par·a·site

en·do·par·a·sit·ic

en·do·par·a·sit·ism

en·do·pep·ti·dase

en·do·per·ox·ide

en·do·phil·ic

en·do·phle·bi·tis
    pl en·do·phle·bi·tis·es
    or en·do·phle·bit·i·des

en·doph·thal·mi·tis

en·do·phyt·ic

en·do·plasm

en·do·plas·mic

en·do·poly·ploid

en·do·poly·ploi·dy
    pl en·do·poly·ploi·dies

en·do·pros·the·sis
    pl en·do·pros·the·ses

en·do·ra·dio·sonde

en·dor·phin

β-en·dor·phin
    var of beta-endorphin

en·do·sal·pinx
    pl en·do·sal·pin·ges

en·do·scope

en·do·scop·ic

en·do·scop·i·cal·ly

en·dos·co·pist

en·dos·co·py
    pl en·dos·co·pies

en·do·skel·e·tal

en·do·skel·e·ton

end·os·mo·sis

end·os·mot·ic

end·os·mot·i·cal·ly

en·do·spore

en·do·spor·u·la·tion

end·os·te·al

end·os·te·itis
    or end·os·ti·tis

end·os·te·um
    pl end·os·tea

en·do·sym·bi·o·sis
    pl en·do·sym·bi·o·ses

en·do·sym·bi·ot·ic

en·do·the·li·al

en·do·the·li·o·ma
    pl en·do·the·li·o·mas
    or en·do·the·li·o·ma·ta

en·do·the·li·um
    pl en·do·the·lia

en·do·therm

en·do·ther·mic
    also en·do·ther·mal

en·do·ther·my
    pl en·do·ther·mies

en·do·tox·emia

en·do·tox·ic

en·do·tox·in

en·do·tox·oid

en·do·tra·che·al

en·e·ma
    pl en·e·mas
    also ene·ma·ta

en·er·get·ic

en·er·get·ics

en·er·gid
en·er·giz·er
en·er·gy
  pl en·er·gies

en·er·vate
  en·er·vat·ed
  en·er·vat·ing
en·er·va·tion
  weakening (see inner-
    vation)

en·flur·ane
en·gorge
  en·gorged
  en·gorg·ing
en·gorge·ment
en·gram
  also en·gramme

en·gram·mic
en·keph·a·lin
en·keph·a·lin·er·
  gic
en·large
  en·larged
  en·larg·ing
en·large·ment
enol
eno·lase
eno·lic
en·oph·thal·mos
  also en·oph·thal·mus

en·os·to·sis
  pl en·os·to·ses

en·si·form
en·tad

ent·ame·ba
  also ent·amoe·ba
  pl ent·ame·bas
  or ent·ame·bae
  also ent·amoe·bas
  or ent·amoe·bae

ent·am·e·bi·a·sis
  also ent·am·oe·bi·a·
    sis
  pl ent·am·e·bi·a·ses
  also ent·am·oe·bi·a·
    ses

ent·ame·bic
  also ent·amoe·bic

Ent·amoe·ba
en·ter·al
en·ter·al·gia
en·ter·ec·to·my
  pl en·ter·ec·to·mies

en·ter·ic
en·ter·i·tis
  pl en·ter·it·i·des
  or en·ter·i·tis·es

En·tero·bac·ter
En·tero·bac·te·ri·
  a·ce·ae
en·tero·bac·te·ri·
  al
en·tero·bac·te·ri·
  um
en·tero·bi·a·sis
  pl en·tero·bi·a·ses

En·te·ro·bi·us
en·ter·o·cele
  hernia (see entero-
    coele)

en·tero·chro·maf·
  fin
en·tero·coc·cal

en·tero·coc·cus
  pl en·tero·coc·ci

En·ter·o·coc·us
en·tero·coele
  or en·tero·coel
  coelom (see entero-
    cele)

en·tero·co·li·tis
en·ter·o·cri·nin
en·tero·en·te·ros·
  to·my
  pl en·tero·en·te·ros·
    to·mies

en·tero·gas·tric
en·tero·gas·trone
en·ter·og·e·nous
en·tero·he·pat·ic
en·tero·hep·a·ti·
  tis
en·tero·ki·nase
en·ter·o·lith
en·ter·on
en·tero·patho·gen
en·tero·patho·gen·
  ic
en·ter·op·a·thy
  pl en·ter·op·a·thies

en·ter·op·to·sis
  pl en·ter·op·to·ses

en·ter·op·tot·ic
en·ter·or·rha·gia
en·tero·ste·no·sis
  pl en·tero·ste·no·ses

en·ter·os·to·mal
en·ter·os·to·my
  pl en·ter·os·to·mies

en·tero·tome

en·te·rot·o·my
 pl en·te·rot·o·mies

en·tero·tox·emia

en·tero·toxi·gen·ic

en·tero·tox·in

en·tero·vi·ral

en·tero·vi·rus

en·ti·ty
 pl en·ti·ties

en·to·blast

en·to·blas·tic

en·to·cone

en·to·co·nid

en·to·derm

en·to·der·mal
 or en·to·der·mic

en·to·mi·on
 pl en·to·mia

en·to·mo·log·i·cal

en·to·mol·o·gist

en·to·mol·o·gy
 pl en·to·mol·o·gies

en·to·mo·pho·bia

en·top·ic

en·top·i·cal·ly

ent·op·tic

en·to·ret·i·na

en·to·zoa
 sing en·to·zo·on

en·to·zo·ic

en·trails

en·train

en·train·ment

en·tro·pic

en·tro·pi·cal·ly

en·tro·pi·on

en·tro·py
 pl en·tro·pies

enu·cle·ate

 enu·cle·at·ed

 enu·cle·at·ing

enu·cle·ation

enu·cle·a·tor

en·ure·sis
 pl en·ure·ses

en·uret·ic

en·ven·om·ation

en·ven·om·iza·
 tion

en·vi·ron·ment

en·vi·ron·men·tal

en·vi·ron·men·tal·
 ism

en·zo·ot·ic

en·zy·got·ic

en·zy·mat·ic
 also en·zy·mic

en·zy·mat·i·cal·ly
 also en·zy·mi·cal·ly

en·zyme

en·zy·mo·log·i·cal

en·zy·mol·o·gist

en·zy·mol·o·gy
 pl en·zy·mol·o·gies

eo·sin
 or eo·sine

eo·sin·o·cyte

eo·sin·o·pe·nia

eo·sin·o·pe·nic

eo·sin·o·phil
 also eo·sin·o·phile

eo·sin·o·phil·ia

eo·sin·o·phil·ic

ep·ar·te·ri·al

ep·ax·i·al

ep·en·dy·ma

ep·en·dy·mal

ep·en·dy·mi·tis
 pl ep·en·dy·mit·i·
 des

ep·en·dy·mo·ma
 pl ep·en·dy·mo·mas
 also ep·en·dy·mo·
 ma·ta

eph·apse

eph·ap·tic

ephed·ra

ephed·rine

ephe·lis
 pl ephe·li·des

epi·an·dros·ter·
 one

epi·blast

epi·blas·tic

epib·o·ly
 pl epib·o·lies

epi·bul·bar

epi·can·thic

epi·can·thus

epi·car·dia
 part of the esophagus

epi·car·di·al

epi·car·di·um
 pl epi·car·dia
 *part of a membrane
 around the heart*

epi·cen·tral

epi·chord·al

epi·con·dy·lar

epi·con·dyle

epi·con·dy·li·tis

epi·cra·ni·al
epi·cra·ni·um
pl epi·cra·nia

epi·cra·ni·us
pl epi·cra·nii

epic·ri·sis
pl epic·ri·ses
summation

epi·cri·sis
pl epi·cri·ses
secondary crisis

ep·i·crit·ic
ep·i·dem·ic
also ep·i·dem·i·cal

ep·i·dem·i·cal·ly
ep·i·de·mic·i·ty
pl ep·i·de·mic·i·ties

ep·i·de·mi·o·log·i·cal
also ep·i·de·mi·o·log·ic

ep·i·de·mi·ol·o·gist
ep·i·de·mi·ol·o·gy
pl ep·i·de·mi·ol·o·gies

ep·i·derm
epi·der·mal
also epi·der·mic

ep·i·der·mat·ic
ep·i·der·mi·dal·iza·tion
epi·der·mis
epi·der·mi·tis
pl epi·der·mi·tis·es
or epi·der·mit·i·des

epi·der·mi·za·tion
epi·der·moid

ep·i·der·mol·y·sis
pl ep·i·der·mol·y·ses

ep·i·der·mo·my·co·sis
pl ep·i·der·mo·my·co·ses

Ep·i·der·moph·y·ton

ep·i·der·moph·y·to·sis
pl ep·i·der·moph·y·to·ses

ep·i·did·y·mal
ep·i·did·y·mec·to·my
pl ep·i·did·y·mec·to·mies

ep·i·did·y·mis
pl ep·i·did·y·mi·des

ep·i·did·y·mi·tis
ep·i·did·y·mo-or·chi·tis
ep·i·did·y·mo·vas·os·to·my
pl ep·i·did·y·mo·vas·os·to·mies

epi·du·ral
epi·fol·li·cu·li·tis
epi·gas·tric
epi·gas·tri·um
pl epi·gas·tria

epi·gas·tri·us
epi·gen·e·sis
pl epi·gen·e·ses

epi·ge·net·ic
epi·ge·net·i·cal·ly

epi·glot·tic
or epi·glot·tal

epi·glot·tid·e·an
epi·glot·ti·dec·to·my
pl epi·glot·ti·dec·to·mies

epi·glot·tis
ep·i·glot·ti·tis
epi·hy·al
ep·i·la·tion
ep·i·lem·ma
ep·i·lep·sy
pl ep·i·lep·sies

ep·i·lep·tic
ep·i·lep·ti·cal·ly
ep·i·lep·ti·form
ep·i·lep·to·gen·ic
ep·i·lep·toid
ep·i·loia
epi·mer
ep·i·mere
epi·mer·ic
epi·my·si·um
pl epi·my·sia

epi·neph·rine
also epi·neph·rin

epi·neu·ri·um
epi·phe·nom·e·non
epiph·o·ra
epiph·y·se·al
also ep·i·phys·i·al

epiph·y·si·od·e·sis
pl epiph·y·si·od·e·ses

epiph·y·si·ol·y·sis
  pl epiph·y·si·ol·y·ses

epiph·y·sis
  pl epiph·y·ses

epiph·y·si·tis

epi·pi·al

epi·plo·ec·to·my
  pl epi·plo·ec·to·mies

ep·i·plo·ic

epi·plo·on
  pl ep·i·plo·a

epi·pter·ic

epi·sclera

epi·scler·al

epi·scle·ri·tis

epi·si·or·rha·phy
  pl epi·si·or·rha·phies

epi·si·ot·o·my
  pl epi·si·ot·o·mies

epi·som·al

epi·some

ep·i·spa·di·as

ep·i·spas·tic

epis·ta·sis
  pl epis·ta·ses

epi·stat·ic

ep·i·stax·is
  pl ep·i·stax·es

epi·ster·nal

ep·i·stro·phe·us

epi·ten·din·e·um

epi·thal·a·mus
  pl epi·thal·a·mi

ep·i·the·li·al

ep·i·the·li·oid

ep·i·the·li·o·ma
  pl ep·i·the·li·o·mas
  or ep·i·the·li·o·ma·
    ta

ep·i·the·li·o·ma·
  tous

ep·i·the·li·um
  pl ep·i·the·lia

ep·i·the·li·za·tion
  or ep·i·the·lial·iza·
    tion

ep·i·the·lize
  or ep·i·the·li·al·ize
  ep·i·the·lized
    or ep·i·the·li·al·
      ized
  ep·i·the·liz·ing
    or ep·i·the·li·al·
      iz·ing

ep·i·thet

ep·i·troch·lea

epi·troch·le·ar

epi·tu·ber·cu·lo·
  sis
  pl epi·tu·ber·cu·lo·
    ses

epi·tu·ber·cu·lous

epi·tym·pan·ic

epi·tym·pa·num

ep·i·typh·li·tis

epi·zoa

epi·zo·ic

epi·zo·ot·ic

epi·zo·ot·i·cal·ly

epi·zo·oti·o·log·i·
  cal
  also epi·zo·ooti·o·log·
    ic

epi·zo·oti·ol·o·gy
  also epi·zo·ootol·o·gy
  pl epi·zo·ot·i·ol·o·
    gies
  also epi·zo·ootol·o·
    gies

ep·o·nych·i·um

ep·ooph·o·ron

Ep·som salts
  or Ep·som salt

Ep·stein-Barr vi·
  rus

epu·lis
  pl epu·li·des

equa·tion·al

equa·tor

equa·to·ri·al

equi·an·al·ge·sic

equi·ca·lo·ric

equi·len·in

equil·i·brate
  equil·i·brat·ed
  equil·i·brat·ing

equil·i·bra·tion

equil·i·bra·to·ry

equi·lib·ri·um
  pl equi·lib·ri·ums
  or equi·lib·ria

eq·ui·lin

equi·po·tent

equi·po·ten·tial

equiv·a·lence

equiv·a·lent

era·sion

er·bi·um

erect

erec·tile

erec·til·i·ty
  pl erec·til·i·ties
erec·tion
erec·tor
erec·tor pi·li
erec·tor spi·nae
erep·sin
ereth·ic
er·e·thism
er·ga·sia
er·gas·to·plasm
er·gas·to·plas·mic
er·go·cal·cif·er·ol
er·go·gen·ic
er·go·graph
er·go·graph·ic
er·go·ma·nia
er·go·ma·ni·ac
er·gom·e·ter
er·go·met·ric
er·go·met·rine
er·go·nom·ic
er·go·nom·i·cal·ly
er·go·nom·ics
er·gon·o·mist
er·go·no·vine
er·go·phobe
er·go·pho·bia
er·gos·ter·ol
er·got
er·got·a·mine
er·go·ther·a·py
  pl er·go·ther·a·pies
er·go·thi·o·ne·ine
er·got·ic
er·got·ism
er·got·ized

er·go·tox·ine
Er·len·mey·er flask
er·o·ge·ne·ity
  pl er·o·ge·ne·ities
erog·e·nous
  also er·o·gen·ic
Eros
erose
ero·sion
ero·sive
erot·ic
  also erot·i·cal
erot·i·ca
erot·i·cism
er·o·tism
er·o·ti·za·tion
er·o·tize
  er·o·tized
  er·o·tiz·ing
ero·to·gen·e·sis
  pl ero·to·gen·e·ses
er·o·to·log·i·cal
er·o·tol·o·gy
  pl er·o·tol·o·gies
ero·to·ma·nia
ero·to·ma·ni·ac
ero·to·path
er·o·top·a·thy
  pl er·o·top·a·thies
er·rhine
eru·cic
eruct
eruc·tate
  eruc·tat·ed
  eruc·tat·ing
eruc·ta·tion
erupt

erup·tion
erup·tive
er·y·sip·e·las
er·y·si·pel·a·tous
er·y·sip·e·loid
er·y·sip·e·lo·thrix
er·y·the·ma
er·y·the·mal
er·y·the·ma mul·
  ti·for·me
er·y·the·ma no·do·
  sum
er·y·the·ma·to·ge·
  nic
er·y·them·a·tous
  also er·y·the·mic
er·y·thor·bate
er·y·thras·ma
eryth·re·de·ma
er·y·thre·mia
er·y·thrism
er·y·thris·tic
  also er·y·thris·mal
eryth·ri·tyl tet·ra·
  ni·trate
eryth·ro·blast
eryth·ro·blas·te·
  mia
eryth·ro·blas·tic
eryth·ro·blas·to·
  pe·nia
eryth·ro·blas·to·
  sis
  pl eryth·ro·blas·to·
  ses
eryth·ro·blas·to·
  sis fe·ta·lis

eryth·ro·blas·to·
sis ne·o·na·to·
rum
eryth·ro·blas·tot·
ic
eryth·ro·cyte
eryth·ro·cy·the·
mia
eryth·ro·cyt·ic
eryth·ro·cy·tom·e·
ter
eryth·ro·cy·to·pe·
nia
eryth·ro·cy·to·poi·
e·sis
  pl eryth·ro·cy·to·poi·
  e·ses
eryth·ro·cy·tor·
rhex·is
  pl eryth·ro·cy·tor·
  rhex·es
eryth·ro·cy·to·sis
  eryth·ro·cy·to·
  ses
eryth·ro·der·ma
  pl eryth·ro·der·mas
  or eryth·ro·der·ma·
  ta
eryth·ro·der·mia
eryth·ro·don·tia
eryth·ro·gen·e·sis
  pl eryth·ro·gen·e·ses
eryth·ro·gen·ic
eryth·ro·gone
ery·throid
er·y·thro·i·dine

eryth·ro·leu·ke·
mia
eryth·ro·leu·ke·
mic
eryth·ro·mel·al·
gia
eryth·ro·my·cin
er·y·thron
eryth·ro·pe·nia
eryth·ro·phage
eryth·ro·pha·gia
eryth·ro·phago·cy·
to·sis
  pl eryth·ro·phago·cy·
  to·ses
er·y·throph·i·lous
eryth·ro·pla·sia
eryth·ro·poi·e·sis
  pl eryth·ro·poi·e·ses
eryth·ro·poi·et·ic
eryth·ro·poi·e·tin
er·y·throp·sia
  or er·y·thro·pia
eryth·ro·sin
  also eryth·ro·sine
er·y·thro·sis
  pl er·y·thro·ses
es·cape
  es·caped
  es·cap·ing
es·cap·ism
es·cap·ist
es·char
es·cha·rot·ic
Esch·e·rich·ia
es·cutch·eon
es·er·ine

Es·march ban·
dage
  or Es·march's ban·
  dage
es·od·ic
esoph·a·ge·al
esoph·a·gec·to·my
  pl esoph·a·gec·to·
  mies
esoph·a·gi·tis
esoph·a·go·gas·
trec·to·my
  pl esoph·a·go·gas·
  trec·to·mies
esoph·a·go·gas·
tric
esoph·a·go·gas·
tros·co·py
  pl esoph·a·go·gas·
  tros·co·pies
esoph·a·go·gas·
tros·to·my
  pl esoph·a·go·gas·
  tros·to·mies
esoph·a·go·je·ju·
nos·to·my
  pl esoph·a·go·je·ju·
  nos·to·mies
esoph·a·go·my·ot·
o·my
  pl esoph·a·go·my·ot·
  o·mies
esoph·a·go·plas·ty
  pl esoph·a·go·plas·
  ties
esoph·a·go·scope
esoph·a·go·scop·ic

esoph·a·gos·co·pist

esoph·a·gos·co·py
pl esoph·a·gos·co·pies

esoph·a·gos·to·my
pl esoph·a·gos·to·mies

esoph·a·got·o·my
pl esoph·a·got·o·mies

esoph·a·gus
pl esoph·a·gi

es·o·pho·ria

es·o·tro·pia

es·o·trop·ic

es·pun·dia

es·sence

es·sen·tial

es·ter

es·ter·ase

es·ter·i·fi·able

es·ter·ifi·ca·tion

es·ter·i·fy
es·ter·i·fied
es·ter·i·fy·ing

es·the·sia

es·the·si·om·e·ter

es·the·si·om·e·try
pl es·the·si·om·e·tries

es·the·sio·phys·i·ol·o·gy
pl es·the·sio·phys·i·ol·o·gies

es·thi·o·mene

es·ti·val

es·ti·vate
es·ti·vat·ed
es·ti·vat·ing

es·tra·di·ol

es·tral

es·trin

es·trin·iza·tion

es·tri·ol

es·tro·gen

es·tro·gen·ic

es·tro·gen·i·cal·ly

es·tro·gen·ic·i·ty
pl es·tro·gen·ic·i·ties

es·trone

es·trous

es·tru·al

es·tru·ate
es·tru·at·ed
es·tru·at·ing

es·tru·a·tion

es·trus
or es·trum

eth·a·cryn·ic

eth·am·bu·tol

etha·mi·van

eth·a·nol

eth·a·nol·amine

eth·chlor·vy·nol

ether

ethe·re·al

ether·iza·tion

ether·ize
ether·ized
ether·iz·ing

eth·i·cal
also eth·ic

eth·ics

ethid·ium

ethi·nyl
var of ethynyl

eth·i·on·amide

ethi·o·nine

ethis·ter·one

eth·moid
or eth·moi·dal

eth·moid·ec·to·my
pl eth·moid·ec·to·mies

eth·moid·itis

eth·mo·max·il·lary

eth·mo·tur·bi·nal

eth·no·log·i·cal
also eth·no·log·ic

eth·nol·o·gy
pl eth·nol·o·gies

etho·hexa·di·ol

etho·log·i·cal

ethol·o·gy
pl ethol·o·gies

etho·sux·i·mide

eth·yl

eth·yl·ene

eth·yl·ene·di·amine·tetra·ac·e·tate

eth·yl·ene·di·amine·tetra·ace·tic

eth·yl·enic

eth·yl·eni·cal·ly

eth·yl·mor·phine

ethy·nyl
also ethi·nyl

ethy·nyl·es·tra·di·
  ol

ethy·nyl·oes·tra·di·
  ol

etio·chol·an·ol·
  one

eti·o·late
  eti·o·lat·ed
  eti·o·lat·ing
eti·o·la·tion
eti·o·log·ic
  or eti·o·log·i·cal
eti·o·log·i·cal·ly
eti·ol·o·gy
  pl eti·ol·o·gies

etio·patho·gen·e·
  sis
  pl etio·patho·gen·e·
  ses

etio·por·phy·rin
etor·phine
Eu·bac·te·ri·a·les
eu·ca·lyp·tol
  also eu·ca·lyp·tole

eu·ca·lyp·tus
  pl eu·ca·lyp·ti
  or eu·ca·lyp·tus·es

eu·cary·ote
  var of eu·kary·ote

eu·cary·ot·ic
  var of eu·kary·ot·ic

euc·at·ro·pine
Eu·ces·to·da
eu·chlor·hyd·ria
eu·chro·mat·ic

eu·chro·ma·tin
eu·di·om·e·ter
eu·dio·met·ric
eu·gen·ic
eu·gen·i·cal·ly
eu·gen·i·cist
eu·gen·ics
eu·ge·nol
eu·gle·na
eu·gle·noid
eu·glob·u·lin
eu·gon·ic
eu·kary·ote
  also eu·cary·ote

eu·kary·ot·ic
  also eu·cary·ot·ic

eu·my·cete
Eu·my·ce·tes
eu·nuch
eu·nuch·ism
eu·nuch·oid
  also eu·nuch·oi·dal

eu·nuch·oid·ism
eu·pep·sia
eu·pep·tic
eu·phen·ic
eu·phen·ics
eu·pho·ria
eu·pho·ri·ant
eu·phor·ic
eu·phor·i·cal·ly
eu·phor·i·gen·ic
eu·plas·tic
eu·ploid
eu·ploi·dy
  pl eu·ploi·dies

eup·nea

eup·ne·ic
eu·prax·ia
eu·ro·pi·um
Eu·ro·ti·a·les
eu·ryg·nath·ic
eu·ryg·na·thism
eu·ry·on
eu·sta·chian
eu·tha·na·sia
eu·than·a·tize
  also eu·tha·nize

eu·than·a·tized
  also eu·tha·nized

eu·than·a·tiz·
  ing
  also eu·tha·niz·ing

eu·then·ics
Eu·the·ria
eu·the·ri·an
eu·thy·roid
eu·thy·roid·ism
eu·to·cia
evac·u·ant
evac·u·ate
  evac·u·at·ed
  evac·u·at·ing
evac·u·a·tion
evac·u·a·tive
evag·i·nate
  evag·i·nat·ed
  evag·i·nat·ing
evag·i·na·tion
Ev·ans blue
even·tra·tion
ever·si·ble
ever·sion
evert

evir·a·tion
evis·cer·ate
  evis·cer·at·ed
  evis·cer·at·ing
evis·cer·a·tion
evo·ca·tion
evo·ca·tor
evo·lu·tion
evo·lu·tion·ari·ly
evo·lu·tion·ary
evo·lu·tio·nist
evulse
  evulsed
  evuls·ing
evul·sion
ewe-necked
Ew·ing's sar·co·
  ma
ex·ac·er·bate
  ex·ac·er·bat·ed
  ex·ac·er·bat·ing
ex·ac·er·ba·tion
ex·al·ta·tion
ex·am·i·na·tion
ex·am·ine
  ex·am·ined
  ex·am·in·ing
ex·am·in·er
ex·an·them
  also ex·an·the·ma
  pl ex·an·thems
  also ex·an·them·a·ta
  or ex·an·the·mas

ex·an·them·a·tous
  or ex·an·the·mat·ic

ex·ca·vate
  ex·ca·vat·ed
  ex·ca·vat·ing
ex·ca·va·tion
ex·ca·va·tor
ex·ce·men·to·sis
  pl ex·ce·men·to·ses
  or ex·ce·men·to·sis·
    es
ex·cip·i·ent
ex·cise
  ex·cised
  ex·cis·ing
ex·ci·sion
ex·ci·sion·al
ex·cit·abil·i·ty
  pl ex·cit·abil·i·ties
ex·cit·able
ex·ci·tant
ex·ci·ta·tion
ex·cit·ato·ry
ex·cite
  ex·cit·ed
  ex·cit·ing
ex·cite·ment
ex·ci·tor
ex·clude
  ex·clud·ed
  ex·clud·ing
ex·clu·sion
ex·coch·le·a·tion
ex·co·ri·ate
  ex·co·ri·at·ed
  ex·co·ri·at·ing
ex·co·ri·a·tion
ex·cre·ment
ex·cre·men·tal

ex·cre·men·ti·
  tious
ex·cres·cence
ex·cres·cent
ex·cre·ta
ex·cre·tal
ex·crete
  ex·cret·ed
  ex·cret·ing
ex·cret·er
ex·cre·tion
ex·cre·to·ry
ex·cur·sion
ex·cyst
ex·cys·ta·tion
  or ex·cyst·ment
ex·en·ter·ate
  ex·en·ter·at·ed
  ex·en·ter·at·ing
ex·en·ter·a·tion
ex·er·cise
  ex·er·cised
  ex·er·cis·ing
ex·er·e·sis
  pl ex·er·e·ses
ex·er·gon·ic
ex·flag·el·late
  ex·flag·el·lat·ed
  ex·flag·el·lat·ing
ex·flag·el·la·tion
ex·fo·li·ate
  ex·fo·li·at·ed
  ex·fo·li·at·ing
ex·fo·li·a·tion
ex·fo·li·a·tive
ex·ha·la·tion

ex·hale
  ex·haled
  ex·hal·ing
ex·haust
ex·haus·tion
ex·hib·it
ex·hi·bi·tion·ism
ex·hi·bi·tion·ist
ex·hi·bi·tion·is·tic
ex·hi·bi·tion·is·ti·
  cal·ly
ex·hu·ma·tion
ex·hume
  ex·humed
  ex·hum·ing
ex·i·tus
  pl ex·i·tus

exo·bi·o·log·i·cal
exo·bi·ol·o·gist
exo·bi·ol·o·gy
  pl exo·bi·ol·o·gies

exo·crine
exo·cri·nol·o·gy
  pl exo·cri·nol·o·gies

exo·cy·to·sis
  pl exo·cy·to·ses

exo·cy·tot·ic
ex·od·ic
ex·odon·tia
ex·odon·tist
exo·en·zyme
exo·eryth·ro·cyt·ic
exo·gam·ic
ex·og·a·mous
ex·og·a·my
  pl ex·og·a·mies

exo·gas·tru·la
  pl exo·gas·tru·las
  or exo·gas·tru·lae

exo·gas·tru·la·tion
ex·og·e·nous
  or ex·o·gen·ic
ex·om·pha·los
  pl ex·om·pha·li

ex·on
ex·on·ic
exo·nu·cle·ase
exo·pep·ti·dase
exo·phil·ic
  pl ex·oph·i·lies

ex·o·pho·ria
ex·o·phor·ic
ex·oph·thal·mia
ex·oph·thal·mic
ex·oph·thal·mos
  also ex·oph·thal·mus

exo·phyt·ic
exo·skel·e·tal
exo·skel·e·ton
ex·os·mo·sis
  pl ex·os·mo·ses

ex·os·mot·ic
exo·spore
ex·os·tec·to·my
  pl ex·os·tec·to·mies

ex·os·to·sis
  pl ex·os·to·ses

ex·os·tot·ic
exo·ther·mic
  also exo·ther·mal
exo·ther·mi·cal·ly

exo·ther·mi·ci·ty
  pl exo·ther·mi·ci·
  ties

exo·tox·ic
exo·tox·in
exo·tro·pia
ex·pan·der
ex·pan·sion
ex·pan·sive
ex·pan·sive·ness
ex·pect
ex·pec·tan·cy
  pl ex·pec·tan·cies

ex·pec·tant
ex·pec·to·rant
ex·pec·to·rate
  ex·pec·to·rat·ed
  ex·pec·to·rat·
  ing
ex·pec·to·ra·tion
ex·per·i·ment
ex·per·i·men·tal
ex·per·i·men·tal·
  ist
ex·per·i·men·ta·
  tion
ex·per·i·ment·er
ex·pi·ra·tion
ex·pi·ra·to·ry
ex·pire
  ex·pired
  ex·pir·ing
ex·plant
ex·plant
ex·plan·ta·tion
ex·plo·ra·tion
ex·plor·ato·ry

ex·plore
  ex·plored
  ex·plor·ing
ex·plor·er
ex·plo·sion
ex·pose
  ex·posed
  ex·pos·ing
ex·po·sure
ex·press
ex·pres·sion
ex·pres·siv·i·ty
  pl ex·pres·siv·i·ties
ex·pul·sion
ex·pul·sive
ex·san·gui·nate
  ex·san·gui·nat·ed
  ex·san·gui·nat·ing
ex·san·gui·na·tion
ex·san·guine
ex·san·guin·i·ty
  pl ex·san·guin·i·ties
ex·san·gui·no·trans·fu·sion
ex·sect
ex·sec·tion
ex·sic·cate
  ex·sic·cat·ed
  ex·sic·cat·ing
ex·sic·ca·tion
ex·sic·co·sis
  pl ex·sic·co·ses
ex·stro·phy
  pl ex·stro·phies
ex·tend

ex·tend·er
ex·ten·si·bil·i·ty
  pl ex·ten·si·bil·i·ties
ex·ten·si·ble
ex·ten·sion
ex·ten·sor
ex·ten·sor car·pi ra·di·al·is brev·is
ex·ten·sor car·pi ra·di·al·is lon·gus
ex·ten·sor car·pi ul·na·ris
ex·ten·sor dig·i·ti min·i·mi
ex·ten·sor dig·i·to·rum brev·is
ex·ten·sor dig·i·to·rum com·mu·nis
ex·ten·sor di·gi·to·rum lon·gus
ex·ten·sor hal·lu·cis brev·is
ex·ten·sor hal·lu·cis lon·gus
ex·ten·sor in·di·cis
ex·ten·sor pol·li·cis brev·is
ex·ten·sor pol·li·cis lon·gus
ex·te·ri·or
ex·te·ri·or·iza·tion

ex·te·ri·or·ize
  ex·te·ri·or·ized
  ex·te·ri·or·iz·ing
ex·tern
  also ex·terne
ex·ter·nal
ex·ter·nal·ize
  ex·ter·nal·ized
  ex·ter·nal·iz·ing
ex·tern·ship
ex·tero·cep·tive
ex·tero·cep·tor
ex·tero·fec·tive
ex·tinct
ex·tinc·tion
ex·tin·guish
ex·tir·pate
  ex·tir·pat·ed
  ex·tir·pat·ing
ex·tir·pa·tion
ex·tor·sion
ex·tra·bul·bar
ex·tra·cap·su·lar
ex·tra·cel·lu·lar
ex·tra·chro·mo·som·al
ex·tra·cor·po·re·al
ex·tra·cor·pus·cu·lar
ex·tra·cra·ni·al
ex·tract
ex·tract·abil·i·ty
  pl ex·tract·abil·i·ties
ex·tract·able
  also ex·tract·ible
ex·tract·ant

ex·trac·tion
ex·trac·tive
ex·trac·tor
ex·tra·cys·tic
ex·tra·du·ral
ex·tra·em·bry·on·ic
ex·tra·en·ter·ic
ex·tra·eryth·ro·cyt·ic
ex·tra·fu·sal
ex·tra·gen·i·tal
ex·tra·he·pat·ic
ex·tra·in·tes·ti·nal
ex·tra·mac·u·lar
ex·tra·mas·toid
ex·tra·med·ul·lary
ex·tra·mi·to·chon·dri·al
ex·tra·mu·ral
ex·tra·nu·cle·ar
ex·tra·oc·u·lar
ex·tra·or·al
ex·tra·peri·to·ne·al
ex·tra·pi·tu·itary
ex·tra·pla·cen·tal
ex·tra·py·ra·mi·dal
ex·tra·re·nal
ex·tra·ret·i·nal
ex·tra·sen·so·ry
ex·tra·sys·to·le
ex·tra·sys·tol·ic
ex·tra·tu·bal
ex·tra·uter·ine
ex·tra·vag·i·nal

ex·trav·a·sate
   ex·trav·a·sat·ed
   ex·trav·a·sat·ing
ex·trav·a·sa·tion
ex·tra·vas·cu·lar
ex·tra·ven·tric·u·lar
ex·trem·i·ty
   pl ex·trem·i·ties
ex·trin·sic
ex·trin·si·cal·ly
ex·tro·ver·sion
   or ex·tra·ver·sion
ex·tro·ver·sive
   or ex·tra·ver·sive
ex·tro·vert
   or ex·tra·vert
ex·tro·vert·ed
   or ex·tra·vert·ed
ex·trude
   ex·trud·ed
   ex·trud·ing
ex·tru·sion
ex·tu·bate
   ex·tu·bat·ed
   ex·tu·bat·ing
ex·tu·ba·tion
ex·u·date
ex·u·da·tion
ex·u·da·tive
ex·ude
   ex·ud·ed
   ex·ud·ing
eye·ball
eye·brow
eye·cup
eyed

eyed·ness
eye·drop·per
eye·drop·per·ful
eye·drops
eye·glass·es
eye·ground
eye·hole
eye·lash·es
eye·lid
eye·piece
eye·sight
eye·spot
eye·strain
eye·tooth
   pl eye·teeth
eye·wash
eye·wink

F

fa·bel·la
   pl fa·bel·lae
fab·ri·ca·tion
Fa·bry's dis·ease
fab·u·la·tion
face·bow
face-lift
face-lift·ing
fac·et
fac·et·ec·to·my
   pl fac·et·ec·to·mies
fac·et·ed
   or fac·et·ted
fa·cial
   of the face (see fascial)
fa·cies
   pl fa·cies

fa·cies Hip·po·crat·ica

fa·cil·i·tate
 fa·cil·i·tat·ed
 fa·cil·i·tat·ing
fa·cil·i·ta·tion
fa·cil·i·ta·to·ry
fa·cil·i·ty
 pl fa·cil·i·ties

fac·ing
fa·cio·scap·u·lo·hu·mer·al
F-ac·tin
fac·ti·tious
fac·tor
fac·to·ri·al
fac·ul·ta·tive
fac·ul·ty
 pl fac·ul·ties

fag·o·py·rism
 also fag·o·py·ris·mus
 pl fag·o·py·risms
 also fag·o·py·ris·mus·es

Fahr·en·heit
fail·ure
fal·cate
 also fal·cat·ed
fal·ces
 pl of falx
fal·cial
fal·ci·form
fal·cip·a·rum ma·lar·ia
fal·cu·lar
fal·lo·pi·an
Fal·lot's te·tral·o·gy

fall·out
fal·si·fi·ca·tion
fal·si·fy
 fal·si·fied
 fal·si·fy·ing
falx
 pl fal·ces
falx ce·re·bel·li
falx cer·e·bri
fa·mes
fa·mil·ial
fam·i·ly
 pl fam·i·lies

Fan·co·ni's ane·mia
Fan·co·ni syn·drome
fan·go
Fan·nia
fan·ta·size
 fan·ta·sized
 fan·ta·siz·ing
fan·tast
fan·ta·sy
 also phan·ta·sy
 pl fan·ta·sies
 also phan·ta·sies

fan·ta·sy
 also phan·ta·sy
fan·ta·sied
 also phan·ta·sied
fan·ta·sy·ing
 also phan·ta·sy·ing

fan·tom
 var of phantom

far·ad
far·a·day

fa·rad·ic
 also far·a·da·ic

far·a·dism
far·a·di·za·tion
far·a·dize
 far·a·dized
 far·a·diz·ing
far·a·diz·er
far·cy
 pl far·cies

far·fa·ra
fa·ri·na
far·i·na·ceous
farm·er's lung
far·ne·sol
far·row
far·sight·ed
fas·cia
 pl fas·ci·ae
 or fas·cias

fas·cial
 of a sheet of connective tissue (*see* facial)

fas·cia la·ta
 pl fas·ci·ae la·tae

fas·ci·cle
fas·ci·cled
fas·cic·u·lar
fas·cic·u·late
 or fas·cic·u·lat·ed

fas·cic·u·la·tion
fas·cic·u·lus
 pl fas·cic·u·li

fas·cic·u·lus cu·ne·atus
fas·cic·u·lus grac·i·lis

fas·ci·ec·to·my
pl fas·ci·ec·to·mies

fas·ci·i·tis
or fas·ci·tis

fas·ci·o·la
pl fas·ci·o·lae
or fas·ci·o·las

fas·ci·o·lar

fa·sci·o·li·a·sis
pl fa·sci·o·li·a·ses

fas·ci·o·li·cid·al

fas·ci·o·li·cide

Fas·ci·ol·i·dae

Fas·ci·o·loi·des

fas·ci·o·lop·si·a·sis
pl fas·ci·o·lop·si·a·ses

Fas·ci·o·lop·sis

fas·ci·ot·o·my
pl fas·ci·ot·o·mies

fas·ci·tis
var of fasciitis

fas·tid·i·ous

fas·tid·i·um

fas·tig·ial

fas·tig·i·um

fast·ness

fa·tal

fa·tal·i·ty
pl fa·tal·i·ties

fa·ti·ga·bil·i·ty
also fa·ti·gua·bil·i·ty
pl fa·ti·ga·bil·i·ties
also fa·ti·gua·bil·i·ties

fa·ti·ga·ble
also fa·ti·gua·ble

fa·tigue

fa·tigued

fa·tigu·ing

fat-sol·u·ble

fat·ti·ness

fat·ty

fat·ti·er

fat·ti·est

fau·ces

fau·cial

fau·na
pl fau·nas
also fau·nae

fau·nal

fa·va bean

fa·ve·o·late

fa·vic

fa·vism

fa·vus

feath·er

feath·ered

fea·ture

fe·bric·u·la

fe·bri·fa·cient

fe·brif·ic

fe·brif·u·gal

feb·ri·fuge

fe·brile

fe·bris

fe·cal

fe·ca·lith

fe·cal·oid

fe·ces

Fech·ner's law

fec·u·la
pl fec·u·lae

fe·cu·lence

fec·u·lent

fe·cund

fe·cun·date

fe·cun·dat·ed

fe·cun·dat·ing

fe·cun·da·tion

fe·cun·di·ty
pl fe·cun·di·ties

fee·ble·mind·ed

feed·back

feel·er

feel·ing

fee split·ter

fee split·ting

Feh·ling's so·lu·tion
or Feh·ling so·lu·tion

fel

feld·sher

Fe·li·dae

fe·line

fel·late

fel·lat·ed

fel·lat·ing

fel·la·tio
also fel·la·tion
pl fel·la·tios
also fel·la·tions

fel·la·tor

fel·la·tory

fel·la·trice

fel·la·trix
pl fel·la·trix·es
or fel·la·tri·ces

felo-de-se
pl fe·lo·nes-de-se
or felos-de-se

fel·on
Fel·ty's syn·drome
fe·male
fem·i·nine
fem·i·nin·i·ty
    pl fem·i·nin·i·ties
fem·i·nism
fem·i·ni·za·tion
fem·i·nize
    fem·i·nized
    fem·i·niz·ing
fem·o·ral
fem·o·ro·pop·li·te·al
fe·mur
    pl fe·murs
    or fem·o·ra
fe·nes·tra
    pl fe·nes·trae
fe·nes·tral
fe·nes·tra coch·le·ae
fe·nes·tra oval·is
fe·nes·tra ro·tun·da
fen·es·trat·ed
fen·es·tra·tion
fe·nes·tra ves·ti·bu·li
fen·flur·amine
fen·ta·nyl
fenu·greek
    also foenu·greek
fer·ment
fer·ment·able
fer·men·ta·tion
fer·men·ta·tive

fer·men·ter
    or fer·men·tor
fer·mi·um
fer·ric
fer·ri·he·mo·glo·bin
fer·ri·tin
fer·rous
fer·tile
fer·til·i·ty
    pl fer·til·i·ties
fer·til·iza·tion
fer·til·ize
    fer·til·ized
    fer·til·iz·ing
fer·til·i·zin
fer·u·la
fes·cue foot
fes·ter
    fes·tered
    fes·ter·ing
fes·ti·nat·ing
fes·ti·na·tion
fe·tal
fe·ta·tion
fe·ti·ci·dal
fe·ti·cide
fet·id
fe·tish
    also fe·tich
fe·tish·ism
    also fe·tich·ism
fet·ish·ist
    also fet·ich·ist
fe·tish·is·tic
    also fe·tich·is·tic
fe·tish·is·ti·cal·ly

fet·lock
fe·tol·o·gist
fe·tol·o·gy
    pl fe·tol·o·gies
fe·tom·e·try
    pl fe·tom·e·tries
fe·to·pro·tein
fe·tor
    also foe·tor
fe·tor he·pat·i·cus
fe·to·scope
fe·tos·co·py
    pl fe·tos·co·pies
fe·tus
    pl fe·tus·es
Feul·gen
fe·ver
    fe·vered
    fe·ver·ing
fe·ver·ish
fi·ber
    or fi·bre
fi·ber of Mül·ler
fi·ber-op·tic
fi·ber op·tics
fi·ber·scope
fi·bril
fi·bril·la
    pl fi·bril·lae
fi·bril·lar
fi·bril·lary
fi·bril·late
    fi·bril·lat·ed
    fi·bril·lat·ing
fi·bril·la·tion
fi·bril·lo·gen·e·sis
    pl fi·bril·lo·gen·e·ses

fi·brin
fi·brin·ase
fi·brin·o·gen
fi·brin·o·gen·o·pe·
 nia
fi·bri·noid
fi·bri·no·ly·sin
fi·bri·no·ly·sis
 pl fi·bri·no·ly·ses
fi·bri·no·lyt·ic
fi·bri·no·pe·nia
fi·bri·no·pep·tide
fi·bri·no·pu·ru·lent
fi·bri·nous
fi·bro·ad·e·no·ma
 pl fi·bro·ad·e·no·mas
 or fi·bro·ad·e·no·ma·
 ta
fi·bro·are·o·lar
fi·bro·blast
fi·bro·blas·tic
fi·bro·car·ti·lage
fi·bro·car·ti·lag·i·
 nous
fi·bro·cys·tic
fi·bro·cyte
fi·bro·cyt·ic
fi·bro·elas·tic
fi·bro·elas·to·sis
 pl fi·bro·elas·to·ses
fi·bro·gen·e·sis
 pl fi·bro·gen·e·ses
fi·bro·gen·ic
fi·broid
fi·bro·ma
 pl fi·bro·mas
 also fi·bro·ma·ta

fi·bro·ma·to·gen·ic
fi·bro·ma·toid
fi·bro·ma·to·sis
 pl fi·bro·ma·to·ses
fi·bro·ma·tous
fi·bro·my·o·ma
 pl fi·bro·my·o·mas
 also fi·bro·my·o·ma·ta
fi·bro·my·o·ma·
 tous
fi·bro·my·o·si·tis
fi·bro·myx·o·ma
 pl fi·bro·myx·o·mas
 or fi·bro·myx·o·ma·ta
fi·bro·pla·sia
fi·bro·plas·tic
fi·bro·sar·co·ma
 pl fi·bro·sar·co·mas
 or fi·bro·sar·co·ma·ta
fi·brose
 fi·brosed
 fi·bros·ing
fi·bro·se·rous
fi·bro·sis
 pl fi·bro·ses
fi·bro·sit·ic
fi·bro·si·tis
fi·brot·ic
fi·brous
fib·u·la
 pl fib·u·lae
 or fib·u·las
fib·u·lar
fib·u·lo·cal·ca·ne·al
fi·cin
Fick prin·ci·ple

fièvre bou·ton·
 neuse
fig·ure
fig·ure-ground
fi·la
 pl of filum
fil·a·ment
fil·a·men·tous
fi·lar·ia
 pl fi·lar·i·ae
fi·lar·i·al
fil·a·ri·a·sis
 also fil·a·ri·o·sis
 pl fil·a·ri·a·ses
 also fil·a·ri·o·ses
fil·ar·i·at·ed
fi·lar·i·cid·al
fi·lar·i·cide
fi·lar·i·form
fi·lar·i·id
 or fi·lar·id
Fil·a·ri·idae
fi·lar·i·oid
Fi·lar·i·oi·dea
fil·ial
fi·lic·ic
fil·i·cin
fi·li·form
fil·i·pin
fil·let
fill·ing
fil·o·po·di·um
 also fil·o·pod
 pl fil·o·po·di·a
 also fil·o·pods

fil·ter
　　fil·tered
　　fil·ter·ing
fil·ter·abil·i·ty
　　pl fil·ter·abil·i·ties
fil·ter·able
　　also fil·tra·ble
fil·trate
　　fil·trat·ed
　　fil·trat·ing
fil·tra·tion
fi·lum
　　pl fi·la
fi·lum ter·mi·na·le
　　pl fi·la ter·mi·na·lia
fim·bria
　　pl fim·bri·ae
fim·bri·al
fim·bri·at·ed
　　also fim·bri·ate
first-de·gree burn
fish-liv·er
fish·skin dis·ease
fis·sion
　　fis·sioned
　　fis·sion·ing
fis·sion·al
fis·su·ra
　　pl fis·su·rae
fis·sur·al
fis·su·ra·tion
fis·sure
fis·sured
fis·sure of Ro·lan·
　　do
fis·sure of Syl·vi·us

fis·tu·la
　　pl fis·tu·las
　　or fis·tu·lae
fis·tu·lec·to·my
　　pl fis·tu·lec·to·mies
fis·tu·li·za·tion
fis·tu·lous
fix·ate
　　fix·at·ed
　　fix·at·ing
fix·a·tion
fix·a·tive
flac·cid
flac·cid·i·ty
　　pl flac·cid·i·ties
fla·gel·lant
fla·gel·lant·ism
fla·gel·lar
fla·gel·late
flag·el·lat·ed
flag·el·la·tion
fla·gel·li·form
fla·gel·lin
flag·el·lo·sis
　　pl flag·el·lo·ses
fla·gel·lum
　　pl fla·gel·la
　　also fla·gel·lums
flail
flare
　　flared
　　flar·ing
flare-up
flat·foot
　　pl flat·feet
flat-foot·ed
flat·u·lence

flat·u·lent
fla·tus
flat·worm
fla·va·none
fla·vin
fla·vine
fla·vone
fla·vo·pro·tein
fla·vor
　　fla·vored
　　fla·vor·ing
flax·seed
flea·bite
fleam
flea·seed
flea·wort
flec·tion
　　var of flexion
Fletch·er·ism
fletch·er·ize
　　fletch·er·ized
　　fletch·er·iz·ing
flews
flex·i·bil·i·ty
　　pl flex·i·bil·i·ties
flex·i·ble
flex·ion
　　also flec·tion
flex·or
flex·or car·pi ra·di·
　　al·is
flex·or car·pi ul·
　　nar·is
flex·or dig·i·ti min·
　　i·mi brev·is
flex·or dig·i·to·rum
　　brev·is

flex·or dig·i·to·rum lon·gus

flex·or dig·i·to·rum pro·fund·us

flex·or dig·i·to·rum su·per·fi·ci·al·is

flex·or hal·lu·cis brev·is

flex·or hal·lu·cis lon·gus

flex·or pol·li·cis brev·is

flex·or pol·li·cis lon·gus

flex·or ret·in·ac·u·lum

flex·u·ous

flex·ur·al

flex·ure

float·er

float·ing

floc·cil·la·tion

floc·cu·lar

floc·cu·late
  floc·cu·lat·ed
  floc·cu·lat·ing

floc·cu·la·tion

floc·cule

floc·cu·lent

floc·cu·lo·nod·u·lar

floc·cu·lus
  pl floc·cu·li

flo·ra
  pl flo·ras
  also flo·rae

flo·ral

Flor·ence flask

flor·id

floss

flow·er·ing dog·wood

flow·ers

flow·me·ter

flu

fluc·tu·ant

fluc·tu·ate
  fluc·tu·at·ed
  fluc·tu·at·ing

fluc·tu·a·tion

flu·cy·to·sine

flu·dro·cor·ti·sone

flu·id

flu·id·ex·tract

flu·id·glyc·er·ate

flu·id·i·ty
  pl flu·id·i·ties

flu·id·ounce

flu·idram
  or flu·idrachm

fluke

flu·o·cin·o·lone ac·e·to·nide

flu·o·resce
  flu·o·resced
  flu·o·resc·ing

flu·o·res·ce·in

flu·o·res·cence

flu·o·res·cent

flu·o·ri·date
  flu·o·ri·dat·ed
  flu·o·ri·dat·ing

flu·o·ri·da·tion

flu·o·ri·da·tion·ist

flu·o·ride

flu·o·ri·di·za·tion

flu·o·ri·dize
  flu·o·ri·dized
  flu·o·ri·diz·ing

flu·o·rine

flu·o·ro·chrome

flu·o·rom·e·ter
  or flu·o·rim·e·ter

flu·o·ro·met·ric
  or flu·o·ri·met·ric

flu·o·rom·e·try
  or flu·o·rim·e·try
  pl flu·o·rom·e·tries
  or flu·o·rim·e·tries

flu·o·ro·roent·gen·og·ra·phy
  pl flu·o·ro·roent·gen·og·ra·phies

flu·o·ro·scope
  flu·o·ro·scoped
  flu·o·ro·scop·ing

flu·o·ro·scop·ic

flu·o·ro·scop·i·cal·ly

flu·o·ros·co·pist

flu·o·ros·co·py
  pl flu·o·ros·co·pies

flu·o·ro·sis

flu·o·rot·ic

flu·o·ro·ura·cil

flu·phen·azine

flur·az·e·pam

flur·o·thyl

flut·ter

flux

fly·blow
  fly·blew
  fly·blown
fly-strike
  fly-struck
fo·cal
fo·cal·iza·tion
fo·cal·ize
  fo·cal·ized
  fo·cal·iz·ing
fo·cus
  pl fo·ci
  also fo·cus·es
fo·cus
  fo·cused
    also fo·cussed
  fo·cus·ing
    also fo·cus·sing
fo·cus·able
foenu·greek
  var of fenugreek
foe·tor
  var of fetor
fo·la·cin
fo·late
Fo·ley cath·e·ter
fo·li·ate
fo·lic
fo·lie
fo·lie à deux
  pl fo·lies à deux
fo·lie du doute
  pl fo·lies du doute
fo·lin·ic
fo·li·um
  pl fo·lia
fol·li·cle

fol·li·cle-stim·u·lat·
  ing hor·mone
fol·lic·u·lar
fol·lic·u·lin
fol·lic·u·li·tis
fol·lic·u·lus
  pl fol·lic·u·li
fol·low-up
  adjective or noun
follow up
  verb
fo·ment
fo·men·ta·tion
fomi·tes
fon·ta·nel
  or fon·ta·nelle
food·stuff
foot-and-mouth
  dis·ease
foot·can·dle
foot·plate
foot-pound
  pl foot-pounds
foot-pound-sec·
  ond
fo·ra·men
  pl fo·ram·i·na
  or fo·ra·mens
fo·ra·men ce·cum
fo·ra·men lac·er·
  um
fo·ra·men mag·
  num
fo·ra·men of
  Lusch·ka
fo·ra·men of Ma·
  gen·die

fo·ra·men of Mon·
  ro
fo·ra·men of Wins·
  low
fo·ra·men ova·le
fo·ra·men ro·tun·
  dum
fo·ra·men spin·o·
  sum
fo·ram·i·nal
for·ceps
  pl for·ceps
for·ci·pres·sure
For·dyce's dis·ease
  also For·dyce dis·ease
fore·arm
fore·brain
fore·fin·ger
fore·foot
  pl fore·feet
fore·gut
fore·head
for·eign
fore·leg
fore·limb
fore·milk
fo·ren·sic
fore·play
fore·plea·sure
fore·skin
fore·stom·ach
fore·wa·ters
form·al·de·hyde
for·ma·lin
for·mate
for·ma·tion
for·ma·tive

forme fruste
  pl formes frustes

for·mic

for·mi·ca·tion

for·mol·ized

for·mu·la
  pl for·mu·las
  or for·mu·lae

for·mu·lary
  pl for·mu·lar·ies

for·myl

for·ni·cate
  for·ni·cat·ed
  for·ni·cat·ing

for·ni·ca·tion

for·ni·ca·tor

for·ni·ca·trix
  pl for·ni·ca·tri·ces

for·nix
  pl for·ni·ces

fos·sa
  pl fos·sae

fos·sa na·vic·u·lar·is

fos·sa oval·is

Fos·sar·ia

fos·sate

fos·su·la
  pl fos·su·lae

fou·droy·ant

fo·vea
  pl fo·ve·ae

fo·vea cen·tra·lis

fo·ve·al

fo·ve·ate

fo·ve·a·tion

fo·ve·o·la
  pl fo·ve·o·lae
  or fo·ve·o·las

fo·ve·o·lar

fo·ve·o·late

Fow·ler's so·lu·tion

fox·glove

frac·tion

frac·tion·ate
  frac·tion·at·ed
  frac·tion·at·ing

frac·tion·a·tion

frac·ture
  frac·tured
  frac·tur·ing

frag·ile

fra·gil·i·tas os·si·um

fra·gil·i·ty
  pl fra·gil·i·ties

fraise

fram·be·sia

fran·ci·um

Frank·fort hor·i·zon·tal plane

fra·ter·nal

freck·le
  freck·led
  freck·ling

free-as·so·ci·ate
  free-as·so·ci·at·ed
  free-as·so·ci·at·ing

free·base
  free·based
  free·bas·ing

free-float·ing

free-liv·ing

free·mar·tin

freeze
  froze
  fro·zen
  freez·ing

freeze-dry
  freeze-dried
  freeze-dry·ing

freeze-etch

freeze-etched

freeze-etch·ing

freeze frac·ture
  also freeze-frac·tur·ing
  noun

freeze-frac·ture
  verb
  freeze-frac·tured
  freeze-frac·tur·ing

Frei test

frem·i·tus

fre·nal

fren·ec·to·my
  pl fren·ec·to·mies

fren·u·lum
  pl fren·u·la

fre·num
  pl fre·nums
  or fre·na

fren·zied

fren·zy
  pl fren·zies

fre·quen·cy
  pl fre·quen·cies

Freud·ian
Freud·ian·ism
Freund's ad·ju·
vant
FR flocculation
reaction
fri·a·bil·i·ty
pl fri·a·bil·i·ties

fri·a·ble
fri·ar's bal·sam
Fried·länd·er's ba·
cil·lus
also Fried·länd·er ba·
cil·lus

Fried·man test
also Fried·man's test

Fried·reich's atax·
ia
frig·id
fri·gid·i·ty
pl fri·gid·i·ties

Fröh·lich's syn·
drome
or Froeh·lich's syn·
drome
also Fröh·lich syn·
drome

frons
pl fron·tes

front·ad
fron·tal
fron·ta·lis
fron·to·oc·cip·i·tal
fron·to·pa·ri·etal
fron·to·tem·po·ral

frost·bite
frost·bit
frost·bit·en
frost·bit·ing
frot·tage
frot·teur
fruc·to·kin·ase
fruc·to·san
fruc·tose
fruc·tose-1,6-di·
phos·phate
fruc·tose-6-phos·
phate
fruc·to·side
fruc·tos·uria
fruit·ing body
fru·se·mide
frus·trate
frus·trat·ed
frus·trat·ing
frus·tra·tion
fuch·sin
or fuch·sine

fuch·sin·o·phil
also fuch·sin·o·phile
or fuch·si·no·phil·ic

fu·cose
fu·co·si·dase
fu·co·si·do·sis
pl fu·co·si·do·ses

fu·cus
fu·gu
fugue
ful·gu·rate
ful·gu·rat·ed
ful·gu·rat·ing
ful·gu·ra·tion

ful·mi·nant
ful·mi·nat·ing
ful·mi·na·tion
fu·ma·gil·lin
fu·ma·rase
fu·ma·rate
fu·mar·ic
fu·mi·gant
fu·mi·gate
fu·mi·gat·ed
fu·mi·gat·ing
fu·mi·ga·tion
fu·mi·ga·tor
func·tion
func·tioned
func·tion·ing
func·tion·al
fun·da·ment
fun·dec·to·my
pl fun·dec·to·mies

fun·dic
fun·dus
pl fun·di

fun·du·scop·ic
also fun·do·scop·ic

fun·dus·co·py
also fun·dos·co·py
pl fun·dus·co·pies
also fun·dos·co·
pies

fun·gal
fun·gate
fun·gat·ed
fun·gat·ing
fun·ga·tion
fun·ge·mia

fun·gi
pl of fungus

Fun·gi
*division or other group
of lower plants*

fun·gi·cid·al

fun·gi·cide

fun·gi·ci·din

fun·gi·form

Fun·gi Im·per·fec·ti

fun·gi·sta·sis
pl fun·gi·sta·ses

fun·gi·stat

fun·gi·stat·ic

fun·gi·stat·i·cal·ly

fun·gi·tox·ic

fun·gi·tox·ic·i·ty
pl fun·gi·tox·ic·i·ties

fun·goid

fun·gous

fun·gus
pl fun·gi
also fun·gus·es

fu·nic

fu·nic·u·lar

fu·nic·u·li·tis

fu·nic·u·lus
pl fu·nic·u·li

fu·nis

fun·ny bone

fu·ra·nose

fu·ra·zol·i·done

fur·co·cer·cous

fur·cu·la

fur·fur

fur·fu·ra·ceous

fur·fu·ral

fu·ro·se·mide

furred

fur·row

fur·se·mide

fu·run·cle
boil (see carbuncle,
caruncle)

fu·run·cu·lar

fu·run·cu·loid

fu·run·cu·lo·sis
pl fu·run·cu·lo·ses

fu·run·cu·lous

fu·run·cu·lus
pl fu·run·cu·li

fu·sar·i·um
pl fu·sar·ia

fu·si·form

fu·sion

fu·sion·al

fu·so·bac·te·ri·um
pl fu·so·bac·te·ria

fu·so·cel·lu·lar

fu·so·spi·ro·chet·al

fu·so·spi·ro·chet·o·sis
pl fu·so·spi·ro·chet·o·ses

G

G-ac·tin

gad·fly
pl gad·flies

gad·o·lin·i·um

Ga·dus

gage
var of gauge

ga·lac·ta·gogue
or ga·lac·to·gogue

ga·lac·tan

ga·lac·tin

ga·lac·to·cele

ga·lac·to·ki·nase

ga·lac·to·lip·id

ga·lac·to·phore

gal·ac·toph·o·rous

ga·lac·to·poi·e·sis
pl ga·lac·to·poi·e·ses

ga·lac·to·poi·et·ic

ga·lac·tor·rhea

ga·lac·tos·amine

ga·lac·tose

ga·lac·tos·emia

ga·lac·tos·emic

ga·lac·to·si·dase

ga·lac·to·side

gal·ac·to·sis
pl gal·ac·to·ses

ga·lac·tos·uria

ga·lact·uron·ic

Gal·ba

ga·lea

ga·len·ic
also ga·len·i·cal
adjective

ga·len·i·cal
noun

Ga·len's vein

gal·la

gal·la·mine tri·eth·io·dide

gall·blad·der

gal·lic
gal·li·um
gal·lon
gal·lop·ing
gall·stone
gal·van·ic
gal·van·i·cal·ly
gal·va·nism
gal·va·ni·za·tion
gal·va·nize
  gal·va·nized
  gal·va·niz·ing
gal·va·nom·e·ter
gal·va·no·met·ric
gal·va·no·scope
gal·va·no·tax·is
  pl gal·va·no·tax·es
gal·va·no·ther·a·py
  pl gal·va·no·ther·a·pies
gal·va·no·tro·pic
gal·va·not·ro·pism
gal·ziek·te
gam·boge
gam·etan·gi·um
  pl gam·etan·gia
ga·mete
ga·met·ic
ga·met·i·cal·ly
ga·me·to·cide
ga·me·to·cyte
ga·me·to·gen·e·sis
  pl ga·me·to·gen·e·ses
gam·etog·e·nous
gam·etog·e·ny
  pl gam·etog·enies

gam·etog·o·ny
  pl gam·etog·o·nies
gam·ic
gam·ma
gam·ma-ami·no·bu·tyr·ic ac·id
  also γ-ami·no·bu·tyr·ic ac·id
gam·ma glob·u·lin
gam·mop·a·thy
  pl gam·mop·a·thies
gamo·gen·e·sis
  pl gamo·gen·e·ses
gamo·ge·net·ic
gamo·ge·net·i·cal·ly
gam·ont
gan·gli·al
gan·gli·at·ed
gan·gli·form
gan·gli·o·blast
gan·gli·o·cyte
gan·gli·o·ma
  pl gan·gli·o·mas
  or gan·gli·o·ma·ta
gan·gli·on
  pl gan·glia
  also gan·gli·ons
gan·gli·on·at·ed
gan·gli·on·ec·to·my
  pl gan·gli·on·ec·to·mies
gan·glio·neu·ro·ma
  pl gan·glio·neu·ro·mas
  or gan·glio·neu·ro·ma·ta
gan·gli·on·ic

gan·gli·on·it·is
gan·gli·o·side
gan·gli·o·si·do·sis
  pl gan·gli·o·si·do·ses
gan·go·sa
gan·grene
  gan·grened
  gan·gren·ing
gan·gre·nous
Gan·ser syn·drome
  or Gan·ser's syn·drome
gar·den he·lio·trope
gar·get
gar·gety
gar·gle
  gar·gled
  gar·gling
gar·goyl·ism
Gärt·ner's ba·cil·lus
Gart·ner's duct
gas·eous
gas·kin
gas-liq·uid
gas·se·ri·an
gas·ter·oph·i·lo·sis
  pl gas·ter·oph·i·lo·ses
Gas·ter·oph·i·lus
gas·tral
gas·tral·gia
gas·tral·gic
gas·trec·to·my
  pl gas·trec·to·mies
gas·tric
gas·trin

gas·tri·no·ma
pl gas·tri·no·mas
or gas·tri·no·ma·ta

gas·tri·tis

gas·tro·anas·to·mo·sis
pl gas·tro·anas·to·mo·ses

gas·troc·ne·mi·al

gas·troc·ne·mi·us
pl gas·troc·ne·mii

gas·tro·coel
also gas·tro·coele

gas·tro·co·lic
Gas·tro·dis·coi·des
gas·tro·du·o·de·nal
gas·tro·du·o·de·ni·tis

gas·tro·du·o·de·nos·to·my
pl gas·tro·du·o·de·nos·to·mies

gas·tro·en·ter·ic
gas·tro·en·ter·i·tis
pl gas·tro·en·ter·it·i·des

gas·tro·en·ter·o·log·i·cal
or gas·tro·en·ter·o·log·ic

gas·tro·en·ter·ol·o·gist

gas·tro·en·ter·ol·o·gy
pl gas·tro·en·ter·ol·o·gies

gas·tro·en·ter·op·a·thy
pl gas·tro·en·ter·op·a·thies

gas·tro·en·ter·os·to·my
pl gas·tro·en·ter·os·to·mies

gas·tro·ep·i·plo·ic
gas·tro·esoph·a·ge·al
gas·tro·gen·ic
or gas·trog·e·nous
gas·tro·in·tes·ti·nal
gas·tro·je·ju·nal
gas·tro·je·ju·nos·to·my
pl gas·tro·je·ju·nos·to·mies

gas·tro·lith
gas·trol·o·gist
gas·trol·o·gy
pl gas·trol·o·gies

gas·trol·y·sis
pl gas·trol·y·ses

gas·tro·ma·la·cia
gas·trop·a·thy
pl gas·trop·a·thies

gas·tro·pexy
pl gas·tro·pex·ies

gas·tro·phren·ic
gas·tro·pli·ca·tion
gas·tro·pod
Gas·tro·poda
gas·trop·to·sis
pl gas·trop·to·ses

gas·tros·chi·sis
pl gas·tros·chi·ses

gas·tro·scope
gas·tro·scop·ic
gas·tros·co·pist
gas·tros·co·py
pl gas·tros·co·pies

gas·tro·splen·ic
gas·tros·to·my
pl gas·tros·to·mies

gas·trot·o·my
pl gas·trot·o·mies

gas·tru·la
pl gas·tru·las
or gas·tru·lae

gas·tru·lar
gas·tru·late
gas·tru·lat·ed
gas·tru·lat·ing
gas·tru·la·tion
Gatch bed
Gau·cher's dis·ease
gauge
also gage
gauged
also gaged
gaug·ing
also gag·ing
gaul·the·ria
gaul·the·rin
gauss
pl gauss
also gauss·es
gauze
ga·vage
geel·dik·kop
Gei·ger count·er

Gei·ger-Mül·ler
  count·er
gel
  gelled
  gel·ling
gel·able
gel·ate
  gel·at·ed
  gel·at·ing
gel·a·tin
  also gel·a·tine
ge·la·ti·ni·za·tion
ge·la·ti·nize
  ge·la·ti·nized
  ge·la·ti·niz·ing
ge·lat·i·nous
gel·ation
geld
gel·ose
ge·mel·lus
  pl ge·mel·li
  also ge·mel·lus·es
gem·i·nate
gem·i·na·tion
gem·ma
  pl gem·mae
gem·ma·tion
gem·mule
ge·na
  pl ge·nae
ge·nal
gen·der
gene
gen·era
  pl of genus
gen·er·al
gen·er·al·iza·tion

gen·er·al·ize
gen·er·al·ized
gen·er·al·iz·ing
gen·er·al·ized
gen·er·ate
  gen·er·at·ed
  gen·er·at·ing
gen·er·a·tion
gen·er·a·tion·al
gen·er·a·tive
ge·ner·ic
ge·ner·i·cal·ly
gen·e·sis
  pl gen·e·ses
gene-splic·ing
ge·net·ic
  also ge·net·i·cal
ge·net·i·cist
ge·net·ics
ge·neto·troph·ic
ge·ni·al
gen·ic
gen·i·cal·ly
ge·nic·u·lar
ge·nic·u·late
ge·nic·u·lo·cal·ca·
  rine
ge·nic·u·lum
  pl ge·nic·u·la
ge·nio·glos·sal
ge·nio·glos·sus
  pl ge·nio·glos·si
ge·nio·hyo·glos·sus
  pl ge·nio·hyo·glos·si
ge·nio·hy·oid
ge·nio·hy·oid·eus
  pl ge·nio·hy·oid·ei

ge·nio·plas·ty
  pl ge·nio·plas·ties
gen·i·tal
gen·i·ta·lia
gen·i·ta·lic
gen·i·tal·i·ty
  pl gen·i·tal·i·ties
gen·i·tal·ly
gen·i·tals
gen·i·to·cru·ral
gen·i·to·fem·o·ral
gen·i·to·uri·nary
ge·nius
  pl ge·nius·es
  or ge·nii
ge·no·der·ma·to·sis
  pl ge·no·der·ma·to·
  ses
ge·nome
  also ge·nom
ge·no·mic
ge·no·type
ge·no·typ·ic
ge·no·typ·i·cal
gen·ta·mi·cin
gen·tian
gen·ti·o·bi·ose
gen·tis·ic
ge·nu
  pl gen·ua
ge·nus
  pl gen·era
ge·nu val·gum
ge·nu va·rum
geo·med·i·cal
geo·med·i·cine

geo·pa·thol·o·gy
  pl geo·pa·thol·o·gies

ge·o·pha·gia

ge·oph·a·gism

ge·oph·a·gy
  pl ge·oph·a·gies

geo·tac·tic

geo·tax·is
  pl geo·tax·es

ge·ot·ri·cho·sis
  Ge·ot·ri·chum

geo·tro·pic

geo·tro·pi·cal·ly

ge·ot·ro·pism

ge·ra·ni·ol

ge·rat·ic

ger·a·tol·o·gy
  pl ger·a·tol·o·gies

ger·i·at·ric

ger·i·a·tri·cian

ger·i·a·trist

ger·i·o·psy·cho·sis
  pl ger·i·o·psy·cho·ses

ger·ma·nin

ger·ma·ni·um

germ·free

ger·mi·cid·al

ger·mi·cide

ger·mi·nal

ger·mi·nate
  ger·mi·nat·ed
  ger·mi·nat·ing

ger·mi·na·tion

germ·proof

germy
  germ·i·er
  germ·i·est

ger·o·der·ma

ge·ron·tic
  also ge·ron·tal

ge·ron·to·log·i·cal
  or ge·ron·to·log·ic

ger·on·tol·o·gist

ger·on·tol·o·gy
  pl ger·on·tol·o·gies

ge·ron·to·phil·ia

ge·ron·to·pho·bia

ge·ron·to·ther·a·py
  pl ge·ron·to·ther·a·pies

Gerst·mann's syn·drome

ge·stalt
  pl ge·stalt·en
  or ge·stalts

ge·stalt·ist

ges·tate
  ges·tat·ed
  ges·tat·ing

ges·ta·tion

ges·ta·tion·al

ges·to·sis
  pl ges·to·ses

gi·ant·ism

giar·dia

giar·di·a·sis
  pl giar·di·a·ses

gib·bos·i·ty
  pl gib·bos·i·ties

gib·bous
  adjective
    humpbacked (see gibbus)

gib·bus
  noun
    spinal deformity
    (*see* gibbous)

gid

Gi·em·sa stain
  also Gi·em·sa's stain

gi·gan·tism

gi·gan·to·blast

Gi·la mon·ster

Gil·bert's dis·ease

Gil·christ's dis·ease

gill

gilled

Gilles de la Tou·rette syn·drome
  also Gilles de la Tou·rette's syn·drome

Gim·ber·nat's lig·a·ment

gin·ger

gin·gi·va
  pl gin·gi·vae

gin·gi·val

gin·gi·vec·to·my
  pl gin·gi·vec·to·mies

gin·gi·vi·tis

gin·gi·vo·plas·ty
  pl gin·gi·vo·plas·ties

gin·gi·vo·sto·ma·ti·tis
  pl gin·gi·vo·sto·ma·tit·i·des
  or gin·gi·vo·sto·ma·ti·tis·es

gin·gly·moid

gin·gly·mus
pl gin·gly·mi

gin·seng

gir·dle

gi·tal·in

gi·tox·in

git·ter cell

giz·zard

gla·bel·la
pl gla·bel·lae

gla·bel·lar

gla·brous

gla·cial

glad·i·o·lus
pl glad·i·o·li

glairy
glair·i·er
glair·i·est

glan·dered

glan·der·ous

glan·ders

gland of Bow·man

glan·du·la
pl glan·du·lae

glan·du·lar

glan·du·lous

glans
pl glan·des

glans cli·tor·i·dis

Gla·se·ri·an· fis·sure

Glas·ser's dis·ease

glass·es

Glau·ber's salt
also Glau·ber salt

glau·co·ma

glau·coma·tous

gleet

gleety
gleet·i·er
gleet·i·est

gle·no·hu·mer·al

glen·oid

glia

gli·a·din

gli·al

glid·ing joint

glio·blas·to·ma
pl glio·blas·to·mas
or glio·blas·to·ma·ta

glio·blas·to·ma
mul·ti·for·me

gli·o·ma
pl gli·o·mas
or gli·o·ma·ta

gli·o·ma·to·sis
pl gli·o·ma·to·ses

gli·o·ma·tous

gli·o·sis
pl gli·o·ses

gli·ot·ic

glio·tox·in

Glis·son's cap·sule

glob·al

Glo·bid·i·um

glo·bin

glo·bose

glo·bo·side

glob·u·lar

glob·ule

glob·u·lin

glob·u·lin·uria

glo·bus hys·ter·i·cus

glo·bus pal·li·dus

glo·mal

glom·an·gi·o·ma
pl glom·an·gi·o·mas
or glom·an·gi·o·ma·ta

glo·mec·to·my
pl glo·mec·to·mies

glo·mer·u·lar

glo·mer·u·li·tis

glo·mer·u·lo·ne·phri·tis
pl glo·mer·u·lo·ne·phrit·i·des

glo·mer·u·lo·sa
pl glo·mer·u·lo·sae

glo·mer·u·lo·sal

glo·mer·u·lo·scle·ro·sis
pl glo·mer·u·lo·scle·ro·ses

glo·mer·u·lus
pl glo·mer·u·li

glo·mus
pl glom·era
also glo·mi

glo·mus ca·rot·i·cum

glo·mus coc·cy·ge·um

glo·mus jug·u·la·re

glos·sal

glos·sal·gia

glos·si·na

glos·si·tis

gloss·odyn·ia

glos·so·kin·es·thet·ic

glos·so·la·lia
glos·so·pal·a·tine
glos·so·pal·a·ti·nus
pl glos·so·pal·a·ti·ni
glos·sop·a·thy
pl glos·sop·a·thies
glos·so·pha·ryn·geal
glot·tal
also glot·tic
glot·tis
pl glot·tis·es
or glot·ti·des
glu·ca·gon
glu·can
glu·ca·nase
glu·cide
glu·co·ce·re·bro·si·dase
glu·co·ce·re·bro·side
glu·co·cor·ti·coid
glu·co·gen·e·sis
pl glu·co·gen·e·ses
glu·co·gen·ic
glu·co·ki·nase
glu·co·lip·id
glu·co·neo·gen·e·sis
pl glu·co·neo·gen·e·ses
glu·co·neo·gen·ic
glu·co·pro·tein
glu·cos·amine
glu·cose
glu·cose-1-phos·phate

glu·cose-6-phos·phate
glu·co·si·dase
glu·co·side
glu·co·sid·ic
glu·co·sid·i·cal·ly
glu·cos·uria
glu·co·syl·trans·fer·ase
gluc·uro·nate
gluc·uron·ic
gluc·uron·i·dase
gluc·uro·nide
glu·ta·mate
glu·tam·ic
glu·ta·min·ase
glu·ta·mine
glu·tar·al·de·hyde
glu·ta·thi·one
glu·te·al
glu·ten
glu·te·nin
glu·ten·ous
glu·teth·i·mide
glu·te·us
pl glu·tei
glu·te·us max·i·mus
pl glu·tei max·i·mi
glu·te·us me·di·us
pl glu·tei me·dii
glu·te·us min·i·mus
pl glu·tei min·i·mi
glu·ti·nous
gly·can
gly·ce·mia

gly·ce·mic
glyc·er·al·de·hyde
gly·cer·ic
glyc·er·ide
glyc·er·id·ic
glyc·er·in
or glyc·er·ine
glyc·er·in·ate
glyc·er·in·at·ed
glyc·er·in·at·ing
glyc·er·in·ation
glyc·er·ite
glyc·er·ol
glyc·ero·phos·phate
glyc·ero·phos·phor·ic
glyc·er·yl
gly·cine
gly·cin·uria
gly·co·chol·ate
gly·co·chol·ic
gly·co·coll
gly·co·gen
gly·cog·e·nase
gly·co·gen·e·sis
pl gly·co·gen·e·ses
gly·co·ge·net·ic
gly·co·gen·ic
gly·co·gen·ol·y·sis
pl gly·co·gen·ol·y·ses
gly·co·gen·o·lyt·ic
gly·co·ge·no·sis
pl gly·co·ge·no·ses
gly·col
gly·col·al·de·hyde

gly·co·late
also gly·col·late

gly·col·ic
also gly·col·lic

gly·co·lip·id

gly·col·y·sis
pl gly·col·y·ses

gly·co·lyt·ic

gly·co·lyt·i·cal·ly

gly·co·neo·gen·e·
sis
pl gly·co·neo·gen·e·
ses

gly·co·pep·tide

gly·co·pro·tein

gly·co·pyr·ro·late

gly·cos·ami·no·gly·
can

gly·co·si·dase

gly·co·side

gly·co·sid·ic

gly·co·sid·i·cal·ly

gly·co·sphin·go·lip·
id

gly·cos·uria

gly·cos·uric

gly·co·trop·ic

glycu·re·sis
pl glycu·re·ses

gly·cyl

glyc·yr·rhi·za

glyc·yr·rhi·zic

glyc·yr·rhi·zin

gly·ox·al

gly·ox·a·lase

gly·ox·a·line

gly·ox·yl·ic

gnat

gnath·ic
or gna·thal

gna·thi·on

gna·thob·del·lid

Gna·thob·del·li·da

Gna·thos·to·ma

gna·thos·to·mi·a·
sis
pl gna·thos·to·mi·a·
ses

gno·to·bi·ol·o·gy
pl gno·to·bi·ol·o·gies

gno·to·bi·ote

gno·to·bi·ot·ics

Goa pow·der

goi·ter

goi·tro·gen

goi·tro·gen·e·sis
pl goi·tro·gen·e·ses

goi·tro·gen·ic
also goi·ter·o·gen·ic

goi·tro·ge·nic·i·ty
pl goi·tro·ge·nic·i·ties

goi·trous
also goi·ter·ous

gol·den·seal

Gol·gi

Gol·gi body

go·nad

go·nad·al

go·nad·ec·to·mized

go·nad·ec·to·my
pl go·nad·ec·to·mies

go·nad·o·troph

go·nad·o·trop·ic
or go·nad·o·tro·phic

go·nad·o·tro·pin
or go·nad·o·tro·phin

go·ni·al

go·ni·om·e·ter

go·nio·met·ric

go·ni·on
pl go·nia

go·nio·punc·ture

go·ni·o·scope

go·ni·o·scop·ic

go·ni·os·co·py
pl go·ni·os·co·pies

go·ni·ot·o·my
pl go·ni·ot·o·mies

go·ni·tis

gono·coc·cal
or gono·coc·cic

gono·coc·ce·mia

gono·coc·ce·mic

gono·coc·cus
pl gono·coc·ci

gono·cyte

gon·o·duct

gono·gen·e·sis
pl gono·gen·e·ses

gon·or·rhea

gon·or·rhe·al

go·ny·au·lax

Gooch cru·ci·ble

goose·flesh

goun·dou

gout

gout·i·ness

gouty

Gow·ers's tract

graaf·ian fol·li·cle

grac·ile

grac·i·lis
gra·di·ent
grad·u·ate
  grad·u·at·ed
  grad·u·at·ing
graft-ver·sus-host
Gra·ham's law
gram-atom·ic
  weight
gram·i·ci·din
gram-neg·a·tive
gram-pos·i·tive
Gram's so·lu·tion
Gram's stain
  or Gram stain
gram-vari·able
gra·na
  pl of granum
gra·na·tum
gran·di·ose
gran·di·os·i·ty
  pl gran·di·os·i·ties
gran·u·lar
gran·u·lar·i·ty
  pl gran·u·lar·i·ties
gran·u·late
  gran·u·lat·ed
  gran·u·lat·ing
gran·u·la·tion
gran·ule
gran·u·lo·blast
gran·u·lo·blas·tic
gran·u·lo·blas·to·sis
  pl gran·u·lo·blas·to·ses
gran·u·lo·cyte

gran·u·lo·cyt·ic
gran·u·lo·cy·to·pe·nia
gran·u·lo·cy·to·pe·nic
gran·u·lo·cy·to·poi·e·sis
  pl gran·u·lo·cy·to·poi·e·ses
gran·u·lo·cy·to·sis
  pl gran·u·lo·cy·to·ses
gran·u·lo·ma
  pl gran·u·lo·mas
  or gran·u·lo·ma·ta
gran·u·lo·ma in·gui·na·le
gran·u·lo·ma py·o·gen·i·cum
gran·u·lo·ma·to·sis
  pl gran·u·lo·ma·to·ses
gran·u·lo·ma·tous
gran·u·lo·ma ve·ne·re·um
gran·u·lo·pe·nia
gran·u·lo·poi·e·sis
  pl gran·u·lo·poi·e·ses
gran·u·lo·poi·et·ic
gran·u·lo·sa cell
gra·num
  pl gra·na
graph·ic
gra·phit·ic
graph·o·log·i·cal
gra·phol·o·gist
gra·phol·o·gy
  pl gra·phol·o·gies
grapho·ma·nia

grapho·ma·ni·ac
grapho·mo·tor
graph·or·rhea
grapho·spasm
grat·tage
grav·el
grav·el-blind
Graves' dis·ease
grav·id
grav·i·da
  pl grav·i·das
  or grav·i·dae
gra·vid·ic
gra·vid·i·ty
  pl gra·vid·i·ties
gra·vi·me·ter
gravi·met·ric
gra·vim·e·try
  pl gra·vim·e·tries
gravis
grav·i·ta·tion
grav·i·ta·tion·al
grav·i·ty
  pl grav·i·ties
gray
gray·out
  noun
gray out
  verb
green-blind
green blind·ness
green·sick
green·sick·ness
green·stick
Greg·o·ry's pow·der
grin·de·lia

gripe
  griped
  grip·ing
gripp·al
grippe
grippy
gris·eo·ful·vin
gris·tle
gro·cer's itch
groin
groove
grunt·ing
gry·po·sis
  pl gry·po·ses

guai·ac
guai·a·col
guai·a·cum
gua·nase
gua·neth·i·dine
gua·ni·dine
gua·nine
gua·no·sine
gua·no·sine 3′, 5′-
  mono·phos·
  phate
gua·nyl·ate cy·
  clase
gua·nyl·ic
Guar·nie·ri body
  also Guar·nie·ri's
  body
gu·ber·nac·u·lum
  pl gu·ber·nac·u·la

Guil·lain-Bar·ré
  syn·drome
guil·lo·tine
guin·ea·pig

gul·let
gum·boil
gum·line
gum·ma
  pl gum·mas
  also gum·ma·ta

gum·ma·tous
gur·ney
  pl gur·neys

gus·ta·tion
gus·ta·to·ri·ly
gus·ta·to·ry
Guth·rie test
gut·ta-per·cha
gut·tate
gut·ter
gut·tur·al
Gut·zeit test
gym·nas·tic
gym·nas·tics
Gym·no·din·i·um
gym·no·sperm
gym·no·sper·mous
gyn·an·dro·blas·to·
  ma
  pl gyn·an·dro·blas·to·
  mas
  or gyn·an·dro·blas·to·
  ma·ta

gy·nan·droid
gyn·an·dro·morph
gyn·an·dro·mor·
  phic
gyn·an·dro·mor·
  phism

gyn·an·dro·mor·
  phy
  pl gyn·an·dro·mor·
  phies

gyn·an·dry
  pl gyn·an·dries

gy·ne·cic
gy·ne·co·gen·ic
gy·ne·cog·ra·phy
  pl gy·ne·cog·ra·phies

gy·ne·coid
gy·ne·co·log·ic
  or gy·ne·co·log·i·cal

gy·ne·col·o·gist
gy·ne·col·o·gy
  pl gy·ne·col·o·gies

gy·ne·co·mas·tia
gy·no·gen·e·sis
  pl gy·no·gen·e·ses

gy·no·ge·net·ic
gyp·sum
gy·rase
gy·rate
gy·ra·tion
gy·rec·to·my
  pl gy·rec·to·mies

gy·rose
gy·rus
  pl gy·ri

H

ha·ben·u·la
  pl ha·ben·u·lae

ha·ben·u·lar
hab·it
hab·i·tat

hab·it-form·ing
ha·bit·u·al
ha·bit·u·ate
　ha·bit·u·at·ed
　ha·bit·u·at·ing
ha·bit·u·a·tion
hab·i·tus
　pl hab·i·tus

Hab·ro·ne·ma
hab·ro·ne·mi·a·sis
　pl hab·ro·ne·mi·a·ses
hab·ro·ne·mo·sis
　pl hab·ro·ne·mo·ses
hack
Hae·ma·dip·sa
Hae·ma·phy·sa·lis
Hae·ma·to·pi·nus
hae·ma·tox·y·lon
hae·mo·bar·ton·el·
　la
　pl hae·mo·bar·ton·el·
　　lae
hae·mo·bar·ton·el·
　lo·sis
　also he·mo·bar·ton·el·
　　lo·sis
　pl hae·mo·bar·ton·el·
　　lo·ses
　also he·mo·bar·ton·el·
　　lo·ses
hae·mo·glo·bin
　var of hemoglobin
Hae·mo·greg·a·ri·na
hae·mo·greg·a·rine
hae·mon·cho·sis
　pl hae·mon·cho·ses
Hae·mon·chus

hae·moph·i·lus
　pl hae·moph·i·li
Hae·mo·pro·te·i·
　dae
Hae·mo·pro·te·us
Hae·mo·spo·rid·ia
hae·mo·spo·rid·i·
　an
haf·ni·um
Hag·e·man fac·tor
Hai·ding·er's
　brush·es
hair·i·ness
hair·worm
hairy
　hair·i·er
　hair·i·est
hal·a·zone
half-blood
　or half-blood·ed
half-bred
half-breed
half-life
half-moon
half-val·ue lay·er
ha·lide
hal·i·ste·re·sis
　pl hal·i·ste·re·ses
hal·i·ste·ret·ic
hal·i·to·sis
　pl hal·i·to·ses
hal·lu·ci·nate
　hal·lu·ci·nat·ed
　hal·lu·ci·nat·ing
hal·lu·ci·na·tion
hal·lu·ci·na·tor
hal·lu·ci·na·to·ri·ly

hal·lu·ci·na·to·ry
hal·lu·ci·no·gen
hal·lu·ci·no·gen·ic
hal·lu·ci·no·gen·i·
　cal·ly
hal·lu·ci·no·sis
　pl hal·lu·ci·no·ses
hal·lux
　pl hal·lu·ces
hal·lux rig·id·us
hal·lux val·gus
ha·lo
　pl ha·los
　or ha·loes
halo·gen
ha·lo·ge·nate
　ha·lo·ge·nat·ed
　ha·lo·ge·nat·ing
ha·lo·ge·na·tion
ha·log·e·nous
hal·o·ge·ton
ha·lom·e·ter
halo·per·i·dol
halo·thane
hal·zoun
ham·a·me·lis
ha·mar·tia
ham·ar·to·ma
　pl ham·ar·to·mas
　or ham·ar·to·ma·ta
ham·ar·toma·tous
ha·mate
ha·ma·tum
　pl ha·ma·ta
　or ha·ma·tums
ham·mer·toe

ham·string
  ham·strung
  ham·string·ing
ham·u·lar
ham·u·lus
  pl ham·u·li
hand·i·cap
hand·i·capped
hand·piece
Hand-Schül·ler-
  Chris·tian dis·
  ease
hang·nail
hang·over
han·sen·osis
  pl han·sen·oses
Han·sen's ba·cil·
  lus
  pl Han·sen's ba·cil·li
Han·sen's dis·ease
H an·ti·gen
hap·a·lo·nych·ia
haph·al·ge·sia
haph·e·pho·bia
hap·lo·dont
hap·lo·don·ty
  pl hap·lo·don·ties
hap·loid
hap·loi·dy
  pl hap·loi·dies
hap·lont
hap·lon·tic
hap·lo·scope
hap·lo·scop·ic
hap·lo·type
hap·ten
hap·ten·at·ed

hap·ten·ic
hap·tic
  or hap·ti·cal
hap·to·glo·bin
hap·to·phore
hard·en·ing
har·de·ri·an gland
Har·der's gland
hard-of-hear·ing
Har·dy-Wein·berg
  law
hare·lip
hare·lipped
har·ma·la
  also har·mal
har·ma·line
har·ma·lol
har·mine
har·poon
Hart·nup dis·ease
harts·horn
Har·vei·an
hash
Ha·shi·mo·to's dis·
  ease
hash·ish
Has·sall's cor·pus·
  cle
haus·to·ri·al
haus·to·ri·um
  pl haus·to·ria
haus·tral
haus·tra·tion
haus·trum
  pl haus·tra
ha·ver·sian
haw

head·ache
head·achy
head·shrink·er
health·i·ly
health·i·ness
healthy
  health·i·er
  health·i·est
hear
  heard
  hear·ing
heart·beat
heart·burn
heart-lung ma·
  chine
heart·wa·ter
heart·worm
heat·stroke
heave
  heaved
  heav·ing
he·be·phre·nia
he·be·phre·nic
Heb·er·den's node
heb·e·tude
hec·tic
hec·to·gram
hec·to·li·ter
hec·to·me·ter
he·don·ic
he·don·i·cal·ly
he·do·nism
he·do·nist
he·do·nis·tic
he·do·nis·ti·cal·ly
Heer·fordt's syn·
  drome

Heim·lich ma·neu·ver

Heinz body

hela cell

he·li·cal

hel·i·cine

hel·i·coid
or he·li·coi·dal

hel·i·co·trema

he·lio·phobe

he·lio·tax·is
pl he·lio·tax·es

he·lio·ther·a·py
pl he·lio·ther·a·pies

he·lio·tro·pic

he·li·ot·ro·pism

he·li·um

he·lix
pl he·li·ces
also he·lix·es

hel·le·bore

hel·minth
pl hel·minths

hel·min·thi·a·sis
pl hel·min·thi·a·ses

hel·min·thic

hel·min·thol·o·gy
pl hel·min·thol·o·gies

Helo·der·ma

help·er T cell

he·ma·cy·tom·e·ter

hem·ad·sorb·ing

hem·ad·sorp·tion

he·ma·dy·na·mom·e·ter

hem·ag·glu·ti·nate

hem·ag·glu·ti·nat·ed

hem·ag·glu·ti·nat·ing

hem·ag·glu·ti·na·tion

hem·ag·glu·ti·nin
also he·mo·ag·glu·ti·nin

he·mal

he·man·gi·ec·ta·sis
pl he·man·gi·ec·ta·ses

he·man·gio·en·do·the·li·o·ma
pl he·man·gio·en·do·the·li·o·mas
or he·man·gio·en·do·the·li·o·ma·ta

hem·an·gi·o·ma
pl hem·an·gi·o·mas
or hem·an·gi·o·ma·ta

he·man·gi·o·ma·to·sis
pl he·man·gi·o·ma·to·ses

hem·an·gio·peri·cy·to·ma
pl hem·an·gio·peri·cy·to·mas
or hem·an·gio·peri·cy·to·ma·ta

he·man·gio·sar·co·ma
pl he·man·gio·sar·co·mas
or he·man·gio·sar·co·ma·ta

he·mar·thro·sis
pl he·mar·thro·ses

he·ma·tein

he·ma·tem·e·sis
pl he·ma·tem·e·ses

he·mat·ic

he·ma·ti·dro·sis

he·ma·tin

he·ma·tin·ic

he·ma·to·blast

he·ma·to·cele

he·ma·to·che·zia

he·ma·to·chy·lu·ria

he·ma·to·col·pos

he·mat·o·crit

he·mat·o·cyst

he·ma·to·gen·ic

he·ma·tog·e·nous

hem·a·to·gone

he·ma·toid

he·ma·to·log·ic
also he·ma·to·log·i·cal

he·ma·tol·o·gist

he·ma·tol·o·gy
pl he·ma·tol·o·gies

he·ma·to·ma
pl he·ma·to·mas
or he·ma·to·ma·ta

he·ma·to·me·tra

he·ma·to·my·e·lia

he·ma·to·pa·thol·o·gist

he·ma·to·pa·thol·o·gy
pl he·ma·to·pa·thol·o·gies

he·ma·to·peri·car·
di·um
  pl he·ma·to·peri·car·
  dia
he·ma·toph·a·gous
he·ma·to·phyte
he·ma·to·poi·e·sis
  pl he·ma·to·poi·e·ses
he·ma·to·poi·et·ic
he·ma·to·por·phy·
  rin
he·ma·to·por·phy·
  rin·u·ria
he·ma·tor·rha·chis
he·ma·to·sal·pinx
  pl he·ma·to·sal·pin·
  ges
he·ma·to·scope
he·ma·tox·y·lin
he·ma·to·zo·al
he·ma·to·zo·an
he·ma·tu·ria
heme
hem·er·a·lo·pia
he·me·ryth·rin
hemi·al·ge·sia
hemi·an·al·ge·sia
hemi·an·es·the·sia
hemi·an·op·sia
  or hemi·an·o·pia
hemi·an·op·tic
hemi·at·ro·phy
  pl hemi·at·ro·phies
hemi·a·zy·gos
hemi·bal·lis·mus
  also hemi·bal·lism
hemi·block

he·mic
hemi·cel·lu·lose
hemi·cel·lu·los·ic
hemi·ce·re·brum
  pl hemi·ce·re·brums
  or hemi·ce·re·bra
hemi·cho·lin·ium
hemi·cho·rea
hemi·col·ec·to·my
  pl hemi·col·ec·to·
  mies
hemi·cra·nia
hemi·cra·ni·al
hemi·cra·ni·o·sis
hemi·de·cor·ti·ca·
  tion
hemi·di·a·phragm
hemi·fa·cial
hemi·field
hemi·gas·trac·to·
  my
  pl hemi·gas·trac·to·
  mies
hemi·glos·sec·to·
  my
  pl hemi·glos·sec·to·
  mies
hemi·hy·per·tro·
  phy
  pl hemi·hy·per·tro·
  phies
hemi·lam·i·nec·to·
  my
  pl hemi·lam·i·nec·to·
  mies
hemi·lat·er·al

hemi·man·dib·u·
  lec·to·my
  pl hemi·man·dib·u·
  lec·to·mies
hemi·me·lia
hemi·me·lus
hemi·me·tab·o·
  lous
he·min
hemi·ne·phrec·to·
  my
  pl hemi·ne·phrec·to·
  mies
hemi·o·pia
  or hemi·op·sia
hemi·op·ic
hemi·pa·re·sis
  pl hemi·pa·re·ses
hemi·pa·ret·ic
hemi·pel·vec·to·
  my
  pl hemi·pel·vec·to·
  mies
hemi·ple·gia
hemi·ple·gic
He·mip·tera
he·mip·ter·an
he·mip·ter·ous
hemi·ret·i·na
  pl hemi·ret·i·nas
  or hemi·ret·i·nae
hemi·ret·i·nal
hemi·sect
hemi·sec·tion
hemi·spasm
hemi·sphere

hemi·spher·ec·to·
my
pl hemi·spher·ec·to·
mies
hemi·spher·ic
hemi·tho·rax
pl hemi·tho·rax·es
or hemi·tho·ra·ces
hemi·thy·roid·ec·
to·my
pl hemi·thy·roid·ec·
to·mies
hemi·zy·gote
hemi·zy·gous
he·mo·ag·glu·ti·nin
var of hemagglutinin
he·mo·bar·ton·el·
lo·sis
var of haemobartonel-
losis
he·mo·bil·ia
he·mo·blast
he·mo·blas·to·sis
pl he·mo·blas·to·ses
he·moc·cult
he·mo·cho·ri·al
he·mo·chro·ma·to·
sis
pl he·mo·chro·ma·to·
ses
he·mo·chro·ma·tot·
ic
he·mo·chro·mo·
gen
he·mo·clas·tic
he·mo·co·ag·u·la·
tion

he·mo·coel
also he·mo·coele
he·mo·coel·ic
he·mo·con·cen·tra·
tion
he·mo·co·nia
also he·mo·ko·nia
he·mo·co·ni·o·sis
pl he·mo·co·ni·o·ses
he·mo·cul·ture
he·mo·cu·pre·in
he·mo·cy·a·nin
he·mo·cyte
he·mo·cy·to·blast
he·mo·cy·to·blas·
tic
he·mo·cy·to·gen·e·
sis
pl he·mo·cy·to·gen·e·
ses
he·mo·cy·tol·y·sis
pl he·mo·cy·tol·y·ses
he·mo·cy·tom·e·ter
he·mo·di·al·y·sis
pl he·mo·di·al·y·ses
he·mo·di·a·lyz·er
he·mo·di·lute
he·mo·di·lut·ed
he·mo·di·lut·ing
he·mo·di·lu·tion
he·mo·dy·nam·ic
he·mo·dy·nam·i·
cal·ly
he·mo·fla·gel·late
he·mo·fus·cin
he·mo·glo·bin
also hae·mo·glo·bin

he·mo·glo·bin·
emia
he·mo·glo·bin·ic
he·mo·glo·bin·om·
e·ter
he·mo·glo·bin·om·
e·try
pl he·mo·glo·bin·om·
e·tries
he·mo·glo·bin·op·
a·thy
pl he·mo·glo·bin·op·
a·thies
he·mo·glo·bi·nous
he·mo·glo·bin·uria
he·mo·glo·bin·uric
he·mo·gram
he·mo·his·tio·blast
he·mo·ko·nia
var of hemoconia
he·mo·lymph
he·mol·y·sate
or he·mol·y·zate
he·mo·ly·sin
he·mo·ly·sis
pl he·mo·ly·ses
he·mo·lyt·ic
he·mo·lyze
he·mo·lyzed
he·mo·lyz·ing
he·mom·e·ter
he·mo·met·ric
he·mo·par·a·site
he·mo·par·a·sit·ic
he·mop·a·thy
pl he·mop·a·thies
he·mo·per·fu·sion

he·mo·peri·car·di·
um
    pl he·mo·peri·car·dia

he·mo·peri·to·ne·
um

he·mo·pex·in

he·mo·pha·gia

he·moph·a·gous

he·mo·phile

he·mo·phil·ia

he·mo·phil·i·ac

he·mo·phil·ic

He·moph·i·lus

he·mo·pneu·mo·
tho·rax
    pl he·mo·pneu·mo·
    tho·rax·es
    or he·mo·pneu·mo·
    tho·ra·ces

he·mo·poi·e·sis
    pl he·mo·poi·e·ses

he·mo·poi·et·ic

he·mo·pro·tein

he·mop·to·ic

he·mop·ty·sis
    pl he·mop·ty·ses

he·mo·rhe·ol·o·gy
    pl he·mo·rhe·ol·o·gies

hem·or·rhage
    hem·or·rhaged
    hem·or·rhag·ing
hem·or·rhag·ic
hem·or·rhag·in
hem·or·rhoid
hem·or·rhoid·al

hem·or·rhoid·ec·to·
my
    pl hem·or·rhoid·ec·to·
    mies

he·mo·sal·pinx
    pl he·mo·sal·pin·ges

he·mo·sid·er·in

he·mo·sid·er·o·sis
    pl he·mo·sid·er·o·ses

he·mo·sid·er·ot·ic

He·mo·spo·rid·ia

he·mo·sta·sis
    pl he·mo·sta·ses

he·mo·stat

he·mo·stat·ic

he·mo·ther·a·py
    pl he·mo·ther·a·pies

he·mo·tho·rax
    pl he·mo·tho·rax·es
    or he·mo·tho·ra·ces

he·mo·tox·ic

he·mo·tox·in

he·mot·ro·phe

he·mo·zo·in

hemp

hen·bane

Hen·der·son-Has·
sel·balch equa·
tion

Hen·le's loop

Hen·och-Schön·
lein

He·noch's pur·pu·
ra

hen·ry
    pl hen·rys
    or hen·ries

he·par

hep·a·ran

hep·a·rin

hep·a·rin·iza·tion

hep·a·rin·ize
    hep·a·rin·ized
    hep·a·rin·iz·ing

hep·a·rin·oid

hep·a·ri·tin

hep·a·tec·to·mized

hep·a·tec·to·my
    pl hep·a·tec·to·mies

he·pat·ic

he·pat·i·cos·to·my
    pl he·pat·i·cos·to·
    mies

he·pat·i·cot·o·my
    pl he·pat·i·cot·o·mies

hep·a·tit·ic

hep·a·ti·tis
    pl hep·a·tit·i·des

hep·a·ti·za·tion

hep·a·tized

he·pa·to·bil·i·ary

he·pa·to·car·cin·o·
gen

he·pa·to·car·cin·o·
gen·e·sis
    pl he·pa·to·car·cin·o·
    gen·e·ses

he·pa·to·car·cin·o·
gen·ic

he·pa·to·car·cin·o·
ge·nic·i·ty
    pl he·pa·to·car·cin·o·
    ge·nic·i·ties

he·pa·to·car·ci·no·
ma
pl he·pa·to·car·ci·no·
mas
or he·pa·to·car·ci·no·
ma·ta

he·pa·to·cel·lu·lar

he·pa·to·cyte

he·pa·to·gen·ic
or hep·a·tog·e·nous

hep·a·tog·ra·phy
pl hep·a·tog·ra·phies

he·pa·to·len·tic·u·
lar

he·pa·to·li·en·og·
ra·phy
pl he·pa·to·li·en·og·
ra·phies

hep·a·tol·o·gist

hep·a·tol·o·gy
pl hep·a·tol·o·gies

hep·a·to·ma
pl hep·a·to·mas
or hep·a·to·ma·ta

hep·a·to·ma·tous

he·pa·to·meg·a·lic

he·pa·to·meg·a·ly
pl he·pa·to·meg·a·lies

he·pa·to·pan·cre·at·
ic

hep·a·top·a·thy
pl hep·a·top·a·thies

he·pa·to·por·tal

he·pa·to·re·nal

hep·a·tor·rha·phy
pl hep·a·tor·rha·phies

hep·a·to·sis
pl hep·a·to·ses

he·pa·to·splen·ic

he·pa·to·spleno·
meg·a·ly
pl he·pa·to·spleno·
meg·a·lies

hep·a·tot·o·my
pl hep·a·tot·o·mies

he·pa·to·tox·ic

he·pa·to·tox·ic·i·ty
pl he·pa·to·tox·ic·i·
ties

he·pa·to·tox·in

herb·al

herb·al·ist

her·bi·cid·al

her·bi·vore

her·biv·o·rous

her·biv·o·ry
pl her·biv·o·ries

he·red·i·tar·i·an

he·red·i·tar·i·ly

he·red·i·tary

he·red·i·ty
pl he·red·i·ties

her·e·do·fa·mil·ial

He·ring-Breu·er re·
flex

He·ring the·o·ry

her·i·ta·bil·i·ty
pl her·i·ta·bil·i·ties

her·i·ta·ble

her·maph·ro·dism

her·maph·ro·dite

her·maph·ro·dit·ic

her·maph·ro·dit·
ism

her·met·ic

her·met·i·cal·ly

her·nia
pl her·ni·as
or her·ni·ae

her·ni·al

her·ni·ate

her·ni·at·ed

her·ni·at·ing

her·ni·a·tion

her·nio·plas·ty
pl her·nio·plas·ties

her·ni·or·rha·phy
pl her·ni·or·rha·phies

her·ni·ot·o·my
pl her·ni·ot·o·mies

he·ro·ic

her·o·in

her·o·in·ism

her·pan·gi·na

her·pes

her·pes gen·i·tal·is

her·pes la·bi·al·is

her·pes pro·gen·i·
tal·is

her·pes sim·plex

her·pes·vi·rus

her·pes zos·ter

her·pet·ic

her·pet·i·form

her·pe·to·pho·bia

Hert·wig's sheath

Herx·heim·er re·
ac·tion

Heschl's gy·rus

hes·per·i·din

Hes·sel·bach's tri·
an·gle

het·a·cil·lin
het·er·a·kid
Het·er·a·kis
het·ero·ag·glu·ti·
nin
het·ero·an·ti·body
  pl het·ero·an·ti·bod·
  ies
het·ero·an·ti·gen
het·ero·aux·in
  var of heterokaryon
het·ero·cary·o·sis
  var of heterokaryosis
het·ero·cary·ot·ic
  var of heterokaryotic
het·ero·cel·lu·lar
het·ero·chro·mat·ic
het·ero·chro·ma·
tin
het·ero·chro·ma·ti·
za·tion
  also het·ero·chro·ma·
  tin·iza·tion
het·ero·chro·ma·
tized
het·ero·chro·mia
het·ero·chro·mo·
some
het·ero·crine
het·ero·cy·clic
het·er·odont
het·ero·du·plex
het·er·oe·cious
het·er·oe·cism
het·ero·erot·ic
het·ero·er·o·tism

het·ero·ga·mete
het·ero·ga·met·ic
het·ero·gam·e·ty
  pl het·ero·gam·e·ties
het·er·og·a·mous
het·er·og·a·my
  pl het·er·og·a·mies
het·ero·ge·ne·ity
  pl het·ero·ge·ne·ities
het·ero·ge·neous
het·ero·ge·net·ic
het·ero·gen·ic
het·ero·ge·note
het·ero·ge·not·ic
het·er·og·e·nous
het·ero·gon·ic
het·er·og·o·ny
  pl het·er·og·o·nies
het·ero·graft
het·ero·kary·on
  also het·ero·cary·on
het·ero·kary·o·sis
  also het·ero·cary·o·sis
het·ero·kary·ot·ic
  also het·ero·cary·ot·ic
het·ero·lat·er·al
het·er·ol·o·gous
het·er·ol·o·gy
  pl het·er·ol·o·gies
het·ero·ly·sin
het·ero·ly·sis
  pl het·ero·ly·ses
het·ero·lyt·ic
het·ero·mer·ic
het·ero·mor·phic
  also het·ero·mor·
  phous

het·ero·mor·phism
het·ero·mor·pho·
sis
  pl het·ero·mor·pho·
  ses
het·er·on·o·mous
het·ero·pha·gic
het·ero·phago·
some
het·er·oph·a·gy
  pl het·er·oph·a·gies
het·ero·phe·my
  pl het·ero·phe·mies
het·ero·phile
  or het·er·o·phil
  also het·er·o·phil·ic
het·ero·pho·ria
het·ero·phor·ic
Het·ero·phy·es
het·ero·phy·id
het·ero·pla·sia
het·ero·plasm
het·ero·plas·tic
het·ero·plas·ty
  pl het·ero·plas·ties
het·ero·ploid
het·ero·ploi·dy
  pl het·ero·ploi·dies
het·ero·poly·mer
het·ero·poly·mer·ic
het·ero·poly·sac·
cha·ride
Het·er·op·tera
het·er·op·ter·ous
het·ero·pyk·no·sis
  also het·ero·pyc·no·sis

het·ero·pyk·not·ic
also het·ero·pyc·not·ic

het·ero·scope

het·er·os·co·py
pl het·er·os·co·pies

het·ero·sex·u·al

het·ero·sex·u·al·i·
ty
pl het·ero·sex·u·al·i·
ties

het·er·o·sis
pl het·er·o·ses

het·ero·sug·ges·
tion

het·ero·tax·ia

het·ero·tax·is
pl het·ero·tax·es

het·ero·thal·lic

het·ero·thal·lism

het·er·ot·ic

het·ero·to·pia

het·ero·top·ic

het·ero·top·i·cal·ly

het·er·ot·opy
pl het·er·ot·opies

het·ero·trans·plant

het·ero·trans·plant·
abil·i·ty
pl het·ero·trans·plant·
abil·i·ties

het·ero·trans·plant·
able

het·ero·trans·plan·
ta·tion

het·ero·trans·plant·
ed

het·ero·tri·cho·sis
pl het·ero·tri·cho·ses

het·ero·troph

het·ero·tro·phic

het·ero·tro·phism

het·ero·tro·phy
pl het·ero·tro·phies

het·ero·tro·pia

het·ero·tro·pic

het·ero·typ·ic

het·ero·zy·go·sis
pl het·ero·zy·go·ses

het·ero·zy·gos·i·ty
pl het·ero·zy·gos·i·ties

het·ero·zy·gote

het·ero·zy·got·ic

het·ero·zy·gous

hex·a·canth

hexa·chlo·ro·eth·
ane
or hexa·chlor·eth·ane

hexa·chlo·ro·
phene

hexa·dac·ty·ly
pl hexa·dac·ty·lies

hex·a·dec·a·no·ic

hexa·flu·o·re·ni·
um

hex·a·mer

hex·a·mer·ic

hexa·me·tho·ni·
um

hexa·meth·y·lene·
tet·ra·mine

hex·amine

hex·a·no·ic

hexa·ploid

hexa·ploi·dy
pl hexa·ploi·dies

hexa·pod

Hex·ap·o·da

hex·es·trol

hexo·bar·bi·tal

hexo·cy·cli·um me·
thyl·sul·fate

hexo·ki·nase

hex·os·a·mine

hex·os·a·min·i·
dase

hex·o·san

hex·ose

hex·u·ron·ic

hex·yl·res·or·cin·ol

hi·a·tal

hi·a·tus

hi·a·tus semi·lu·
nar·is

hi·ber·nate

hi·ber·nat·ed

hi·ber·nat·ing

hi·ber·na·tion

hi·ber·na·tor

hi·ber·no·ma
pl hi·ber·no·mas
or hi·ber·no·ma·ta

hic·cup
also hic·cough

hic·cuped
also hic·cupped
or hic·coughed

hic·cup·ing
also hic·cup·ping
or hic·cough·ing

hic·cup·er
also hic·cough·er

hide·bound
hi·drad·e·ni·tis
hi·drad·e·ni·tis
　sup·pur·a·ti·va
hi·drad·e·no·ma
　pl hi·drad·e·no·mas
　or hi·drad·e·no·ma·ta
hi·dro·sis
　pl hi·dro·ses
hi·drot·ic
hi·lar
hill·ock
hi·lum
　pl hi·la
hi·lus
　pl hi·li
hind·brain
hind·foot
　pl hind·feet
hind·gut
hip·bone
Hip·pe·la·tes
Hip·po·bos·ca
hip·po·bos·cid
Hip·po·bos·ci·dae
hip·po·cam·pal
hip·po·cam·pus
　pl hip·po·cam·pi
Hip·po·crat·ic
Hip·poc·ra·tism
hip·pu·ran
hip·pu·rate
hip·pu·ric
hip·pus
Hirsch·sprung's
　dis·ease
hir·sute

hir·sut·ism
hi·ru·din
Hir·u·din·ea
hir·u·di·ni·a·sis
　pl hir·u·di·ni·a·ses
Hir·u·din·i·dae
Hi·ru·do
His bun·dle
his·ta·mi·nase
his·ta·mine
his·ta·min·er·gic
his·ta·min·ic
his·ta·mi·no·lyt·ic
his·ti·dase
his·ti·dine
his·ti·di·ne·mia
his·ti·di·ne·mic
his·ti·din·uria
his·tio·cyte
his·tio·cyt·ic
his·tio·cy·to·ma
　pl his·tio·cy·to·mas
　also his·tio·cy·to·ma·
　ta
his·tio·cy·to·sis
　pl his·tio·cy·to·ses
his·to·chem·i·cal
his·to·chem·is·try
　pl his·to·chem·is·tries
his·to·com·pat·i·
　bil·i·ty
　pl his·to·com·pat·i·
　bil·i·ties
his·to·com·pat·ible
his·to·dif·fer·en·ti·
　a·tion

his·to·flu·o·res·
　cence
his·to·flu·o·res·cent
his·to·gen·e·sis
　pl his·to·gen·e·ses
his·to·ge·net·ic
his·to·ge·net·i·cal·
　ly
his·to·gram
his·toid
his·to·in·com·pat·i·
　bil·i·ty
　pl his·to·in·com·pat·i·
　bil·i·ties
his·to·in·com·pat·
　ible
his·to·log·i·cal
　or his·to·log·ic
his·to·log·i·cal·ly
his·tol·o·gist
his·tol·o·gy
　pl his·tol·o·gies
his·tol·y·sis
　pl his·tol·y·ses
his·to·lyt·ic
his·tol·y·zate
　or his·tol·y·sate
his·tom·o·nad
his·tom·o·nal
His·tom·o·nas
his·to·mo·ni·a·sis
　pl his·to·mo·ni·a·ses
his·to·mor·pho·log·
　ic
　or his·to·mor·pho·log·
　i·cal

his·to·mor·phol·o·
gy
pl his·to·mor·phol·o·
gies

his·tone

his·to·patho·gen·e·
sis
pl his·to·patho·gen·e·
ses

his·to·path·o·log·ic
or his·to·path·o·log·i·
cal

his·to·pa·thol·o·gist

his·to·pa·thol·o·gy
pl his·to·pa·thol·o·
gies

his·to·phys

his·to·phys·i·o·log·
i·cal
also his·to·phys·i·o·
log·ic

his·to·phys·i·ol·o·
gy
pl his·to·phys·i·ol·o·
gies

his·to·plas·ma

his·to·plas·min

his·to·plas·mo·ma
pl his·to·plas·mo·mas
or his·to·plas·mo·ma·
ta

his·to·plas·mo·sis
pl his·to·plas·mo·ses

his·to·ra·dio·graph·
ic

his·to·ra·di·og·ra·
phy
pl his·to·ra·di·og·ra·
phies

his·to·ry
pl his·to·ries

his·to·tox·ic

his·to·trophe
or his·to·troph

his·to·tro·pic

his·tot·ro·pism

his·to·zo·ic

hoarse
hoars·er
hoars·est

Hodg·kin's dis·
ease

Hoff·mann's drops

Hof·meis·ter se·
ries

hol·an·dric

Hol·ger Niel·sen
meth·od

ho·lism

ho·lis·tic

ho·lis·ti·cal·ly

Hol·land·er test

hol·low

Holm·gren yarn
test

hol·mi·um

ho·lo·blas·tic

ho·lo·blas·ti·cal·ly

ho·lo·crine

ho·lo·en·dem·ic

ho·lo·en·zyme

ho·log·a·mous

ho·lo·gram

ho·lo·graph

ho·log·ra·pher

ho·lo·graph·ic

ho·lo·graph·i·cal·ly

ho·log·ra·phy
pl ho·log·ra·phies

ho·lo·gy·nic

ho·log·y·ny
pl ho·log·y·nies

ho·lo·me·tab·o·
lism

ho·lo·me·tab·o·lous

ho·lo·phyt·ic

ho·lo·sys·tol·ic

ho·lo·zo·ic

Ho·mans' sign

hom·at·ro·pine

ho·meo·path

ho·meo·path·ic

ho·meo·path·i·cal·
ly

ho·me·op·a·thy
pl ho·me·op·a·thies

ho·meo·pla·sia

ho·meo·plas·tic

ho·meo·sis
var of homoeosis

ho·meo·sta·sis

ho·meo·stat·ic

ho·meo·therm
or ho·moio·therm

ho·meo·ther·mic
or ho·moio·ther·mic
or ho·moio·ther·mal

ho·meo·ther·my
or ho·moio·ther·my
pl ho·meo·ther·mies
or ho·moio·ther·mies

ho·me·ot·ic
var of homoeotic

ho·mi·cid·al
ho·mi·cid·al·ly
ho·mi·cide
hom·i·nid
Ho·min·i·dae
hom·i·nine
hom·i·ni·za·tion
hom·i·nized
hom·i·noid
Hom·i·noi·dea
ho·mo
  pl ho·mos
ho·mo·cary·on
  var of homokaryon
ho·mo·cary·ot·ic
  var of homokaryotic
ho·mo·cys·te·ine
ho·mo·cys·tine
ho·mo·cys·tin·uria
ho·mo·cys·tin·uric
ho·mo·cy·to·tro·pic
ho·moe·ol·og·ous
ho·moeo·logue
  or ho·moeo·log
ho·moe·osis
  or ho·me·osis
ho·moe·ot·ic
  also ho·me·ot·ic
ho·mo·erot·ic
ho·mo·erot·i·cism
  also ho·mo·erot·ism
ho·mo·fer·men·ta·tive
ho·mo·fer·ment·er
ho·mo·ga·met·ic
ho·mog·a·mous
  or ho·mo·gam·ic

ho·mog·a·my
  pl ho·mog·a·mies
ho·mo·ge·nate
ho·mo·ge·ne·ity
  pl ho·mo·ge·ne·ities
ho·mo·ge·neous
ho·mo·ge·ni·za·tion
ho·mo·ge·nize
  ho·mog·e·nized
  ho·mog·e·niz·ing
ho·mog·e·niz·er
ho·mog·e·nous
ho·mo·gen·tis·ic
ho·mo·graft
ho·moio·therm
  var of homeotherm
ho·moio·ther·mic
  var of homeothermic
ho·moio·ther·my
  var of homeothermy
ho·mo·kary·on
  also ho·mo·cary·on
ho·mo·kary·ot·ic
  also ho·mo·cary·ot·ic
ho·mo·lat·er·al
ho·mo·lec·i·thal
ho·mol·o·gize
  ho·mol·o·gized
  ho·mol·o·giz·ing
ho·mol·o·gous
ho·mo·logue
  also ho·mo·log
ho·mol·o·gy
  pl ho·mol·o·gies
ho·mol·y·sis
  pl ho·mol·y·ses

ho·mo·lyt·ic
ho·mon·o·mous
hom·on·y·mous
ho·mo·phile
ho·mo·pho·bia
ho·mo·pho·bic
ho·mo·plas·tic
ho·mo·plasty
  pl ho·mo·plas·ties
ho·mo·poly·nu·cleo·tide
ho·mo·poly·pep·tide
ho·mo·poly·sac·char·ide
Ho·mop·tera
ho·mop·ter·an
ho·mop·ter·ous
ho·mos
  pl of homo
ho·mo·sal·ate
Ho·mo sa·pi·ens
ho·mo·ser·ine
ho·mo·sex·u·al
ho·mo·sex·u·al·i·ty
  pl ho·mo·sex·u·al·i·ties
ho·mo·spo·rous
ho·mo·thal·lism
ho·mo·top·ic
ho·mo·trans·plant
ho·mo·trans·plant·abil·i·ty
  pl ho·mo·trans·plant·abil·i·ties
ho·mo·trans·plant·able

ho·mo·trans·plan·
ta·tion
ho·mo·tro·pic
ho·mo·type
ho·mo·typ·ic
  or ho·mo·typ·i·cal
ho·mo·va·nil·lic
ho·mo·zy·go·sis
  pl ho·mo·zy·go·ses
ho·mo·zy·gos·i·ty
  pl ho·mo·zy·gos·i·ties
ho·mo·zy·gote
ho·mo·zy·gous
ho·mun·cu·lus
  pl ho·mun·cu·li

hoof
  pl hooves
  or hoofs

Hooke's law
hook·let
hook·worm
hor·de·o·lum
  pl hor·de·o·la

hore·hound
  also hoar·hound

hor·i·zon·tal
hor·mon·al
hor·mone
hor·mo·no·gen·e·
  sis
  pl hor·mo·no·gen·e·
  ses
hor·mo·no·gen·ic
hor·mo·nol·o·gy
  pl hor·mo·nol·o·gies
hor·mo·no·poi·et·
  ic

hor·mo·no·ther·a·
  py
  pl hor·mo·no·ther·a·
  pies
Hor·ner's syn·
  drome
horn·i·fied
ho·rop·ter
hor·op·ter·ic
hor·rip·i·late
  hor·rip·i·lat·ed
  hor·rip·i·lat·ing
hor·rip·i·la·tion
horse·fly
  pl horse·flies

horse·pox
Hor·ton's syn·
  drome
hos·pice
hos·pi·tal
hos·pi·tal·ism
hos·pi·tal·iza·tion
hos·pi·tal·ize
  hos·pi·tal·ized
  hos·pi·tal·iz·ing
hos·tel
hos·tile
hos·til·i·ty
  pl hos·til·i·ties
Ho·tis test
house·break
  house·broke
  house·bro·ken
  house·break·ing
house·fly
  pl house·flies
house·maid's knee

house·man
  pl house·men
Hous·ton's valve
How·ard test
How·ell-Jol·ly
  body
How·ship's la·cu·
  na
  pl How·ship's la·cu·
  nae
Hr fac·tor
H-sub·stance
Hub·bard tank
Huh·ner test
hu·man·iza·tion
hu·man·oid
hu·man T-cell leu·
  ke·mia vi·rus
hu·man T-cell
  lym·pho·tro·pic
  vi·rus
hu·man T-lym·
  pho·tro·pic vi·
  rus
hu·mec·tant
hu·mer·al
hu·mer·us
  pl hu·meri
hu·mid
hu·mid·i·fi·ca·tion
hu·mid·i·fi·er
hu·mid·i·fy
  hu·mid·i·fied
  hu·mid·i·fy·ing
hu·mid·i·ty
  pl hu·mid·i·ties
hu·mor

hydrocodone

hu·mor·al
hump·back
hump·backed
hunch·back
hunch·backed
hun·ger
Hun·ner's ul·cer
Hun·ter's ca·nal
Hun·ter's syn·
drome
  or Hun·ter syn·drome
Hun·ting·ton's cho·
rea
Hur·ler's syn·
drome
  or Hur·ler syn·drome
hutch·in·so·ni·an
Hutch·in·son's
teeth
Hutch·in·son's tri·
ad
Hux·ley's lay·er
Huy·ge·ni·an eye·
piece
  also Huy·gens eye·
piece
hy·a·line
  or hy·a·lin
hy·a·lin·iza·tion
hy·a·lin·ized
hy·a·li·tis
Hy·a·lom·ma
hy·a·lo·plasm
hy·a·lo·plas·mic
hy·al·uro·nate
hy·al·uron·ic
hy·al·uron·i·dase

hy·brid
hy·brid·i·ty
  pl hy·brid·i·ties
hy·brid·iza·tion
hy·brid·ize
  hy·brid·ized
  hy·brid·iz·ing
hy·brid·iz·er
hy·brid·oma
hy·can·thone
hy·dan·to·in
hy·dan·to·in·ate
hy·da·tid
hy·da·tid·i·form
hy·da·tid of Mor·
ga·gni
hy·da·tid·o·sis
  pl hy·da·tid·o·ses
hy·dra·gogue
  also hy·dra·gog
hy·dral·azine
hy·dram·ni·os
  also hy·dram·ni·on
hy·dram·ni·ot·ic
hy·dran·en·ceph·a·
ly
  pl hy·dran·en·ceph·a·
  lies
hy·drar·thro·sis
  pl hy·drar·thro·ses
hy·drase
hy·dras·tine
hy·dras·ti·nine
hy·dras·tis
hy·dra·tase

hy·drate
  hy·drat·ed
  hy·drat·ing
hy·dra·tion
hy·dra·zide
hy·dra·zine
hy·dre·mia
hy·dre·mic
hy·dren·ceph·a·lo·
cele
hy·dren·ceph·a·lus
  pl hy·dren·ceph·a·li
hy·dren·ceph·a·ly
  pl hy·dren·ceph·a·lies
hy·dride
hy·droa
hy·dro·bro·mic
hy·dro·bro·mide
hy·dro·car·bon
hy·dro·cele
hy·dro·ce·lec·to·my
  pl hy·dro·ce·lec·to·
  mies
hy·dro·ce·phal·ic
hy·dro·ceph·a·lus
  pl hy·dro·ceph·a·li
hy·dro·ceph·a·ly
  pl hy·dro·ceph·a·lies
hy·dro·chlo·ric
hy·dro·chlo·ride
hy·dro·chlo·ro·thi·
a·zide
hy·dro·cho·le·re·sis
  pl hy·dro·cho·le·re·
  ses
hy·dro·cho·le·ret·ic
hy·dro·co·done

hy·dro·col·loid
hy·dro·col·loi·dal
hy·dro·col·pos
hy·dro·cor·ti·sone
hy·dro·cy·an·ic
hy·dro·flu·me·thi·
  a·zide
hy·dro·gel
hy·dro·gen
hy·drog·e·nase
hy·dro·ge·nate
  hy·dro·ge·nat·ed
  hy·dro·ge·nat·ing
hy·dro·ge·na·tion
hy·drog·e·nous
hy·dro·lase
hy·drol·o·gy
  pl hy·drol·o·gies
hy·dro·ly·sate
  or hy·dro·ly·zate
hy·dro·ly·sis
hy·dro·lyt·ic
hy·dro·lyt·i·cal·ly
hy·dro·lyz·able
hy·dro·lyze
  hy·dro·lyzed
  hy·dro·lyz·ing
hy·dro·me·tra
hy·dro·me·tro·col·
  pos
hy·dro·mor·phone
hy·dro·ne·phro·sis
  pl hy·dro·ne·phro·ses
hy·dro·ne·phrot·ic
hy·dro·ni·um
hy·dro·os·mot·ic
hy·dro·path·ic

hy·dro·path·i·cal·ly
hy·drop·a·thy
  pl hy·drop·a·thies
hy·dro·pe·nia
hy·dro·pe·nic
hy·dro·peri·car·di·
  um
  pl hy·dro·peri·car·dia
hy·dro·peri·to·ne·
  um
  pl hy·dro·peri·to·nea
  or hy·dro·peri·to·ne·
    ums
hy·dro·phil·ia
hy·dro·phil·ic
hy·dro·phi·lic·i·ty
  pl hy·dro·phi·lic·i·ties
hy·dro·pho·bia
hy·dro·pho·bic
hy·droph·thal·mos
hy·drop·ic
hy·dro·pneu·mo·
  tho·rax
  pl hy·dro·pneu·mo·
    tho·rax·es
  or hy·dro·pneu·mo·
    tho·ra·ces
hy·drops
  pl hy·drop·ses
hy·drops fe·tal·is
hy·dro·qui·nine
hy·dro·qui·none
hy·dro·rrhea
hy·dro·sal·pinx
  pl hy·dro·sal·pin·ges
hy·dro·sol
hy·dro·sol·ic
hy·dro·sol·u·ble

hy·dro·tac·tic
hy·dro·tax·is
  pl hy·dro·tax·es
hy·dro·ther·a·peu·
  tic
hy·dro·ther·a·pist
hy·dro·ther·a·py
  pl hy·dro·ther·a·pies
hy·dro·ther·mal
hy·dro·tho·rax
  pl hy·dro·tho·rax·es
  or hy·dro·tho·ra·ces
hy·dro·tro·pic
hy·dro·tro·pism
hy·dro·ure·ter
hy·drous
hy·drox·ide
hy·droxo·co·bal·
  amin
hy·droxy·ace·tic
hy·droxy·am·phet·
  amine
hy·droxy·ap·a·tite
  or hy·drox·yl·ap·a·tite
hy·droxy·ben·zene
hy·droxy·bu·ty·rate
hy·droxy·bu·tyr·ic
hy·droxy·chlor·o·
  quine
25-hy·droxy·cho·le·
  cal·cif·er·ol
17-hy·droxy·cor·ti·
  co·ste·roid
hy·droxy·di·one
6-hy·droxy·do·pa·
  mine

5-hy·droxy·in·dole·
   ace·tic ac·id
hy·drox·yl
hy·drox·yl·amine
hy·drox·y·lase
hy·drox·yl·ic
hy·droxy·ly·sine
hy·droxy·pro·ges·
   ter·one
   or 17α-hy·droxy·pro·
   ges·ter·one

hy·droxy·pro·line
8-hy·droxy·quin·o·
   line
hy·droxy·ste·roid
5-hy·droxy·tryp·ta·
   mine
hy·droxy·urea
hy·droxy·zine
Hy·dro·zoa
hy·dro·zo·an
hy·giene
hy·gien·ic
hy·gien·i·cal·ly
hy·gien·ist
hy·gric
hy·gro·ma
   pl hy·gro·mas
   or hy·gro·ma·ta

hy·grom·e·ter
hy·gro·met·ric
hy·grom·e·try
   pl hy·grom·e·tries

hy·gro·my·cin B
hy·gro·scope
hy·gro·scop·ic
hy·men

hy·men·al
hy·men·ec·to·my
   pl hy·men·ec·to·mies
hy·me·no·le·pi·a·
   sis
   pl hy·me·no·le·pi·a·
   ses

Hy·me·nol·e·pis
Hy·me·nop·tera
hy·men·ot·o·my
   pl hy·men·ot·o·mies
hyo·epi·glot·tic
hyo·glos·sal
hyo·glos·sus
   pl hyo·glos·si

hy·oid
hyo·man·dib·u·lar
hyo·scine
hyo·scy·a·mine
hyo·scy·a·mus
hyo·thy·roid
hyp·acu·sic
   also hyp·acou·sic

hyp·al·ge·sia
hyp·al·ge·sic
hyp·ar·te·ri·al
hyp·ax·i·al
hy·per·ac·id
hy·per·acid·i·ty
   pl hy·per·acid·i·ties

hy·per·ac·tive
hy·per·ac·tiv·i·ty
   pl hy·per·ac·tiv·i·ties
hy·per·acu·sis
hy·per·acute
hy·per·adren·a·lin·
   emia

hy·per·ad·re·no·
   cor·ti·cism
hy·per·ag·gres·sive
hy·per·al·do·ste·
   ron·emia
hy·per·al·do·ste·
   ron·ism
hy·per·al·ge·sia
hy·per·al·ge·sic
hy·per·al·i·men·ta·
   tion
hy·per·ami·no·ac·
   id·uria
hy·per·am·mo·ne·
   mia
   also hy·per·am·mon·i·
   emia

hy·per·am·mo·ne·
   mic
hy·per·am·y·las·
   emia
hy·per·arous·al
hy·per·azo·te·mia
hy·per·bar·ic
hy·per·bar·i·cal·ly
hy·per·be·ta·li·po·
   pro·tein·emia
hy·per·bil·i·ru·bin·
   emia
hy·per·cal·ce·mia
hy·per·cal·ce·mic
hy·per·cal·ci·uria
   also hy·per·cal·cin·
   uria

hy·per·cap·nia
hy·per·cap·nic
hy·per·car·bia

hy·per·ca·thex·is
  pl hy·per·ca·thex·es

hy·per·cel·lu·lar

hy·per·cel·lu·lar·i·ty
  pl hy·per·cel·lu·lar·i·ties

hy·per·ce·men·to·sis
  pl hy·per·ce·men·to·ses

hy·per·chlor·emia

hy·per·chlor·emic

hy·per·chlor·hy·dria

hy·per·cho·les·ter·ol·emia
  or hy·per·cho·les·ter·emia

hy·per·cho·les·ter·ol·emic
  or hy·per·cho·les·ter·emic

hy·per·chro·mat·ic

hy·per·chro·ma·tism

hy·per·chro·ma·to·sis
  pl hy·per·chro·ma·to·ses

hy·per·chro·mia

hy·per·chro·mic

hy·per·chro·mic·i·ty
  pl hy·per·chro·mic·i·ties

hy·per·chy·lo·mi·cro·ne·mia

hy·per·co·ag·u·la·bil·i·ty
  pl hy·per·co·ag·u·la·bil·i·ties

hy·per·co·ag·u·la·ble

hy·per·cor·ti·sol·ism

hy·per·cry·al·ge·sia

hy·per·dip·loid

hy·per·dip·loi·dy
  pl hy·per·dip·loi·dies

hy·per·eme·sis
  pl hy·per·eme·ses

hy·per·eme·sis grav·i·dar·um

hy·per·emia

hy·per·emic

hy·per·en·dem·ic

hy·per·en·de·mic·i·ty
  pl hy·per·en·de·mic·i·ties

hy·per·er·gic

hy·per·er·gy
  pl hy·per·er·gies

hy·per·es·the·sia

hy·per·es·thet·ic

hy·per·es·trin·ism

hy·per·es·tro·gen·ism

hy·per·ex·cit·abil·i·ty
  pl hy·per·ex·cit·abil·i·ties

hy·per·ex·cit·ed

hy·per·ex·cite·ment

hy·per·ex·tend

hy·per·ex·ten·si·bil·i·ty
  pl hy·per·ex·ten·si·bil·i·ties

hy·per·ex·ten·si·ble

hy·per·ex·ten·sion

hy·per·func·tion

hy·per·func·tion·al

hy·per·func·tion·ing

hy·per·gam·ma·glob·u·lin·emia

hy·per·gam·ma·glob·u·lin·emic

hy·per·glob·u·lin·emia

hy·per·glob·u·lin·emic

hy·per·glu·ca·gon·emia

hy·per·gly·ce·mia

hy·per·gly·ce·mic

hy·per·go·nad·ism

hy·per·hep·a·rin·emia

hy·per·hep·a·rin·emic

hy·per·hi·dro·sis
  also hy·peri·dro·sis
  pl hy·per·hi·dro·ses
  also hy·peri·dro·ses

hy·per·hy·dra·tion

hy·per·i·cin

hy·per·i·cism
hy·per·im·mune
hy·per·im·mu·ni·
za·tion
hy·per·im·mu·nize
hy·per·im·mu·
nized
hy·per·im·mu·
niz·ing
hy·per·in·fec·tion
hy·per·in·fla·tion
hy·per·in·su·lin·
emia
hy·per·in·su·lin·
emic
hy·per·in·su·lin·
ism
hy·per·in·vo·lu·
tion
hy·per·ir·ri·ta·bil·i·
ty
  pl hy·per·ir·ri·ta·bil·i·
  ties
hy·per·ir·ri·ta·ble
hy·per·ka·le·mia
hy·per·ka·le·mic
hy·per·ke·ra·to·sis
  pl hy·per·ke·ra·to·ses
hy·per·ker·a·tot·ic
hy·per·ki·ne·sia
hy·per·ki·ne·sis
hy·per·ki·net·ic
hy·per·lex·ia
hy·per·lex·ic
hy·per·li·pe·mia
hy·per·li·pe·mic
hy·per·lip·id·emia

hy·per·lip·id·emic
hy·per·li·po·pro·
tein·emia
hy·per·lu·cen·cy
  pl hy·per·lu·cen·cies
hy·per·lu·cent
hy·per·mag·ne·se·
mia
hy·per·men·or·
rhea
hy·per·meta·bol·ic
hy·per·me·tab·o·
lism
hy·per·me·tria
hy·per·me·tro·pia
hy·per·me·tro·pic
hy·perm·ne·sia
hy·perm·ne·sic
hy·per·mo·bile
hy·per·mo·bil·i·ty
  pl hy·per·mo·bil·i·ties
hy·per·morph
hy·per·mor·phic
hy·per·mo·tile
hy·per·mo·til·i·ty
  pl hy·per·mo·til·i·ties
hy·per·myo·to·nia
hy·per·na·tre·mia
hy·per·na·tre·mic
hy·per·neph·roid
hy·per·ne·phro·ma
  pl hy·per·ne·phro·
  mas
  or hy·per·ne·phro·
  ma·ta
hy·per·nu·tri·tion

hy·per·on·to·
morph
hy·per·ope
hy·per·opia
hy·per·opic
hy·per·os·mia
hy·per·os·mo·lal·i·
ty
  pl hy·per·os·mo·lal·i·
  ties
hy·per·os·mo·lar
hy·per·os·mo·lar·i·
ty
  pl hy·per·os·mo·lar·i·
  ties
hy·per·os·mot·ic
hy·per·os·to·sis
  pl hy·per·os·to·ses
hy·per·os·tot·ic
hy·per·ox·al·uria
hy·per·ox·ia
hy·per·par·a·site
hy·per·par·a·sit·ic
hy·per·par·a·sit·
ism
hy·per·para·thy·
roid·ism
hy·per·path·ia
hy·per·path·ic
hy·per·peri·stal·sis
  pl hy·per·peri·stal·ses
hy·per·pha·gia
hy·per·phag·ic
hy·per·pha·lan·
gism
hy·per·phe·nyl·al·
a·nin·emia

hy·per·phe·nyl·al·a·nin·emic
hy·per·pho·ria
hy·per·phos·pha·te·mia
hy·per·phos·pha·tu·ria
hy·per·pi·e·sia
hy·per·pi·et·ic
hy·per·pig·men·ta·tion
hy·per·pig·ment·ed
hy·per·pi·tu·ita·rism
hy·per·pi·tu·itary
hy·per·pla·sia
hy·per·plas·tic
hy·per·plas·ti·cal·ly
hy·per·ploid
hy·per·ploi·dy
pl hy·per·ploi·dies

hy·per·pnea
hy·per·pne·ic
hy·per·po·lar·iza·tion
hy·per·po·lar·ize
hy·per·po·lar·ized
hy·per·po·lar·iz·ing
hy·per·po·tas·se·mia
hy·per·po·tas·se·mic
hy·per·pro·duc·tion

hy·per·pro·lac·tin·emia
hy·per·pro·lac·tin·emic
hy·per·pro·lin·emia
hy·per·pro·tein·emia
hy·per·pro·throm·bin·emia
hy·per·py·ret·ic
hy·per·py·rex·ia
hy·per·py·rex·ic
hy·per·re·ac·tive
hy·per·re·ac·tiv·i·ty
pl hy·per·re·ac·tiv·i·ties

hy·per·re·ac·tor
hy·per·re·flex·ia
hy·per·re·nin·emia
hy·per·res·o·nance
hy·per·res·o·nant
hy·per·re·spon·sive
hy·per·sal·i·va·tion
hy·per·se·crete
hy·per·se·cret·ed
hy·per·se·cret·ing
hy·per·se·cre·tion
hy·per·se·cre·to·ry
hy·per·sen·si·tive
hy·per·sen·si·tive·ness
hy·per·sen·si·tiv·i·ty
pl hy·per·sen·si·tiv·i·ties

hy·per·sen·si·ti·za·tion
hy·per·sen·si·tize
hy·per·sen·si·tized
hy·per·sen·si·tiz·ing
hy·per·sid·er·emia
hy·per·sid·er·e·mic
hy·per·som·nia
hy·per·splen·ic
hy·per·sple·nism
hy·per·sthen·ic
hy·per·sus·cep·ti·bil·i·ty
pl hy·per·sus·cep·ti·bil·i·ties

hy·per·sus·cep·ti·ble
hy·per·tel·or·ism
hy·per·tense
hy·per·ten·sin·ase
hy·per·ten·sin·o·gen
hy·per·ten·sion
hy·per·ten·sive
hy·per·ten·sor
hy·per·ther·mia
hy·per·ther·mic
hy·per·thy·re·o·sis
pl hy·per·thy·re·o·ses

hy·per·thy·roid
hy·per·thy·roid·ism
hy·per·to·nia
hy·per·ton·ic

hy·per·to·nic·i·ty
pl hy·per·to·nic·i·ties

hy·per·to·nus

hy·per·to·ny
pl hy·per·to·nies

hy·per·tri·cho·sis
pl hy·per·tri·cho·ses

hy·per·tri·glyc·er·i·
de·mia

hy·per·tri·glyc·er·i·
de·mic

hy·per·tro·phic

hy·per·tro·phy
pl hy·per·tro·phies

hy·per·tro·phy
hy·per·tro·phied
hy·per·tro·phy·
ing

hy·per·tro·pia

hy·per·uri·ce·mia

hy·per·uri·ce·mic

hy·per·uri·cos·uria

hy·per·ven·ti·late
hy·per·ven·ti·lat·
ed
hy·per·ven·ti·lat·
ing

hy·per·ven·ti·la·
tion

hy·per·vi·ta·min·
osis
pl hy·per·vi·ta·min·
oses

hy·per·vi·ta·min·
ot·ic

hy·per·vol·emia

hy·per·vol·emic

hyp·es·the·sia
or hy·po·es·the·sia

hyp·es·thet·ic
or hy·po·es·thet·ic

hy·pha
pl hy·phae

hy·phal

hy·phe·ma

hyp·na·go·gic
also hyp·no·go·gic

hyp·na·go·gi·cal·ly

hyp·no·anal·y·sis
pl hyp·no·anal·y·ses

hyp·no·an·a·lyt·ic

hyp·no·an·es·the·
sia

hyp·no·gen·ic

hyp·noid
or hyp·noi·dal

hyp·nol·o·gy

hyp·none

hyp·no·pe·dia

hyp·no·pe·dic

hyp·no·pom·pic

hyp·no·sis
pl hyp·no·ses

hyp·no·ther·a·peu·
tic

hyp·no·ther·a·pist

hyp·no·ther·a·py
pl hyp·no·ther·a·pies

hyp·not·ic

hyp·not·i·cal·ly

hyp·no·tism

hyp·no·tist

hyp·no·tiz·abil·i·ty
pl hyp·no·tiz·abil·i·
ties

hyp·no·tiz·able

hyp·no·tize
hyp·no·tized
hyp·no·tiz·ing

hyp·no·tox·in

hy·po·acid·i·ty
pl hy·po·acid·i·ties

hy·po·ac·tive

hy·po·ac·tiv·i·ty
pl hy·po·ac·tiv·i·ties

hy·po·acu·sis

hy·po·adren·al·ism

hy·po·ad·re·no·cor·
ti·cism

hy·po·al·bu·min·
emia

hy·po·al·bu·min·
emic

hy·po·al·ge·sia

hy·po·al·ler·gen·ic

hy·po·ami·no·ac·
id·emia

hy·po·bar·ic

hy·po·bar·ism

hy·po·blast

hy·po·blas·tic

hy·po·bu·lia

hy·po·bu·lic

hy·po·cal·ce·mia

hy·po·cal·ce·mic

hy·po·cal·ci·fi·ca·
tion

hy·po·cap·nia

hy·po·cap·nic

hy·po·cel·lu·lar
hy·po·cel·lu·lar·i·ty
  pl hy·po·cel·lu·lar·i·ties

hy·po·chlor·emia
hy·po·chlor·emic
hy·po·chlor·hy·dria
hy·po·chlor·hy·dric
hy·po·chlo·rite
hy·po·chlo·rous
hy·po·cho·les·ter·ol·emia
  or hy·po·cho·les·ter·emia

hy·po·cho·les·ter·ol·emic
  or hy·po·cho·les·ter·emic

hy·po·chon·dria
hy·po·chon·dri·ac
hy·po·chon·dri·a·cal
hy·po·chon·dri·a·cal·ly
hy·po·chon·dri·a·sis
  pl hy·po·chon·dri·a·ses

hy·po·chon·dri·um
  pl hy·po·chon·dria

hy·po·chro·ma·sia
hy·po·chro·mat·ic
hy·po·chro·mia
hy·po·chro·mic

hy·po·co·ag·u·la·bil·i·ty
  pl hy·po·co·ag·u·la·bil·i·ties

hy·po·co·ag·u·la·ble
hy·po·com·ple·men·te·mia
hy·po·com·ple·men·te·mic
hy·po·con·dy·lar
hy·po·cone
hy·po·con·id
hy·po·con·u·lid
hy·po·cor·ti·cism
hy·po·cy·the·mia
hy·po·der·ma
hy·po·der·mal
hy·po·der·mat·ic
hy·po·der·ma·to·sis
hy·po·der·mi·a·sis
  pl hy·po·der·mi·a·ses

hy·po·der·mic
hy·po·der·mi·cal·ly
hy·po·der·mis
hy·po·der·moc·ly·sis
  pl hy·po·der·moc·ly·ses

hy·po·der·mo·sis
  pl hy·po·der·mo·ses

hy·po·dip·loid
hy·po·dip·loi·dy
  pl hy·po·dip·loi·dies

hy·po·don·tia
hy·po·don·tic
hy·po·dy·nam·ic

hy·po·er·gic
hy·po·er·gy
  pl hy·po·er·gies

hy·po·es·the·sia
  var of hypesthesia

hy·po·es·thet·ic
  var of hypesthetic

hy·po·fer·re·mia
hy·po·fer·re·mic
hy·po·fi·brin·o·gen·emia
hy·po·fi·brin·o·gen·emic
hy·po·func·tion
hy·po·ga·lac·tia
hy·po·gam·ma·glob·u·lin·emia
hy·po·gam·ma·glob·u·lin·emic
hy·po·gas·tric
hy·po·gas·tri·um
  pl hy·po·gas·tria

hy·po·gen·i·tal·ism
hy·po·geu·sia
hy·po·glos·sal
hy·po·glos·sus
  pl hy·po·glos·si

hy·po·glot·tis
  pl hy·po·glot·tis·es
  or hy·po·glot·ti·des

hy·po·glu·ce·mia
hy·po·gly·ce·mia
hy·po·gly·ce·mic
hy·po·go·nad·al
hy·po·go·nad·ism

hy·po·go·nad·o·
trop·ic
or hy·po·go·nad·o·tro·
phic
hy·po·hi·dro·sis
pl hy·po·hi·dro·ses
hy·po·his·ti·di·ne·
mia
hy·po·his·ti·di·ne·
mic
hy·po·hy·dra·tion
hy·po·in·su·lin·ism
hy·po·ka·le·mia
hy·po·ka·le·mic
hy·po·ki·ne·sia
hy·po·ki·ne·sis
pl hy·po·ki·ne·ses
hy·po·ki·net·ic
hy·po·li·pe·mia
hy·po·lip·id·emia
hy·po·lip·id·emic
hy·po·mag·ne·se·
mia
hy·po·mag·ne·se·
mic
hy·po·mag·ne·sia
hy·po·ma·nia
hy·po·ma·ni·ac
hy·po·man·ic
hy·po·mas·tia
hy·po·men·or·rhea
hy·po·mere
hy·po·meta·bol·ic
hy·po·me·tab·o·
lism
hy·po·me·tria

hy·po·min·er·al·
ized
hy·po·mo·bile
hy·po·morph
hy·po·mor·phic
hy·po·mo·til·i·ty
pl hy·po·mo·til·i·ties
hy·po·na·tre·mia
hy·po·na·tre·mic
hy·po·nych·i·al
hy·po·nych·i·um
hy·po·ovar·i·an·
ism
hy·po·para·thy·
roid
hy·po·para·thy·
roid·ism
hy·po·per·fu·sion
hy·po·pha·lan·
gism
hy·po·pha·ryn·geal
hy·po·phar·ynx
pl hy·po·pha·ryn·ges
also hy·po·phar·ynx·
es

hy·po·pho·nia
hy·po·phos·pha·ta·
sia
hy·po·phos·phate
hy·po·phos·pha·te·
mia
hy·po·phos·pha·te·
mic
hy·po·phos·phite
hy·po·phos·phor·ic
hy·po·phos·pho·
rous

hy·po·phy·se·al
also hy·po·phy·si·al

hy·poph·y·sec·to·
mize
hy·poph·y·sec·to·
mized
hy·poph·y·sec·to·
miz·ing
hy·poph·y·sec·to·
my
pl hy·poph·y·sec·to·
mies

hy·po·phys·io·tro·
pic
or hy·po·phys·io·tro·
phic
also hy·po·phys·eo·
tro·pic
or hy·po·phys·eo·tro·
phic

hy·poph·y·sis
pl hy·poph·y·ses

hy·poph·y·sis ce·
re·bri
hy·po·pig·men·ta·
tion
hy·po·pig·ment·ed
hy·po·pi·tu·ita·
rism
hy·po·pi·tu·itary
hy·po·pla·sia
hy·po·plas·tic
hy·po·ploid
hy·po·ploi·dy
pl hy·po·ploi·dies

hy·po·pnea

hy·po·po·tas·se·
mia
hy·po·po·tas·se·
mic
hy·po·pro·sex·ia
hy·po·pro·tein·
emia
hy·po·pro·tein·
emic
hy·po·pro·throm·
bin·emia
hy·po·pro·throm·
bin·emic
hy·po·py·on
hy·po·re·ac·tive
hy·po·re·ac·tiv·i·ty
  pl hy·po·re·ac·tiv·i·
  ties

hy·po·re·ac·tor
hy·po·re·flex·ia
hy·po·re·spon·sive
hy·po·ri·bo·fla·vin·
o·sis
  pl hy·po·ri·bo·fla·vin·
  o·ses

hy·po·sal·i·va·tion
hy·po·se·cre·tion
hy·po·sen·si·tive
hy·po·sen·si·tiv·i·ty
  pl hy·po·sen·si·tiv·i·
  ties

hy·po·sen·si·ti·za·
tion

hy·po·sen·si·tize
hy·po·sen·si·
  tized
hy·po·sen·si·tiz·
  ing
hy·pos·mia
hy·po·spa·dia
hy·po·spa·di·ac
hy·po·spa·di·as
hy·po·spa·dy
  pl hy·po·spa·dies

hy·pos·ta·sis
  pl hy·pos·ta·ses

hy·po·stat·ic
hy·po·sthe·nia
hy·po·sthen·ic
hy·pos·the·nu·ria
hy·pos·the·nu·ric
hy·po·styp·sis
hy·po·styp·tic
hy·po·ten·sion
hy·po·ten·sive
hy·po·tha·lam·ic
hy·po·tha·lam·i·
  cal·ly
hy·po·tha·lam·ico-
  hy·po·phy·se·al
  also hy·po·tha·lam·
  ico-hy·po·phy·si·al

hy·po·thal·a·mo-
  hy·po·phy·se·al
  also hy·po·thal·a·mo-
  hy·po·phy·si·al

hy·po·thal·a·mo-pi·
tu·itary

hy·po·thal·a·mot·o·
my
  pl hy·po·thal·a·mot·o·
  mies

hy·po·thal·a·mus
  pl hy·po·thal·a·mi

hy·po·the·nar
hy·po·ther·mia
hy·po·ther·mic
hy·po·ther·my
  pl hy·po·ther·mies

hy·poth·e·sis
  pl hy·poth·e·ses

hy·po·thy·mia
hy·po·thy·reo·sis
  or hy·po·thy·ro·sis

hy·po·thy·roid
hy·po·thy·roid·ism
hy·po·thy·rox·in·
  emia
hy·po·thy·rox·in·
  emic
hy·po·to·nia
hy·po·ton·ic
hy·po·ton·i·cal·ly
hy·po·to·nic·i·ty
  pl hy·po·to·nic·i·ties

hy·po·to·nus
hy·pot·o·ny
  pl hy·pot·o·nies

hy·po·trich·ia
hy·po·tri·cho·sis
  pl hy·po·tri·cho·ses

hy·po·tri·chot·ic

hy·pot·ro·phy
pl hy·pot·ro·phies

hy·po·tro·pia
hy·po·tym·pan·ic
hy·po·tym·pa·num
pl hy·po·tym·pa·na
also hy·po·tym·pa·nums

hy·po·uri·ce·mia
hy·po·uri·ce·mic
hy·po·uri·cos·uria
hy·po·ven·ti·lat·ed
hy·po·ven·ti·la·tion
hy·po·vi·ta·min·osis
hy·po·vi·ta·min·ot·ic
hy·po·vo·le·mia
hy·po·vo·le·mic
hy·po·xan·thine
hy·po·xan·thine-gua·nine
hyp·ox·emia
hyp·ox·emic
hyp·ox·ia
hyp·ox·ic
hyps·ar·rhyth·mia
or hyps·arhyth·mia

hyps·ar·rhyth·mic
or hyps·arhyth·mic

hyp·si·ce·phal·ic
hyp·si·ceph·a·ly
pl hyp·si·ceph·a·lies

hyp·so·chrome

hyp·so·chro·mic
hyp·so·dont
hyp·so·don·ty
pl hyp·so·don·ties

hys·sop
hys·ter·ec·to·mized
hys·ter·ec·to·my
pl hys·ter·ec·to·mies

hys·ter·e·sis
pl hys·ter·e·ses

hys·te·ria
hys·te·ri·a·gen·ic
hys·ter·ic
noun

hys·ter·i·cal
also hys·ter·ic
adjective

hys·ter·i·form
hys·tero·col·pec·to·my
pl hys·tero·col·pec·to·mies

hys·tero-ep·i·lep·sy
pl hys·tero-ep·i·lep·sies

hys·tero-ep·i·lep·tic
hys·ter·o·gen·ic
hys·ter·o·gram
hys·ter·o·graph
hys·ter·o·graph·ic
hys·ter·og·ra·phy
pl hys·ter·og·ra·phies

hys·ter·oid
hys·tero·oo·pho·rec·to·my
pl hys·tero·oo·pho·rec·to·mies

hys·ter·o·pexy
pl hys·ter·o·pex·ies

hys·ter·o·plas·ty
pl hys·ter·o·plas·ties

hys·ter·or·rha·phy
pl hys·ter·or·rha·phies

hys·ter·or·rhex·is
pl hys·ter·or·rhex·es

hys·ter·o·sal·pin·gog·ra·phy
pl hys·ter·o·sal·pin·gog·ra·phies

hys·ter·o·sal·pin·gos·to·my
pl hys·ter·o·sal·pin·gos·to·mies

hys·ter·o·scope
hys·ter·o·scop·ic
hys·ter·os·co·py
pl hys·ter·os·co·pies

hys·ter·o·sto·mat·o·my
pl hys·ter·o·sto·mat·o·mies

hys·ter·ot·o·my
pl hys·ter·ot·o·mies

I

iat·ric
iat·ro·chem·i·cal
iat·ro·chem·ist
iat·ro·chem·is·try
  pl iat·ro·chem·is·tries
iat·ro·gen·e·sis
  pl iat·ro·gen·e·ses
iat·ro·gen·ic
iat·ro·ge·nic·i·ty
  pl iat·ro·ge·nic·i·ties
iat·ro·math·e·mat·ics
iatro·phys·i·cal
iat·ro·phys·i·cist
iat·ro·phys·ics
ibo·ga·ine
ibu·pro·fen
ichor
ichor·ous
ich·tham·mol
ich·thyo·acantho·tox·ism
ich·thyo·col·la
  or ich·thyo·col
  or ich·thyo·coll
ich·thyo·he·mo·tox·ism
ich·thy·oid
ich·thy·oph·a·gous
ich·thyo·sar·co·tox·in
ich·thyo·sar·co·tox·ism
ich·thy·o·si·form

ich·thy·o·sis
  pl ich·thy·o·ses
ich·thy·o·sis hys·trix gra·vi·or
ich·thy·o·sis sim·plex
ich·thy·o·sis vul·gar·is
ich·thy·ot·ic
ich·thyo·tox·in
ich·thyo·tox·ism
ic·tal
ic·ter·ic
ic·tero·ane·mia
ic·ter·o·gen·ic
ic·ter·oid
ic·ter·us
ic·ter·us gra·vis
ic·ter·us gra·vis neo·na·tor·um
ic·ter·us neo·na·tor·um
ic·tus
id
idea
ide·al·iza·tion
ide·al·ize
  ide·al·ized
  ide·al·iz·ing
ide·ation
ide·ation·al
idée fixe
  pl idées fixes
iden·ti·fi·ca·tion
iden·ti·fy
  iden·ti·fied
  iden·ti·fy·ing

iden·ti·ty
  pl iden·ti·ties
ideo·mo·tor
ideo·pho·bia
id·io·blap·sis
  pl id·io·blap·sis·es
id·io·blap·tic
id·io·chro·mo·some
id·i·o·cy
  pl id·i·o·cies
id·io·gen·e·sis
  pl id·io·gen·e·ses
idio·ge·net·ic
id·io·glos·sia
id·io·gram
id·io·ki·net·ic
id·io·mus·cu·lar
id·io·path·ic
id·io·path·i·cal·ly
id·i·op·a·thy
  pl id·i·op·a·thies
id·io·plasm
id·io·ret·i·nal
id·io·some
id·io·syn·cra·sy
  pl id·io·syn·cra·sies
id·io·syn·crat·ic
id·i·ot
id·i·ot sa·vant
  pl id·i·ots sa·vants
  or id·i·ot sa·vants
id·io·type
id·io·typ·ic
id·io·ven·tric·u·lar
idox·uri·dine
ig·na·tia

Ig·na·tius bean
ig·ni·punc·ture
il·ea
   pl of ileum
il·e·al
   also il·e·ac
il·e·itis
   pl il·e·it·i·des
il·eo·ce·cal
il·eo·co·lic
il·eo·co·li·tis
il·eo·co·los·to·my
   pl il·eo·co·los·to·mies
il·eo·cyto·plas·ty
   pl il·eo·cyto·plas·ties
il·eo·il·e·al
il·eo·proc·tos·to·
  my
   pl il·eo·proc·tos·to·
   mies
il·eo·sig·moid·os·
  to·my
   pl il·eo·sig·moid·os·
   to·mies
il·e·os·to·my
   pl il·e·os·to·mies
il·eo·trans·verse
il·e·um
   pl il·ea
il·e·us
il·ia
   pl of ilium
il·i·ac
   also il·i·al
ili·a·cus
   pl ili·a·ci

il·i·al
   var of iliac
il·io·coc·cy·ge·us
   pl il·io·coc·cy·gei
il·io·cos·ta·lis
il·io·cos·ta·lis cer·
  vi·cis
il·io·cos·ta·lis dor·
  si
il·io·cos·ta·lis lum·
  bor·um
il·io·cos·tal·is tho·
  ra·cis
il·io·fem·o·ral
il·io·hy·po·gas·tric
il·io·in·gui·nal
il·io·lum·bar
il·io·pec·tin·e·al
il·io·pso·as
il·io·tib·i·al
il·i·um
   pl il·ia
ill
il·lin·i·um
il·lu·mi·nant
il·lu·mi·nate
  il·lu·mi·nat·ed
  il·lu·mi·nat·ing
il·lu·mi·na·tion
il·lu·mi·na·tor
il·lu·sion
il·lu·sion·al
il·lu·so·ry
image
  im·aged
  im·ag·ing

im·ag·ery
   pl im·ag·eries
imag·i·nal
imag·i·nary
imag·i·na·tion
imag·ine
  imag·ined
  imag·in·ing
ima·go
   pl ima·goes
   or ima·gi·nes
im·bal·ance
im·bal·anced
im·be·cile
   noun
im·be·cile
   or im·be·cil·ic
   adjective
im·be·cil·i·ty
   pl im·be·cil·i·ties
im·bed
   var of embed
im·bibe
  im·bibed
  im·bib·ing
im·bi·bi·tion
im·bri·cate
  im·bri·cat·ed
  im·bri·cat·ing
im·bri·ca·tion
im·id·az·ole
im·id·az·o·line
im·ide
im·i·do
im·ine
im·i·no
im·i·no·di·ace·tic

im·i·no·gly·cin·
uria
imip·ra·mine
im·ma·ture
im·ma·tu·ri·ty
pl im·ma·tu·ri·ties
im·me·di·ate
im·med·i·ca·ble
im·mer·sion
im·mis·ci·bil·i·ty
pl im·mis·ci·bil·i·ties
im·mis·ci·ble
im·mo·bi·li·za·tion
im·mo·bile
im·mo·bil·i·ty
pl im·mo·bil·i·ties
im·mo·bi·lize
im·mo·bi·lized
im·mo·bi·liz·ing
im·mune
im·mu·ni·ty
pl im·mu·ni·ties
im·mu·ni·za·tion
im·mu·nize
im·mu·nized
im·mu·niz·ing
im·mu·no·ab·sor·
bent
or im·mu·no·ab·sor·
bant
im·mu·no·ad·ju·
vant
im·mu·no·ad·sor·
bent
im·mu·no·ad·sorp·
tion
im·mu·no·as·say

im·mu·no·as·say·
able
im·mu·no·bi·o·log·
i·cal
or im·mu·no·bi·o·log·
ic
im·mu·no·bi·ol·o·
gist
im·mu·no·bi·ol·o·
gy
pl im·mu·no·bi·ol·o·
gies
im·mu·no·blast
im·mu·no·blas·tic
im·mu·no·chem·i·
cal
im·mu·no·chem·
ist
im·mu·no·chem·is·
try
pl im·mu·no·chem·is·
tries
im·mu·no·che·mo·
ther·a·py
pl im·mu·no·che·mo·
ther·a·pies
im·mu·no·com·pe·
tence
im·mu·no·com·pe·
tent
im·mu·no·com·
pro·mised
im·mu·no·con·glu·
ti·nin
im·mu·no·cyte
im·mu·no·cy·to·
chem·i·cal

im·mu·no·cy·to·
chem·is·try
pl im·mu·no·cy·to·
chem·is·tries
im·mu·no·de·fi·
cien·cy
pl im·mu·no·de·fi·
cien·cies
im·mu·no·de·fi·
cient
im·mu·no·de·pres·
sant
im·mu·no·de·pres·
sion
im·mu·no·de·pres·
sive
im·mu·no·di·ag·no·
sis
pl im·mu·no·di·ag·
no·ses
im·mu·no·di·ag·
nos·tic
im·mu·no·dif·fu·
sion
im·mu·no·elec·tro·
pho·re·sis
pl im·mu·no·elec·tro·
pho·re·ses
im·mu·no·elec·tro·
pho·ret·ic
im·mu·no·fer·ri·
tin
im·mu·no·flu·o·
res·cence
im·mu·no·flu·o·
res·cent
im·mu·no·gen

im·mu·no·gen·e·sis
  pl im·mu·no·gen·e·ses

im·mu·no·ge·net·ic
im·mu·no·ge·net·i·cal·ly
im·mu·no·ge·net·i·cist
im·mu·no·gen·ic
im·mu·no·ge·nic·i·ty
  pl im·mu·no·ge·nic·i·ties

im·mu·no·glob·u·lin
im·mu·no·he·ma·to·log·ic
  or im·mu·no·he·ma·to·log·i·cal

im·mu·no·he·ma·tol·o·gist
im·mu·no·he·ma·tol·o·gy
  pl im·mu·no·he·ma·tol·o·gies

im·mu·no·he·mo·ly·sis
  pl im·mu·no·he·mo·ly·ses

im·mu·no·he·mo·lyt·ic
im·mu·no·his·to·chem·i·cal
im·mu·no·his·to·chem·is·try
  pl im·mu·no·his·to·chem·is·tries

im·mu·no·his·to·log·i·cal
  also im·mu·no·his·to·log·ic

im·mu·no·his·tol·o·gy
  pl im·mu·no·his·tol·o·gies

im·mu·no·log·ic
  or im·mu·no·log·i·cal

im·mu·nol·o·gist
im·mu·nol·o·gy
  pl im·mu·nol·o·gies

im·mu·no·par·a·si·tol·o·gist
im·mu·no·par·a·si·tol·o·gy
  pl im·mu·no·par·a·si·tol·o·gies

im·mu·no·patho·gen·e·sis
  pl im·mu·no·patho·gen·e·ses

im·mu·no·path·o·log·ic
  or im·mu·no·path·o·log·i·cal

im·mu·no·pa·thol·o·gist
im·mu·no·pa·thol·o·gy
  pl im·mu·no·pa·thol·o·gies

im·mu·no·phar·ma·col·o·gy
  pl im·mu·no·phar·ma·col·o·gies

im·mu·no·po·ten·ti·at·ing
im·mu·no·po·ten·ti·a·tion
im·mu·no·po·ten·ti·a·tor
im·mu·no·pre·cip·i·ta·ble
im·mu·no·pre·cip·i·tate
  im·mu·no·pre·cip·i·tat·ed
  im·mu·no·pre·cip·i·tat·ing

im·mu·no·pre·cip·i·ta·tion
im·mu·no·pro·lif·er·a·tive
im·mu·no·pro·phy·lac·tic
im·mu·no·pro·phy·lax·is
  pl im·mu·no·pro·phy·lax·es

im·mu·no·ra·dio·met·ric
im·mu·no·re·ac·tion
im·mu·no·re·ac·tive
im·mu·no·re·ac·tiv·i·ty
  pl im·mu·no·re·ac·tiv·i·ties

im·mu·no·reg·u·la·tion

im·mu·no·reg·u·la·to·ry
im·mu·no·se·lec·tion
im·mu·no·sor·bent
im·mu·no·stim·u·lant
im·mu·no·stim·u·la·ting
im·mu·no·stim·u·la·tion
im·mu·no·sup·press
im·mu·no·sup·pres·sant
im·mu·no·sup·pres·sion
im·mu·no·sup·pres·sive
im·mu·no·sup·pres·sor
im·mu·no·sur·veil·lance
im·mu·no·sym·pa·thec·to·mized
im·mu·no·sym·pa·thec·to·my
pl im·mu·no·sym·pa·thec·to·mies
im·mu·no·ther·a·peu·tic
im·mu·no·ther·a·pist
im·mu·no·ther·a·py
pl im·mu·no·ther·a·pies

im·pact·ed
im·pac·tion
im·pair
im·pair·ment
im·pal·pa·ble
im·par
im·ped·ance
im·ped·i·ment
im·per·cep·tion
im·per·fo·rate
im·per·me·abil·i·ty
pl im·per·me·abil·i·ties
im·per·me·able
im·pe·tig·i·ni·za·tion
im·pe·tig·i·nized
im·pe·tig·i·nous
im·pe·ti·go
im·pe·ti·go con·ta·gi·o·sa
im·plant
im·plant·able
im·plan·ta·tion
im·plant·ee
im·plan·tol·o·gist
im·plan·tol·o·gy
pl im·plan·tol·o·gies
im·plo·sive ther·a·py
im·po·tence
im·po·ten·cy
pl im·po·ten·cies
im·po·tent
im·preg·nate
im·preg·nat·ed
im·preg·nat·ing

im·preg·na·tion
im·pres·sion
im·print
im·print·er
im·print·ing
im·pulse
im·pul·sion
im·pul·sive
im·pul·siv·i·ty
pl im·pul·siv·i·ties
im·pure
in·ac·ti·vate
in·ac·ti·vat·ed
in·ac·ti·vat·ing
in·ac·ti·va·tion
in·ac·ti·va·tor
in·ac·tive
in·ac·tiv·i·ty
pl in·ac·tiv·i·ties
in·ad·e·qua·cy
pl in·ad·e·qua·cies
in·ad·e·quate
in·ag·glu·ti·na·bil·i·ty
pl in·ag·glu·ti·na·bil·i·ties
in·ag·glu·ti·na·ble
in·a·ni·tion
in·ap·par·ent
in·ap·pe·tence
in ar·ti·cu·lo mor·tis
in·at·tend
in·at·ten·tion
in·at·ten·tive
in·born

in·breed
in·bred
in·breed·ing
in·ca·pac·i·tant
in·car·cer·at·ed
in·car·cer·a·tion
in·cest
in·ces·tu·ous
in·ci·dence
in·cip·i·en·cy
pl in·cip·i·en·cies

in·cip·i·ent
in·ci·sal
in·cise
in·cised
in·cis·ing
in·ci·si·form
in·ci·sion
in·ci·sion·al
in·ci·sive
in·ci·sor
in·ci·su·ra
pl in·ci·su·rae

in·ci·su·ral
in·ci·sure
in·cit·ant
in·cli·na·tion
in·clu·sion
in·co·ag·u·la·bil·i·ty
pl in·co·ag·u·la·bil·i·ties

in·co·ag·u·la·ble
in·co·erc·ible

in·com·pat·i·bil·i·ty
pl in·com·pat·i·bil·i·ties

in·com·pat·i·ble
in·com·pen·sa·tion
in·com·pen·sa·to·ry
in·com·pe·tence
in·com·pe·ten·cy
pl in·com·pe·ten·cies

in·com·pe·tent
in·com·plete
in·con·ti·nence
in·con·ti·nent
in·co·or·di·nat·ed
also in·co·or·di·nate

in·co·or·di·na·tion
in·cor·po·ra·tion
in·cre·ment
in·cre·men·tal
in·cre·to·ry
in·cross
in·crus·ta·tion
in·cu·bate
in·cu·bat·ed
in·cu·bat·ing
in·cu·ba·tion
in·cu·ba·tion·al
in·cu·ba·tor
in·cu·do·mal·le·al
in·cu·do·mal·le·o·lar
in·cu·do·sta·pe·di·al
in·cur·able
in·cur·ably

in·cus
pl in·cu·des

in·dane·di·one
or in·dan·di·one

in·de·cent
in·de·pen·dent
in·de·ter·mi·nate
in·dex
pl in·dex·es
or in·di·ces

in·dia rub·ber
in·di·can
in·di·can·uria
in·di·cate
in·di·cat·ed
in·di·cat·ing
in·di·ca·tion
in·di·ca·tor
in·dif·fer·ent
in·dig·e·nous
in·di·gest·ibil·i·ty
pl in·di·gest·ibil·i·ties

in·di·gest·ible
in·di·ges·tion
in·di·go
pl in·di·gos
or in·di·goes

in·di·rect
in·di·ru·bin
in·dis·posed
in·dis·po·si·tion
in·di·um
in·di·vid·u·ate
in·di·vid·u·at·ed
in·di·vid·u·at·ing
in·di·vid·u·a·tion
in·do·cy·a·nine

in·dole
in·dole·ace·tic
in·dole·amine
in·do·lence
in·do·lent
in·dol·uria
in·do·meth·a·cin
in·do·phe·nol
In·do·pla·nor·bis
in·dox·yl·uria
in·duce
  in·duced
  in·duc·ing
in·duc·er
in·duc·ibil·i·ty
  pl in·duc·ibil·i·ties
in·duc·ible
in·duct
in·duc·tion
in·duc·tive
in·duc·tor
in·duc·to·ri·um
in·duc·to·ther·my
  pl in·duc·to·ther·mies
in·du·rat·ed
in·du·ra·tion
in·du·ra·tive
in·du·si·um
  pl in·du·sia
in·du·si·um gris·e·um
in·dwell·ing
ine·bri·ant
ine·bri·ate
  ine·bri·at·ed
  ine·bri·at·ing
ine·bri·a·tion

in·ebri·ety
  pl in·ebri·eties
in·er·tia
in·ex·tre·mis
in·fan·cy
  pl in·fan·cies
in·fant
in·fan·ti·ci·dal
in·fan·ti·cide
in·fan·tile
in·fan·til·ism
in·farct
in·farct·ed
in·farc·tion
in·fect
in·fec·tant
in·fec·tion
in·fec·tious
in·fec·tive
in·fec·tiv·i·ty
  pl in·fec·tiv·i·ties
in·fec·tor
in·fe·cund
in·fe·cun·di·ty
  pl in·fe·cun·di·ties
in·fe·ri·or
in·fe·ri·or·i·ty
  pl in·fe·ri·or·i·ties
in·fe·ro·me·di·al
in·fer·tile
in·fer·til·i·ty
  pl in·fer·til·i·ties
in·fest
in·fes·ta·tion
in·fib·u·la·tion

in·fil·trate
  in·fil·trat·ed
  in·fil·trat·ing
in·fil·tra·tion
in·fil·tra·tive
in·firm
in·fir·mar·i·an
in·fir·ma·ry
  pl in·fir·ma·ries
in·fir·mi·ty
  pl in·fir·mi·ties
in·flame
  in·flamed
  in·flam·ing
in·flam·ma·tion
in·flam·ma·to·ry
in·flat·able
in·flate
  in·flat·ed
  in·flat·ing
in·fla·tion
in·flec·tion
in·flu·en·za
in·flu·en·zal
in·fold
in·formed
in·for·mo·some
in·fra·cla·vic·u·lar
in·fra·den·ta·le
in·fra·gle·noid
in·fra·glot·tic
in·fra·hu·man
in·fra·hy·oid
in·fra·mam·ma·ry
in·fra·nu·cle·ar
in·fra·oc·clu·sion
in·fra·or·bit·al

in·fra·pa·tel·lar
in·fra·red
in·fra·re·nal
in·fra·sound
in·fra·spi·na·tus
  pl in·fra·spi·na·ti
in·fra·spi·nous
in·fra·tem·po·ral
in·fra·ten·to·ri·al
in·fra·um·bil·i·cal
in·fun·dib·u·lar
in·fun·dib·u·li·
  form
in·fun·dib·u·lo·pel·
  vic
in·fun·dib·u·lum
  pl in·fun·dib·u·la
in·fuse
  in·fused
  in·fus·ing
in·fu·sion
In·fu·so·ria
in·fu·so·ri·an
in·gest
in·ges·ta
in·ges·tant
in·gest·ible
in·ges·tion
in·gest·ive
in·glu·vi·es
  pl in·glu·vi·es
in·glu·vi·itis
  or in·glu·vi·tis
in·gra·ves·cence
in·gre·di·ent
in·grow·ing
in·grown

in·growth
in·guen
  pl ingui·na
in·gui·nal
in·hal·ant
  also in·hal·ent
in·ha·la·tion
in·ha·la·tion·al
in·ha·la·tor
in·hale
  in·haled
  in·hal·ing
in·hal·er
in·her·it
in·her·it·abil·i·ty
  pl in·her·it·abil·i·ties
in·her·it·able
in·her·i·tance
in·hib·it
in·hi·bi·tion
in·hib·i·tor
in·hib·i·to·ry
in·ho·mo·ge·ne·ity
  pl in·ho·mo·ge·ne·
  ities
in·ho·mo·ge·neous
in·i·ac
in·i·en·ce·phal·ic
in·i·en·ceph·a·lus
in·i·en·ceph·a·ly
  pl in·i·en·ceph·a·lies
in·i·on
ini·ti·a·tor
in·ject
in·ject·able
in·jec·tant
in·jec·tion

in·jec·tor
in·jure
  in·jured
  in·jur·ing
in·ju·ri·ous
in·ju·ry
  pl in·ju·ries
in·lay
in·let
in·mate
in·nards
in·nate
in·ner-di·rect·ed
in·ner-di·rec·tion
in·ner·vate
  in·ner·vat·ed
  in·ner·vat·ing
in·ner·va·tion
  nerve supply (see ener·
  vation)
in·noc·u·ous
in·nom·i·nate
in·oc·u·la·bil·i·ty
  pl in·oc·u·la·bil·i·ties
in·oc·u·la·ble
in·oc·u·late
  in·oc·u·lat·ed
  in·oc·u·lat·ing
in·oc·u·la·tion
in·oc·u·la·tor
in·oc·u·lum
  pl in·oc·u·la
in·op·er·a·bil·i·ty
  pl in·op·er·a·bil·i·ties
in·op·er·a·ble
in·or·gan·ic
in·or·gan·i·cal·ly

in·or·gas·mic
in·os·cu·la·tion
ino·se·mia
ino·sin·ate
ino·sine
ino·sin·ic
ino·si·tol
ino·tro·pic
ino·tro·pism
in·pa·tient
in·quest
in·qui·line
in·qui·lin·ism
in·sal·i·vate
  in·sal·i·vat·ed
  in·sal·i·vat·ing
in·sal·i·va·tion
in·sa·lu·bri·ous
in·sane
in·san·i·tary
in·san·i·ty
  pl in·san·i·ties
in·scrip·tion
in·sect
In·sec·ta
in·sec·tan
in·sec·ti·cid·al
in·sec·ti·cide
in·sec·ti·fuge
In·sec·tiv·o·ra
in·sec·ti·vore
in·se·cure
in·se·cu·ri·ty
  pl in·se·cu·ri·ties
in·sem·i·nate
  in·sem·i·nat·ed
  in·sem·i·nat·ing

in·sem·i·na·tion
in·sen·si·bil·i·ty
  pl in·sen·si·bil·i·ties
in·sen·si·ble
in·sert
in·ser·tion
in·sid·i·ous
in·sight
in si·tu
in·so·la·tion
in·sol·u·ble
in·som·nia
in·som·ni·ac
in·spi·ra·tion
in·spi·ra·tor
in·spire
  in·spired
  in·spir·ing
in·spi·rom·e·ter
in·spis·sat·ed
in·spis·sa·tion
in·spis·sa·tor
in·sta·bil·i·ty
  pl in·sta·bil·i·ties
in·step
in·still
  in·stilled
  in·still·ing
in·stil·la·tion
in·stinct
in·stinc·tive
in·stinc·tu·al
in·sti·tu·tion·al·iza·tion

in·sti·tu·tion·al·ize
  in·sti·tu·tion·al·ized
  in·sti·tu·tion·al·iz·ing
in·stru·ment
in·stru·men·tal
in·stru·men·tar·ium
  pl in·stru·men·tar·ia
in·stru·men·ta·tion
in·suf·fi·cien·cy
  pl in·suf·fi·cien·cies
in·suf·fi·cient
in·suf·flate
in·suf·fla·tion
in·suf·fla·tor
in·su·la
  pl in·su·lae
in·su·lar
in·su·lin
in·su·lin·ase
in·su·lin·emia
in·su·li·no·gen·ic
in·su·lin·oid
in·su·lin·o·ma
  pl in·su·lin·o·mas
  or in·su·lin·o·ma·ta
in·su·li·no·tro·pic
in·su·lo·ma
  pl in·su·lo·mas
  or in·su·lo·ma·ta
in·sus·cep·ti·bil·i·ty
  pl in·sus·cep·ti·bil·i·ties
in·sus·cep·ti·ble

in·take
in·te·grate
 in·te·grat·ed
 in·te·grat·ing
in·te·gra·tion
in·te·gra·tive
in·te·gra·tor
in·teg·ri·ty
 pl in·teg·ri·ties
in·teg·u·ment
in·teg·u·men·ta·ry
in·tel·lect
in·tel·lec·tu·al
in·tel·lec·tu·al·iza·tion
in·tel·lec·tu·al·ize
 in·tel·lec·tu·al·ized
 in·tel·lec·tu·al·iz·ing
in·tel·li·gence
in·tel·li·gent
in·tem·per·ance
in·tem·per·ate
in·tense
in·ten·sive
in·ten·tion
in·ter·ac·i·nar
 or in·ter·ac·i·nous
in·ter·al·ve·o·lar
in·ter·atri·al
in·ter·au·ral
in·ter·au·ric·u·lar
in·ter·body
in·ter·brain

in·ter·breed
 in·ter·bred
 in·ter·breed·ing
in·ter·ca·lat·ed
in·ter·cap·il·lary
in·ter·car·pal
in·ter·cav·ern·ous
in·ter·cel·lu·lar
in·ter·ce·re·bral
in·ter·con·dy·lar
in·ter·con·dy·loid
in·ter·cor·o·nary
in·ter·cos·tal
in·ter·cos·to·bra·chi·al
in·ter·course
in·ter·cris·tal
in·ter·crit·i·cal
in·ter·cross
in·ter·cru·ral
in·ter·cur·rent
in·ter·cus·pal
in·ter·cus·pa·tion
 or in·ter·cus·pi·da·tion
in·ter·den·tal
in·ter·dig·i·tal
in·ter·dig·i·tate
 in·ter·dig·i·tat·ed
 in·ter·dig·i·tat·ing
in·ter·dig·i·ta·tion
in·ter·fas·cic·u·lar
in·ter·fem·o·ral
in·ter·fere
 in·ter·fered
 in·ter·fer·ing

in·ter·fer·ence
in·ter·fer·om·e·ter
in·ter·fer·o·met·ric
in·ter·fer·o·met·ri·cal·ly
in·ter·fer·om·e·try
 pl in·ter·fer·om·e·tries
in·ter·fer·on
in·ter·fer·tile
in·ter·fer·til·i·ty
 pl in·ter·fer·til·i·ties
in·ter·fi·bril·lar
 or in·ter·fi·bril·lary
in·ter·fol·lic·u·lar
in·ter·fron·tal
in·ter·gan·gli·on·ic
in·ter·ge·nic
in·ter·glob·u·lar
in·ter·glu·te·al
in·ter·hemi·spher·ic
 also in·ter·hemi·spher·al
in·ter·ic·tal
in·ter·in·di·vid·u·al
in·ter·ki·ne·sis
 pl in·ter·ki·ne·ses
in·ter·ki·net·ic
in·ter·leu·kin
in·ter·lo·bar
in·ter·lob·u·lar
in·ter·max·il·lary
 pl in·ter·max·il·lar·ies
in·ter·me·di·ary
 pl in·ter·me·di·ar·ies

in·ter·me·din
in·ter·me·dio·lat·er·al
in·ter·me·di·us
in·ter·mem·bra·nous
in·ter·men·in·ge·al
in·ter·men·stru·al
in·ter·mis·sion
in·ter·mit·tence
in·ter·mit·tent
in·ter·mus·cu·lar
in·tern
   also in·terne
in·ter·nal
in·ter·nal·iza·tion
in·ter·nal·ize
   in·ter·nal·ized
   in·ter·nal·iz·ing
in·ter·na·sal
in·ter·neu·ron
in·ter·neu·ro·nal
in·ter·nist
in·ter·no·dal
in·ter·node
in·ter·nu·cle·ar
in·ter·nun·ci·al
in·ter·oc·clu·sal
in·tero·cep·tive
in·tero·cep·tor
in·ter·o·fec·tive
in·ter·or·bit·al
in·ter·os·se·ous
in·ter·os·se·us
   pl in·ter·os·sei
in·ter·pa·ri·etal

in·ter·par·ox·ys·mal
in·ter·pe·dun·cu·lar
in·ter·per·son·al
in·ter·pha·lan·ge·al
in·ter·phase
in·ter·pha·sic
in·ter·po·lat·ed
in·ter·pris·mat·ic
in·ter·prox·i·mal
in·ter·pu·pil·lary
in·ter·ra·dic·u·lar
in·ter·scap·u·lar
in·ter·seg·men·tal
in·ter·sen·so·ry
in·ter·sex
in·ter·sex·u·al
in·ter·sex·u·al·i·ty
   pl in·ter·sex·u·al·i·ties
in·ter·space
in·ter·spi·nal
in·ter·spi·na·lis
   pl in·ter·spi·na·les
in·ter·ster·ile
in·ter·ste·ril·i·ty
   pl in·ter·ste·ril·i·ties
in·ter·stice
   pl in·ter·stic·es
in·ter·stim·u·lus
in·ter·sti·tial
in·ter·sti·tium
   pl in·ter·sti·tia
in·ter·tar·sal
in·ter·trans·ver·sa·les

in·ter·trans·ver·sar·ii
in·ter·trig·i·nous
in·ter·tri·go
in·ter·tro·chan·ter·ic
in·ter·tu·ber·cu·lar
in·ter·tu·bu·lar
in·ter·val
in·ter·vene
   in·ter·vened
   in·ter·ven·ing
in·ter·ven·tion
in·ter·ven·tion·al
in·ter·ven·tric·u·lar
in·ter·ver·te·bral
in·ter·vil·lous
in·tes·ti·nal
in·tes·tine
in·ti·ma
   pl in·ti·mae
   or in·ti·mas
in·ti·mal
in·toed
in·toe·ing
in·tol·er·ance
in·tol·er·ant
in·tor·sion
   or in·tor·tion
in·tort·ed
in·tox·i·cant
in·tox·i·cate
   in·tox·i·cat·ed
   in·tox·i·cat·ing
in·tox·i·ca·tion
in·tra·ab·dom·i·nal
in·tra·al·ve·o·lar

in·tra-am·ni·ot·ic
in·tra-am·ni·ot·i·
  cal·ly
in·tra-aor·tic
in·tra-ar·te·ri·al
in·tra-ar·tic·u·lar
in·tra-atri·al
in·tra-ax·o·nal
in·tra-buc·cal
in·tra-can·a·lic·u·
  lar
in·tra-cap·il·lary
in·tra-cap·su·lar
in·tra-car·di·ac
  also in·tra·car·di·al
in·tra-ca·rot·id
in·tra-car·ti·lag·i·
  nous
in·tra-cav·i·tar·i·ly
in·tra-cav·i·tary
in·tra-cel·lu·lar
in·tra-cel·lu·lar·ly
in·tra-cer·e·bel·lar
in·tra-ce·re·bral
in·tra-cis·ter·nal
in·tra-co·ro·nal
in·tra-cor·o·nary
in·tra-cor·po·re·al
in·tra-cor·pus·cu·
  lar
in·tra-cor·ti·cal
in·tra-cra·ni·al
in·trac·ta·bil·i·ty
  pl in·trac·ta·bil·i·ties
in·trac·ta·ble
in·tra-cu·ta·ne·ous

in·tra-cy·to·plas·
  mic
in·tra-der·mal
in·tra-der·mo·re·
  ac·tion
in·tra-duc·tal
in·tra-du·o·de·nal
in·tra-du·ral
in·tra-epi·der·mal
in·tra-ep·i·the·li·al
in·tra-eryth·ro·cyt·
  ic
in·tra-fa·mil·ial
in·tra-fol·lic·u·lar
in·tra-fu·sal
in·tra-gas·tric
in·tra-gen·ic
in·tra-group
in·tra-he·pat·ic
in·tra-he·pat·i·cal·
  ly
in·tra-hos·pi·tal
in·tra-in·di·vid·u·al
in·tra-jug·u·lar
in·tra-la·mel·lar
in·tra-lam·i·nar
in·tra-len·tic·u·lar
in·tra-le·sion·al
in·tra-leu·ko·cyt·ic
in·tra-lo·bar
in·tra-lob·u·lar
in·tra-lu·mi·nal
in·tra-lym·phat·ic
in·tra-mam·ma·ry
in·tra-med·ul·lary
in·tra-mem·brane

in·tra-mem·bra·
  nous
in·tra-mi·to·chon·
  dri·al
in·tra-mo·lec·u·lar
in·tra-mu·co·sal
in·tra-mu·ral
in·tra-mus·cu·lar
in·tra-myo·car·di·
  al
in·tra-na·sal
in·tra-na·tal
in·tra-neu·ral
in·tra-neu·ro·nal
in·tra-nu·cle·ar
in·tra-nu·cle·o·lar
in·tra-oc·u·lar
in·tra-op·er·a·tive
in·tra-oral
in·tra-os·se·ous
in·tra-ovu·lar
in·tra-par·tum
in·tra-pel·vic
in·tra-pleu·ral
in·tra-pop·u·la·tion
in·tra-pul·mo·nar·
  i·ly
in·tra-pul·mo·nary
  also in·tra·pul·mon·ic
in·tra-rec·tal
in·tra-re·nal
in·tra-ret·i·nal
in·tra-scro·tal
in·tra-spi·nal
in·tra-splen·ic
in·tra-sy·no·vi·al
in·tra-tes·tic·u·lar

in·tra·the·cal
in·tra·tho·rac·ic
in·tra·thy·roi·dal
in·tra·tra·che·al
in·tra·tu·bu·lar
in·tra·tym·pan·ic
in·tra·ure·thral
in·tra·uter·ine
in·tra·vag·i·nal
in·trav·a·sa·tion
in·tra·ve·nous
in·tra·ven·tric·u·lar
in·tra·ver·te·bral
in·tra·ves·i·cal
in·tra·vi·tal
in·tra·vi·tam
in·tra·vit·re·ous
in·trin·sic
in·tro·duce
  in·tro·duced
  in·tro·duc·ing
in·tro·duc·tion
in·troi·tal
in·troi·tus
in·tro·ject
in·tro·jec·tion
in·tro·jec·tive
in·tro·mis·sion
in·tro·mit·tent
in·tron
in·tro·pu·ni·tive
in·tro·spect
in·tro·spec·tion
in·tro·spec·tion·ist
in·tro·spec·tion·is·
  tic
in·tro·spec·tive

in·tro·ver·sion
in·tro·ver·sive
in·tro·vert
in·tu·bate
  in·tu·bat·ed
  in·tu·bat·ing
in·tu·ba·tion
in·tu·it
in·tu·ition
in·tu·ition·al
in·tu·itive
in·tu·mesce
  in·tu·mesced
  in·tu·mesc·ing
in·tu·mes·cence
in·tu·mes·cent
in·tus·sus·cept
in·tus·sus·cep·tion
in·tus·sus·cep·tive
in·tus·sus·cep·tum
  pl in·tus·sus·cep·ta
in·tus·sus·cip·i·ens
  pl in·tus·sus·cip·i·en·
  tes
in·u·lase
  also in·u·lin·ase
in·u·lin
in·unc·tion
in utero
in vac·uo
in·vade
  in·vad·ed
  in·vad·ing
in·vad·er
in·vag·i·nate
  in·vag·i·nat·ed
  in·vag·i·nat·ing

in·vag·i·na·tion
in·va·lid
in·va·lid·ism
in·val·id·i·ty
  pl in·val·id·i·ties
in·va·sion
in·va·sive
in·ver·sion
in·vert
in·vert·ase
In·ver·te·bra·ta
in·ver·te·brate
in·vert·in
in·ver·tor
in·vest
in·vet·er·ate
in·vi·a·bil·i·ty
  pl in·vi·a·bil·i·ties
in·vi·a·ble
in vi·tro
in vi·vo
in·vo·lu·crum
  pl in·vo·lu·cra
in·vol·un·tary
in·vo·lute
  in·vo·lut·ed
  in·vo·lut·ing
in·vo·lu·tion
in·vo·lu·tion·al
in·volve
  in·volved
  in·volv·ing
in·volve·ment
Iod·amoe·ba
io·date
  io·dat·ed
  io·dat·ing

iod·ic
io·dide
io·dim·e·try
   var of iodometry
io·din·ate
   io·din·at·ed
   io·din·at·ing
io·din·ation
io·dine
io·dip·amide
io·dism
io·dize
   io·dized
   io·diz·ing
io·do·ace·tic
io·do·al·phi·on·ic
io·do·ca·sein
io·do·chlor·hy·
   droxy·quin
io·do·de·oxy·uri·
   dine
   or 5-io·do·de·oxy·uri·
   dine
io·do·form
io·do·gor·go·ic
io·do·hip·pur·ate
io·dom·e·try
   also io·dim·e·try
   pl io·dom·e·tries
   also io·dim·e·tries
io·do·phile
   noun
io·do·phil·ic
   also io·do·phile
   adjective
io·do·phor
io·do·phtha·lein

io·do·pro·tein
io·dop·sin
io·do·pyr·a·cet
ion
ion·ic
ion·i·cal·ly
io·ni·um
ion·iz·able
ion·iza·tion
ion·ize
   ion·ized
   ion·iz·ing
ion·o·phore
io·noph·or·ous
ion·to·pho·rese
   ion·to·pho·resed
   ion·to·pho·res·
   ing
ion·to·pho·re·sis
   pl ion·to·pho·re·ses
ion·to·pho·ret·ic
io·phen·dyl·ate
io·phen·ox·ic
io·ta·cism
io·thal·a·mate
io·tha·lam·ic
io·thio·ura·cil
ip·e·cac
   or ipe·ca·cu·a·nha
ipo·date
ip·o·mea
   also ip·o·moea
   dried scammony
   root

Ip·o·moea
   genus of morning glo-
   ries

iprin·dole
ipro·ni·a·zid
ip·sa·tion
ip·si·lat·er·al
iri·dal
iri·dec·to·my
   pl iri·dec·to·mies
iri·den·clei·sis
   pl iri·den·clei·ses
iri·de·re·mia
iri·des
   pl of iris
ir·i·des·cence
ir·i·des·cent
iri·di·ag·no·sis
   pl iri·di·ag·no·ses
irid·i·al
irid·ic
iri·din
irid·i·um
iri·do·cap·su·lot·o·
   my
   pl iri·do·cap·su·lot·o·
   mies
iri·do·cho·roid·itis
iri·do·cy·cli·tis
iri·do·cy·clo·cho·
   roid·itis
iri·do·di·al·y·sis
   pl iri·do·di·al·y·ses
iri·do·do·ne·sis
   pl iri·do·do·ne·ses
ir·i·dol·o·gist
ir·i·dol·o·gy
   pl ir·i·dol·o·gies
iri·do·ple·gia

iri·dos·chi·sis
pl iri·dos·chi·ses
or iri·dos·chi·sis·es

iri·do·scle·rot·o·my
pl iri·do·scle·rot·o·mies

iri·dot·a·sis
pl iri·dot·a·ses

iri·dot·o·my
pl iri·dot·o·mies

iris
pl iris·es
or iri·des

iris bom·bé

iri·tis

ir·ra·di·ance

ir·ra·di·ate
ir·ra·di·at·ed
ir·ra·di·at·ing

ir·ra·di·a·tion

ir·ra·di·a·tor

ir·ra·tio·nal

ir·ra·tio·nal·i·ty
pl ir·ra·tio·nal·i·ties

ir·ra·tio·nal·ly

ir·re·duc·ibil·i·ty
pl ir·re·duc·ibil·i·ties

ir·re·duc·ible

ir·reg·u·lar

ir·reg·u·lar·i·ty
pl ir·reg·u·lar·i·ties

ir·re·me·di·a·ble

ir·re·spi·ra·ble

ir·ri·gate
ir·ri·gat·ed
ir·ri·gat·ing

ir·ri·ga·tion

ir·ri·ga·tor

ir·ri·ta·bil·i·ty
pl ir·ri·ta·bil·i·ties

ir·ri·ta·ble

ir·ri·tant

ir·ri·tate
ir·ri·tat·ed
ir·ri·tat·ing

ir·ri·ta·tion

ir·ri·ta·tive

ir·ru·mate
ir·ru·mat·ed
ir·ru·mat·ing

ir·ru·ma·tion

ir·ru·ma·tor

is·aux·e·sis
pl is·aux·e·ses

is·aux·et·ic

isch·emia

isch·emic

is·chi·al

is·chi·at·ic

is·chi·ec·to·my
pl is·chi·ec·to·mies

is·chio·cap·su·lar

is·chio·cav·er·no·sus
pl is·chio·cav·er·no·si

is·chio·coc·cy·geus
pl is·chio·coc·cy·gei

is·chio·fem·o·ral

is·chi·op·a·gus

is·chio·pu·bic

is·chio·rec·tal

is·chi·um
pl is·chia

isch·uria

Ishi·ha·ra test

is·land

is·land of Lang·er·hans

is·land of Reil

is·let

is·let of Lang·er·hans

iso·ag·glu·ti·na·tion

iso·ag·glu·ti·nin

iso·ag·glu·tin·o·gen

iso·al·lele

iso·al·lox·a·zine

iso·am·yl

iso·an·dros·ter·one

iso·an·ti·body
pl iso·an·ti·bod·ies

iso·an·ti·gen

iso·an·ti·gen·ic

iso·an·ti·ge·nic·i·ty
pl iso·an·ti·ge·nic·i·ties

iso·bor·nyl thio·cyano·ace·tate

iso·bu·tyl

iso·ca·lo·ric

iso·ca·lo·ri·cal·ly

iso·car·box·az·id

iso·chro·mat·ic

iso·chro·mo·some

iso·chron·ic

iso·chro·nism

iso·cit·rate

iso·cit·ric

iso·cor·tex

iso·cy·a·nide

iso·cy·clic
iso·dose
iso·elec·tric
iso·elec·tro·fo·cus·
   ing
iso·en·zy·mat·ic
iso·en·zyme
iso·en·zy·mic
iso·eth·a·rine
iso·fluro·phate
iso·ga·mete
iso·ga·met·ic
isog·a·mous
isog·a·my
   pl isog·a·mies
iso·ge·ne·ic
iso·gen·ic
isog·o·ny
   pl isog·o·nies
iso·graft
iso·hem·ag·glu·ti·
   na·tion
iso·hem·ag·glu·ti·
   nin
iso·hem·ag·glu·tin·
   o·gen
iso·he·mo·ly·sin
iso·he·mol·y·sis
   pl iso·he·mol·y·ses
iso·im·mune
iso·im·mu·ni·za·
   tion
iso·lant
iso·late
   iso·lat·ed
   iso·lat·ing
iso·la·tion

iso·lec·i·thal
iso·leu·cine
isol·o·gous
iso·ly·ser·gic
iso·mal·tose
iso·mer
isom·er·ase
isom·er·ic
isom·er·ide
isom·er·ism
isom·er·i·za·tion
isom·er·ize
   isom·er·ized
   isom·er·iz·ing
iso·me·thep·tene
iso·met·ric
iso·met·ri·cal·ly
iso·morph
iso·mor·phic
iso·mor·phism
iso·mor·phous
iso·ni·a·zid
iso·nic·o·tin·ic
iso·nip·e·caine
iso·ni·trile
iso·os·mot·ic
iso·phane
iso·pre·cip·i·tin
iso·preg·nen·one
iso·pro·pa·mide
iso·pro·pa·nol
iso·pro·pyl
iso·pro·pyl·ar·te·re·
   nol
iso·pro·ter·e·nol
isop·ter
iso·pyk·no·sis

iso·pyk·not·ic
is·os·mot·ic
is·os·mot·i·cal·ly
iso·sor·bide
iso·sor·bide di·ni·
   trate
Isos·po·ra
isos·the·nu·ria
iso·therm
iso·ther·mal
iso·thio·pen·dyl
iso·ton·ic
iso·ton·i·cal·ly
iso·to·nic·i·ty
   pl iso·to·nic·i·ties
iso·tope
iso·to·pic
iso·to·pi·cal·ly
iso·to·py
   pl iso·to·pies
iso·trans·plant
iso·trans·plan·ta·
   tion
iso·tro·pic
isot·ro·py
   pl isot·ro·pies
iso·type
iso·typ·ic
iso·va·ler·ic
iso·vol·u·met·ric
is·ox·az·o·lyl
is·ox·su·prine
iso·zyme
iso·zy·mic
is·pa·ghul
isth·mic
isth·mus

it·a·con·ate
it·a·con·ic
itai-itai
itch
itch·i·ness
itchy
  itch·i·er
  itch·i·est
iter
itis
Ix·o·des
ix·od·i·cide
ix·od·id
Ix·od·i·dae
ix·o·doid
Ix·o·doi·dea

J

jaag·siek·te
  also jaag·ziek·te
  or jag·siek·te
  or jag·ziek·te
jab·o·ran·di
jack·et
Jack·so·ni·an ep·i·lep·sy
Ja·cob·son's car·ti·lage
Ja·cob·son's nerve
Ja·cob·son's or·gan
jac·ti·tate
  jac·ti·tat·ed
  jac·ti·tat·ing
jac·ti·ta·tion
Jaf·fé re·ac·tion
  also Jaf·fé's re·ac·tion

jag·siek·te
  var of jaag·siek·te
jag·ziek·te
  var of jaag·siek·te
jake leg
jal·ap
jal·a·pin
ja·mais vu
James-Lange the·o·ry
James·town weed
jani·ceps
Ja·nus green
Jap·a·nese B en·ceph·a·li·tis
Ja·risch-Herx·hei·mer re·ac·tion
Jat·ro·pha
jaun·dice
Ja·velle wa·ter
jaw·bone
je·ju·nal
je·ju·ni·tis
je·ju·no·gas·tric
je·ju·no·il·e·al
je·ju·no·il·e·it·is
je·ju·no·il·e·os·to·my
  pl je·ju·no·il·e·os·to·mies
je·ju·nos·to·my
  pl je·ju·nos·to·mies
je·ju·num
  pl je·ju·na
jel·ly
  pl jel·lies
jel·ly·fish

Jen·ne·ri·an
Jen·ner's stain
je·quir·i·ty bean
jes·sa·mine
Je·su·its' bark
jet lag
jet-lagged
jig·ger
jim·son·weed
  also jimp·son·weed
jit·ter
jit·teri·ness
jit·ters
jit·tery
Jo·cas·ta com·plex
jock itch
jock·strap
Joh·ne's ba·cil·lus
Joh·ne's dis·ease
joh·nin
john·ny
  also john·nie
  pl john·nies
joint·ed
joule
Joule's equiv·a·lent
ju·gal
ju·glone
jug·u·lar
ju·gum
  pl ju·ga
  or ju·gums
ju·jube
jump·ing French·men of Maine
junc·tion

kelp

junc·tion·al
Jung·ian
ju·ni·per
just-no·tice·able
  dif·fer·ence
jus·to ma·jor
jus·to mi·nor
ju·ve·nile
ju·ve·nile-on·set di·
  a·be·tes
jux·ta-ar·tic·u·lar
jux·ta·cor·ti·cal
jux·ta·glo·mer·u·
  lar
jux·ta·med·ul·lary
jux·ta·pose
  jux·ta·posed
  jux·ta·pos·ing
jux·ta·po·si·tion
jux·ta·py·lor·ic
jux·ta·res·ti·form

K

Kahn test
kai·nic
kak·ke
kak·or·rhaph·io·
  pho·bia
kala-azar
ka·li·um
ka·li·ure·sis
  also kal·ure·sis
  pl ka·li·ure·ses
  also kal·ure·ses
ka·li·uret·ic
kal·li·din

kal·li·kre·in
Kall·man's syn·
  drome
ka·ma·la
kana·my·cin
Kan·ner's syn·
  drome
ka·olin
Ka·po·si's sar·co·
  ma
kap·pa
ka·ra·ya
ka·rez·za
Kar·ta·ge·ner's syn·
  drome
karyo·clas·tic
  or karyo·cla·sic
karyo·cyte
karyo·gam·ic
kary·og·a·my
  pl kary·og·a·mies
karyo·gram
karyo·ki·ne·sis
  pl karyo·ki·ne·ses
karyo·ki·net·ic
kary·o·log·i·cal
  also kary·o·log·ic
kary·ol·o·gy
  pl kary·ol·o·gies
karyo·lymph
kary·ol·y·sis
  pl kary·ol·y·ses
karyo·lyt·ic
karyo·met·ric
kary·om·e·try
  pl kary·om·e·tries
karyo·plasm

karyo·pyk·no·sis
karyo·pyk·not·ic
kary·or·rhec·tic
kary·or·rhex·is
  pl kary·or·rhex·es
karyo·some
karyo·the·ca
karyo·tin
karyo·type
karyo·typ·ic
karyo·typ·i·cal·ly
karyo·typ·ing
kat
  var of khat
kata·ther·mom·e·
  ter
Ka·ta·ya·ma
ka·tha·rom·e·ter
kat·zen·jam·mer
ka·va
ka·va ka·va
Ka·wa·sa·ki dis·
  ease
Kay·ser-Flei·scher
  ring
ked
Kee·ley cure
kef
Kell
Kel·ler
kel·lin
  var of khellin
ke·loid
  also che·loid
ke·loi·dal
kelp

kel·vin
*unit of temperature on
Kelvin scale*

Kel·vin scale
ken·nel cough
Ken·ny meth·od
Ke·nya ty·phus
ker·a·sin
ker·a·tan
ker·a·tec·to·my
  pl ker·a·tec·to·mies

ke·rat·ic
ker·a·tin
ker·a·tin·ase
ker·a·ti·ni·za·tion
ker·a·ti·nize
  ker·a·ti·nized
  ker·a·ti·niz·ing
ker·a·ti·no·cyte
ker·a·ti·nol·y·sis
  pl ker·a·ti·nol·y·ses

ker·a·ti·no·lyt·ic
ker·a·ti·no·phil·ic
ker·a·ti·nous
ker·a·ti·tis
  pl ker·a·tit·i·des

ker·a·ti·tis punc·ta·
ta
ker·a·to·ac·an·tho·
ma
  pl ker·a·to·ac·an·tho·
  mas
  or ker·a·to·ac·an·tho·
  ma·ta
ker·a·to·cele
ker·a·to·con·junc·
ti·vi·tis

ker·a·to·con·junc·
ti·vi·tis sic·ca
ker·a·to·co·nus
ker·a·to·der·ma
ker·a·to·der·ma
  blen·nor·rhag·i·
  cum
ker·a·to·der·mia
ker·a·to·gen·ic
ker·a·tog·e·nous
ker·a·to·hy·a·lin
  also ker·a·to·hy·a·line

ker·a·tol·y·sis
  pl ker·a·tol·y·ses

ker·a·to·lyt·ic
ker·a·to·ma
  pl ker·a·to·mas
  or ker·a·to·ma·ta

ker·a·to·ma·la·cia
ker·a·tome
ker·a·tom·e·ter
ker·a·tom·e·try
  pl ker·a·tom·e·tries

ker·at·o·mil·eu·sis
ker·a·top·a·thy
  pl ker·a·top·a·thies

ker·a·to·pha·kia
ker·a·to·plas·tic
ker·a·to·plas·ty
  pl ker·a·to·plas·ties

ker·a·to·pros·the·
sis
  pl ker·a·to·pros·the·
  ses

ker·a·to·scope
ker·a·tos·co·py
  pl ker·a·tos·co·pies

ker·a·to·sis
  pl ker·a·to·ses

ker·a·to·sis blen·
  nor·rhag·i·ca
ker·a·to·sis fol·li·
  cu·lar·is
ker·a·to·sis pi·la·ris
ker·a·to·sul·fate
ker·a·tot·ic
ker·a·tot·o·mist
ker·a·tot·o·my
  pl ker·a·tot·o·mies

ke·rau·no·pho·bia
ke·ri·on
ker·nic·ter·ic
ker·nic·ter·us
Ker·nig sign
  or Ker·nig's sign

ke·ta·mine
ke·tene
ke·to
ke·to·ac·i·do·sis
  pl ke·to·ac·i·do·ses

ke·to·bem·i·done
ke·to·co·na·zole
ke·to·gen·e·sis
  pl ke·to·gen·e·ses

ke·to·gen·ic
ke·to·glu·ta·rate
ke·to·glu·tar·ic
ke·to·hep·tose
ke·to·hex·ose
ke·tol
ke·tol·y·sis
  pl ke·tol·y·ses

ke·to·lyt·ic
ke·tone

ke·to·ne·mia
also ke·to·nae·mia

ke·to·ne·mic
also ke·to·nae·mic

ke·ton·ic

ke·ton·uria

ke·tose

ke·to·sis
pl ke·to·ses

ke·to·ste·roid

ke·tot·ic

khat
also kat
or qat
or quat

khel·lin
also kel·lin

kid·ney
pl kid·neys

ki·lo·base

ki·lo·cal·o·rie

kilo·cy·cle

ki·lo·gram

kilo·li·ter

ki·lo·me·ter

ki·nase

kin·dred

ki·ne·mat·ic
or ki·ne·mat·i·cal

ki·ne·mat·ics

ki·ne·plas·tic
var of cineplastic

ki·ne·plas·ty
var of cineplasty

kin·e·sim·e·ter

ki·ne·si·o·log·ic
or ki·ne·si·o·log·i·cal

ki·ne·si·ol·o·gist

ki·ne·si·ol·o·gy
pl ki·ne·si·ol·o·gies

ki·ne·sis
pl ki·ne·ses

ki·ne·si·ther·a·py
pl ki·ne·si·ther·a·pies

kin·es·the·sia

kin·es·the·sis
pl kin·es·the·ses

kin·es·thet·ic

kin·es·thet·i·cal·ly

ki·net·ic

ki·net·i·cal·ly

ki·net·i·cist

ki·net·ics

ki·net·o·car·dio·gram

ki·net·o·car·dio·graph·ic

ki·net·o·car·di·og·ra·phy
pl ki·net·o·car·di·og·ra·phies

ki·net·o·chore

ki·neto·nu·cle·us

ki·neto·plast

ki·neto·plas·tic

kin·e·to·sis
pl kin·e·to·ses

ki·neto·som·al

ki·neto·some

king's evil

ki·nin

ki·ni·nase

ki·nin·o·gen

ki·nin·o·gen·ic

ki·no

ki·no·cil·i·um
pl ki·no·cil·ia

ki·no·plasm
also ki·no·plas·ma

Kirsch·ner wire

Kjel·dahl

kjel·dahl·iza·tion

kjel·dahl·ize
kjel·dahl·ized
kjel·dahl·iz·ing

kleb·si·el·la

Klebs-Löff·ler ba·cil·lus

Klein·ian

klep·to·lag·nia

klep·to·ma·nia

klep·to·ma·ni·ac

klieg eyes
or kleig eyes

Kline·fel·ter's syn·drome
also Kline·fel·ter syn·drome

Kline test

Klip·pel-Feil syn·drome

Klump·ke's pa·ral·y·sis

knee·cap

knee jerk

knee·pan

Kne·mi·do·kop·tes

knock-knee

knock-kneed

knuck·le

Koch's ba·cil·lus
  or Koch ba·cil·lus

Koch's phe·nom·e·
  non
  also Koch phe·nom·e·
  non

Koch's pos·tu·lates

Kohs blocks

koil·onych·ia

ko·jic

ko·la nut

Kol·mer re·ac·tion

ko·nio·cor·tex

Kop·lik's spots
  or Kop·lik spots

Korff's fi·ber

Ko·rot·koff sounds
  also Ko·rot·kow
    sounds
  or Ko·rot·kov sounds

Kor·sa·koff's psy·
  cho·sis

Kor·sa·koff's syn·
  drome
  or Kor·sa·koff syn·
    drome

kos·so
  or kous·so
  or ko·so

Krab·be's dis·ease

krad
  pl krad
  also krads

Krae·pe·lin·i·an

krait

kra·me·ria

krau·ro·sis
  pl krau·ro·ses

krau·ro·sis vul·vae

krau·rot·ic

Krau·se's cor·pus·
  cle

Krau·se's end-bulb

Krau·se's mem·
  brane

kre·bi·o·zen

Krebs cy·cle

Kro·may·er lamp

Kru·ken·berg tu·
  mor

kryp·ton

Küm·mell's dis·
  ease

Kupf·fer cell
  also Kupf·fer's cell

ku·ru

Kuss·maul breath·
  ing

Kveim test

kwa·shi·or·kor

Kya·sa·nur For·est
  dis·ease

ky·mo·gram

ky·mo·graph

ky·mo·graph·ic

ky·mog·ra·phy
  pl ky·mog·ra·phies

kyn·uren·ic

kyn·uren·ine

ky·pho·sco·li·o·sis
  pl ky·pho·sco·li·o·ses

ky·pho·sco·li·ot·ic

ky·pho·sis
  pl ky·pho·ses

ky·phot·ic

L

lab

La·bar·raque's so·
  lu·tion

la·bel
  la·beled
    or la·belled
  la·bel·ing
    or la·bel·ling

la·bia
  pl of labium

la·bi·al

la·bi·al·ism

la·bia ma·jo·ra

la·bia mi·no·ra

la·bile

la·bil·i·ty
  pl la·bil·i·ties

la·bi·li·za·tion

la·bio-buc·cal

la·bio-cli·na·tion

la·bio-den·tal

la·bio-glos·so·pha·
  ryn·geal

la·bio-lin·gual

la·bio-lin·gual·ly

la·bio-scro·tal

la·bi·um
  pl la·bia

la·bor

lab·o·ra·to·ry
  pl lab·o·ra·to·ries

la·brum

lab·y·rinth

lab·y·rin·thec·to·
mized
lab·y·rin·thec·to·
my
pl lab·y·rin·thec·to·
mies
lab·y·rin·thine
lab·y·rin·thi·tis
lab·y·rin·thot·o·my
pl lab·y·rin·thot·o·
mies
lac·er·ate
lac·er·at·ed
lac·er·at·ing
lac·er·a·tion
la·cer·tus fi·bro·sus
Lach·e·sis
lach·ry·mal
var of lacrimal
lach·ry·mate
var of lacrimate
lach·ry·ma·tion
var of lacrimation
lach·ry·ma·tor
var of lacrimator
lach·ry·ma·to·ry
var of lacrimatory
lac op·er·on
lac·ri·mal
also lach·ry·mal
lac·ri·ma·le
lac·ri·mate
also lach·ry·mate
lac·ri·mat·ed
also lach·ry·mat·ed
lac·ri·mat·ing
also lach·ry·mat·
ing

lac·ri·ma·tion
also lach·ry·ma·tion
lac·ri·ma·tor
also lach·ry·ma·tor
lac·ri·ma·to·ry
also lach·ry·ma·to·ry
lact·aci·de·mia
lac·ta·gogue
lact·al·bu·min
lac·tam
β-lac·tam·ase
lac·tase
lac·tate
lac·tat·ed
lac·tat·ing
lac·ta·tion
lac·te·al
lac·te·nin
lac·tic
lac·tif·er·ous
lac·tim
Lac·to·bac·il·la·ce·
ae
lac·to·ba·cil·lus
pl lac·to·ba·cil·li
lac·to·chrome
lac·to·fer·rin
lac·to·fla·vin
lac·to·gen
lac·to·gen·e·sis
pl lac·to·gen·e·ses
lac·to·gen·ic
lac·to·gen·i·cal·ly
lac·to·glob·u·lin
lac·tom·e·ter
lac·to·met·ric
lac·tone

lac·ton·ic
lac·to·ni·za·tion
lac·to·ovo·veg·e·
tar·i·an
lac·to·per·ox·i·dase
lac·to·phos·phate
lac·to·pro·tein
lac·tose
lac·tos·uria
lac·to·veg·e·tar·i·an
lac·tu·ca·ri·um
lac·tu·lose
la·cu·na
pl la·cu·nae
la·cu·nar
Lae·laps
Laen·nec's cir·rho·
sis
or Laën·nec's cir·rho·
sis
la·e·trile
La·fora body
La·fora's dis·ease
la·ge·na
pl la·ge·nae
Lag·o·chi·las·ca·ris
lag·oph·thal·mos
or lag·oph·thal·mus
la grippe
Laing·ian
laky
lak·i·er
lak·i·est
lal·la·tion
la·lop·a·thy
pl la·lop·a·thies
La·marck·ian

La·marck·ian·ism
La·marck·ism
La·maze
lamb·da
lamb·da·cism
lamb·doid
  or lamb·doi·dal

lam·bert
Lam·blia
lam·bli·a·sis
  pl lam·bli·a·ses
la·mel·la
  pl la·mel·lae
  also la·mel·las

la·mel·lar
la·mel·late
lam·el·lat·ed
la·mel·la·tion
la·mel·li·form
la·mel·li·po·di·um
  pl la·mel·li·po·dia

lam·i·na
  pl lam·i·nae
  also lam·i·nas

lam·i·na cri·bro·sa
  pl lam·i·nae cri·bro·sae

lam·i·na du·ra
lam·i·na·gram
  var of laminogram

lam·i·na·graph
  var of laminograph

lam·i·na·graph·ic
  var of laminographic

lam·i·nag·ra·phy
  var of laminography

lam·i·na pro·pria
  pl lam·i·nae pro·pri·ae

lam·i·nar
lam·i·nar·ia
lam·i·nar·in
lam·i·na spi·ral·is
lam·i·nat·ed
lam·i·na ter·mi·nal·is
lam·i·na·tion
lam·i·nec·to·my
  pl lam·i·nec·to·mies

lam·i·ni·tis
lam·i·no·gram
  or lam·i·na·gram

lam·i·no·graph
  or lam·i·na·graph

lam·i·no·graph·ic
  or lam·i·na·graph·ic

lam·i·nog·ra·phy
  or lam·i·nag·ra·phy
  pl lam·i·nog·ra·phies
  or lam·i·nag·ra·phies

lam·i·not·o·my
  pl lam·i·not·o·mies

lam·pas
lamp·brush
lam·siek·te
  or lam·ziek·te

la·nat·o·side
lance
  lanced
  lanc·ing
Lance·field group
  also Lance·field's group

lan·cet
lan·ci·nat·ing
land·mark
Lan·dolt ring
Lan·dry's pa·ral·y·sis
Lang·er·hans cell
Lang·hans cell
Lang·hans gi·ant cell
Lang·hans' lay·er
lan·o·lin
la·nos·ter·ol
Lan·sing vi·rus
lan·tha·nide
lan·tha·num
lan·tho·pine
la·nu·gi·nous
la·nu·go
la·pac·tic
lap·a·ro·scope
lap·a·ro·scop·ic
lap·a·ros·co·pist
lap·a·ros·co·py
  pl lap·a·ros·co·pies

lap·a·rot·om·ize
  lap·a·rot·om·ized
  lap·a·rot·om·iz·ing

lap·a·rot·o·my
  pl lap·a·rot·o·mies

lap·in·ized
La·place's law
lap·pa
lard·worm
Lar·sen's syn·drome

lar·va
  pl lar·vae
    also lar·vas

lar·val

lar·val mi·grans

lar·va mi·grans
  pl lar·vae mi·gran·tes

lar·vi·cid·al

lar·vi·cid·al·ly

lar·vi·cide
  also lar·va·cide

lar·vi·cid·ing

lar·vip·a·rous

lar·vi·phag·ic

lar·vi·pos·it

lar·vi·po·si·tion

lar·viv·o·rous

la·ryn·geal

la·ryn·geal·ly

lar·yn·gec·to·mee

lar·yn·gec·to·mized

lar·yn·gec·to·my
  pl lar·yn·gec·to·mies

lar·yn·gis·mus stri·du·lus
  pl lar·yn·gis·mi strid·u·li

lar·yn·git·ic

lar·yn·gi·tis
  pl lar·yn·git·i·des

la·ryn·go·cele

la·ryn·go·fis·sure

lar·yn·gog·ra·phy
  pl lar·yn·gog·ra·phies

la·ryn·go·log·i·cal
  also la·ryn·go·log·ic

lar·yn·gol·o·gist

lar·yn·gol·o·gy
  pl lar·yn·gol·o·gies

la·ryn·go·pha·ryn·ge·al

la·ryn·go·phar·yn·gi·tis
  pl la·ryn·go·phar·yn·git·i·des

la·ryn·go·phar·ynx

la·ryn·go·plas·ty
  pl la·ryn·go·plas·ties

la·ryn·go·scope

la·ryn·go·scop·ic
  or la·ryn·go·scop·i·cal

lar·yn·gos·co·py
  pl lar·yn·gos·co·pies

la·ryn·go·spasm

lar·yn·got·o·my
  pl lar·yn·got·o·mies

la·ryn·go·tra·che·al

la·ryn·go·tra·che·itis

la·ryn·go·tra·cheo·bron·chi·tis
  pl la·ryn·go·tra·cheo·bron·chit·i·des

lar·ynx
  pl lar·yn·ges
    or lar·ynx·es
  part of the trachea
  (*see* pharynx)

la·sal·o·cid

la·ser

L-as·par·a·gi·nase

Las·sa fe·ver

Las·sa vi·rus

las·si·tude

la·tah

la·ten·cy
  pl la·ten·cies

la·tent

la·ten·ti·a·tion

lat·er·ad

lat·er·al

lat·er·al·i·ty
  pl lat·er·al·i·ties

lat·er·al·iza·tion

lat·er·al·ize
  lat·er·al·ized
  lat·er·al·iz·ing

la·tex
  pl la·ti·ces
    or la·tex·es

lath·y·rism

lath·y·rit·ic

lath·y·ro·gen

lath·y·ro·gen·ic

la·tis·si·mus dor·si
  pl la·tis·si·mi dor·si

lat·ro·dec·tism

Lat·ro·dec·tus

lat·tice

laud·able pus

lau·dan·i·dine

lau·da·nine

lau·dan·o·sine

lau·da·num

Lau·rence-Moon-Biedl syn·drome

Lau·rer's ca·nal

lau·ric

la·vage
  la·vaged
  la·vag·ing

la·va·tion

lav·en·der
Lav·er·a·nia
law·ren·ci·um
lax·a·tion
lax·a·tive
lax·i·ty
  pl lax·i·ties
lay·er
lay·er of Lang·
  hans
la·zar
laz·a·ret·to
  or laz·a·ret
  pl laz·a·ret·tos
  or laz·a·rets
L-do·pa
leach
leach·abil·i·ty
  pl leach·abil·i·ties
leach·able
leach·ate
leaf·let
learn
  learned
    also learnt
  learn·ing
learn·er
Le·boy·er
LE cell
lec·i·thal
lec·i·thin
lec·i·thin·ase
lec·i·tho·pro·tein
lec·tin
leech
LE fac·tor
left-hand·ed

Legg-Cal·vé-Per·
  thes dis·ease
Legg-Per·thes dis·
  ease
leg·he·mo·glo·bin
Le·gion·el·la
le·gion·el·lo·sis
Le·gion·naires' ba·
  cil·lus
Le·gion·naires' dis·
  ease
  also Le·gion·naire's
    dis·ease
le·gu·min
leio·myo·blas·to·
  ma
  pl leio·myo·blas·to·
    mas
  or leio·myo·blas·to·
    ma·ta
leio·my·o·ma
  pl leio·my·o·mas
  or leio·my·o·ma·ta
leio·my·o·ma·tous
leio·myo·sar·co·ma
  pl leio·myo·sar·co·
    mas
  or leio·myo·sar·co·
    ma·ta
lei·ot·ri·chous
Leish·man body
Leish·man-Don·o·
  van body
leish·man·ia
leish·man·ial
leish·man·i·a·sis
  pl leish·man·i·a·ses
leish·man·i·form

leish·man·i·o·sis
  pl leish·man·i·o·ses
lem·nis·cal
lem·nis·cus
  pl lem·nis·ci
len·i·tive
lens·om·e·ter
Len·te in·su·lin
len·ti·co·nus
len·tic·u·lar
len·tic·u·lo·stri·ate
len·ti·form
len·tig·i·no·sis
len·ti·go
  pl len·tig·i·nes
len·ti·go ma·lig·na
len·ti·go se·nil·is
le·o·nine
le·on·ti·a·sis
  pl le·on·ti·a·ses
le·on·ti·a·sis os·sea
lep·er
Lep·i·dop·tera
lep·i·dop·ter·an
lep·i·dop·ter·ous
lep·o·thrix
  pl lep·o·thrix·es
  also le·pot·ri·ches
lep·ra
lep·re·chaun·ism
lep·rid
lep·ro·lin
lep·rol·o·gist
lep·rol·o·gy
  pl lep·rol·o·gies

lep·ro·ma
  pl lep·ro·mas
  or lep·ro·ma·ta

le·pro·ma·tous
lep·ro·min
lep·ro·pho·bia
lep·ro·sar·i·um
  pl lep·ro·sar·i·ums
  or lep·ro·sar·ia

lep·ro·sery
  or lep·ro·ser·ie
  pl lep·ro·ser·ies

lep·ro·stat·ic
lep·ro·sy
  pl lep·ro·sies

lep·rot·ic
lep·rous
lep·ti
  pl of leptus

lep·to·ceph·a·ly
  pl lep·to·ceph·a·lies

lep·to·men·in·ge·al
lep·to·me·nin·ges
lep·to·men·in·gi·tis
  pl lep·to·men·in·git·i·
  des

lep·to·me·ninx
lep·tom·o·nad
lep·tom·o·nas
lep·to·phos
lep·to·pro·so·pic
lep·tor·rhine
lep·to·scope
lep·to·some
  or lep·to·som·ic
  also lep·to·so·mat·ic

lep·to·spi·ra
  pl lep·to·spi·ra
  or lep·to·spi·ras
  or lep·to·spi·rae

lep·to·spi·ral
lep·to·spire
lep·to·spi·ri·ci·dal
lep·to·spi·ro·sis
  pl lep·to·spi·ro·ses

lep·to·spir·uria
lep·to·tene
lep·to·thrix
  pl lep·to·trich·ia
  also lep·tot·ri·ches

Lep·to·trich·ia
lep·tus
  pl lep·tus·es
  also lep·ti

Le·riche's syn·
  drome
les·bi·an
les·bi·an·ism
Lesch-Ny·han syn·
  drome
le·sion
le·sioned
le·thal
le·thal·i·ty
  pl le·thal·i·ties

le·thar·gic
leth·ar·gy
  pl leth·ar·gies

Let·ter·er-Si·we
  dis·ease
leu·cine
leu·ci·no·sis
  pl leu·ci·no·ses
  or leu·ci·no·sis·es

leu·cin·uria
leu·co·cy·to·zo·on
  pl leu·co·cy·to·zoa

leu·co·cy·to·zoo·no·
  sis
  pl leu·co·cy·to·zoo·
  no·ses

leu·co·nos·toc
leu·cov·o·rin
Leu·en·keph·a·lin
leuk·ane·mia
leu·ka·phe·re·sis
  pl leu·ka·phe·re·ses

leu·ke·mia
leu·ke·mic
leu·ke·mid
leu·ke·mo·gen
leu·ke·mo·gen·e·
  sis
  pl leu·ke·mo·gen·e·
  ses

leu·ke·mo·gen·ic
leu·ke·mo·ge·nic·i·
  ty
  pl leu·ke·mo·ge·nic·i·
  ties

leu·ke·moid
leu·ker·gy
  pl leu·ker·gies

leu·kin
leu·ko·ag·glu·ti·nin
leu·ko·blast
leu·ko·blas·to·sis
  pl leu·ko·blas·to·ses

leu·ko·ci·din
leu·ko·cyte
leu·ko·cy·the·mia

leu·ko·cyt·ic
leu·ko·cy·to·gen·e·
sis
pl leu·ko·cy·to·gen·e·
ses
leu·ko·cy·to·sis
pl leu·ko·cy·to·ses
leu·ko·cy·tot·ic
leu·ko·der·ma
leu·ko·dys·tro·phy
pl leu·ko·dys·tro·
phies
leu·ko·en·ceph·a·li·
tis
pl leu·ko·en·ceph·a·
lit·i·des
leu·ko·en·ceph·a·
lop·a·thy
pl leu·ko·en·ceph·a·
lop·a·thies
leu·ko·ker·a·to·sis
pl leu·ko·ker·a·to·ses
leu·ko·ma
leu·ko·maine
leu·kon
leuk·onych·ia
leu·ko·pe·nia
leu·ko·pe·nic
leu·ko·phe·re·sis
pl leu·ko·phe·re·ses
leu·ko·pla·kia
leu·ko·pla·kic
leu·ko·poi·e·sis
pl leu·ko·poi·e·ses
leu·ko·poi·et·ic
leu·kor·rhea
leu·kor·rhe·al

leu·ko·sar·co·ma
pl leu·ko·sar·co·mas
or leu·ko·sar·co·ma·
ta
leu·ko·sar·co·ma·
to·sis
pl leu·ko·sar·co·ma·
to·ses
leu·ko·sis
pl leu·ko·ses
leu·ko·tac·tic
leu·ko·tac·ti·cal·ly
leu·ko·tax·ine
leu·ko·tax·is
pl leu·ko·tax·es
leu·kot·ic
leu·ko·tome
leu·kot·o·my
pl leu·kot·o·mies
leu·ko·tox·in
leu·ko·trich·ia
leu·ko·tri·ene
leu·ko·vi·rus
leu·ro·cris·tine
lev·al·lor·phan
le·vam·i·sole
lev·an
lev·ar·ter·e·nol
le·va·tor
pl lev·a·to·res
or le·va·tors
lev·a·to·res cos·tar·
um
le·va·tor la·bii su·
pe·ri·or·is

le·va·tor pal·pe·
brae su·pe·ri·or·
is
le·va·tor pros·ta·tae
le·va·tor scap·u·lae
le·va·tor ve·li pal·a·
ti·ni
Le·Veen shunt
lev·i·gate
lev·i·gat·ed
lev·i·gat·ing
lev·i·ga·tion
Le·vin tube
le·vo·car·dia
le·vo·car·dio·gram
le·vo·di·hy·droxy·
phe·nyl·al·a·
nine
levo·do·pa
le·vo·pro·poxy·
phene
le·vo·ro·ta·tion
le·vo·ro·ta·to·ry
or le·vo·ro·ta·ry
lev·or·pha·nol
le·vo·thy·rox·ine
lev·u·li·nate
lev·u·lin·ic
lev·u·lo·san
lev·u·lose
lev·u·los·emia
lev·u·los·uria
Lew·is
lew·is·ite
Ley·dig cell
also Ley·dig's cell
L-form

li·bid·i·nal
li·bid·i·ni·za·tion
li·bid·i·nize
 li·bid·i·nized
 li·bid·i·niz·ing
li·bid·i·nous
li·bi·do
 pl li·bi·dos
Lib·man-Sacks en·do·car·di·tis
lice
 pl of louse
li·cense
 li·censed
 li·cens·ing
li·cen·ti·ate
li·chen
li·chen·i·fi·ca·tion
li·chen·i·fied
li·chen·in
li·chen·oid
li·chen pla·nus
li·chen scle·ro·sus et atro·phi·cus
li·chen sim·plex chron·i·cus
li·chen spi·nu·lo·sus
li·chen trop·i·cus
lic·o·rice
li·do·caine
li·do·fla·zine
Lie·ber·kühn's gland
Lie·ber·mann-Bur·chard re·ac·tion

li·en·cu·lus
 pl li·en·cu·li
li·eno·re·nal
li·en·ter·ic
Lie·se·gang rings
lig·a·ment
lig·a·ment of Coo·per
lig·a·ment of Treitz
lig·a·ment of Zinn
lig·a·men·to·pexy
 pl lig·a·men·to·pex·ies
lig·a·men·tous
lig·a·men·tum
 pl lig·a·men·ta
lig·a·men·tum fla·vum
 pl lig·a·men·ta fla·va
lig·a·men·tum nu·chae
 pl lig·a·men·ta nu·chae
lig·a·men·tum te·res
lig·a·men·tum ve·no·sum
li·gand
li·gand·ed
li·gase
li·gate
 li·gat·ed
 li·gat·ing
li·ga·tion

lig·a·ture
 lig·a·tured
 lig·a·tur·ing
lig·nin
lig·no·caine
lig·no·cel·lu·lose
lig·no·cel·lu·los·ic
lig·no·cer·ic
lig·num vi·tae
 pl lig·num vi·taes
lig·u·la
lim·bal
lim·ber·neck
lim·bic
lim·bus
li·men
lime·wa·ter
lim·i·nal
lin·a·mar·in
lin·co·my·cin
linc·tus
 pl linc·tus·es
lin·dane
Lin·dau's dis·ease
lin·ea
 pl lin·e·ae
lin·ea al·ba
 pl lin·e·ae al·bae
lin·ea as·pe·ra
 pl lin·e·ae as·pe·rae
lin·e·ae al·bi·can·tes
lin·ear
lin·ear·i·ty
 pl lin·ear·i·ties
lin·ear·ly

lin·ea semi·lu·nar·
is
pl lin·e·ae semi·lu·
nar·es

line·breed
line·bred
line·breed·ing

lin·gua
pl lin·guae

lin·gual
Lin·guat·u·la

lin·guat·u·lid

lin·guat·u·lo·sis
pl lin·guat·u·lo·ses

lin·gui·form

lin·gu·la
pl lin·gu·lae

lin·gu·lar

lin·guo·ver·sion

lin·i·ment

li·nin

link·age

Lin·nae·an
or Lin·ne·an

li·no·le·ate

lin·ole·ic

lin·ole·nic

lin·seed

li·o·thy·ro·nine

li·pase

li·pec·to·my
pl li·pec·to·mies

li·pe·mia

li·pe·mic

lip·id
also lip·ide

li·pid·ic

lip·i·do·sis
pl lip·i·do·ses

lip·in

li·po·ate

li·po·atro·phic

li·po·at·ro·phy
pl li·po·at·ro·phies

li·po·blast

li·po·ca·ic

li·po·chon·dri·on
pl li·po·chon·dria

li·po·chon·dro·dys·
tro·phy
pl li·po·chon·dro·dys·
tro·phies

li·po·chrome

li·po·cyte

li·po·dys·tro·phy
pl li·po·dys·tro·phies

li·po·fi·bro·ma
pl li·po·fi·bro·mas
also li·po·fi·bro·ma·ta

li·po·fus·cin

li·po·fus·cin·o·sis

li·po·gen·e·sis
pl li·po·gen·e·ses

li·po·ge·net·ic

li·po·gen·ic
also li·pog·e·nous

li·po·ic.

li·poid
or li·poi·dal

li·poid·o·sis
pl li·poid·o·ses

li·pol·y·sis
pl li·pol·y·ses

li·po·lyt·ic

li·po·ma
pl li·po·mas
or li·po·ma·ta

li·po·ma·to·sis
pl li·po·ma·to·ses

li·po·ma·tous

li·po·mi·cron

li·po·phage

li·po·pha·gic

li·po·phan·er·o·sis
pl li·po·phan·er·o·ses

li·po·phil·ic

li·po·phi·lic·i·ty
pl li·po·phi·lic·i·ties

li·po·poly·sac·cha·
ride

li·po·pro·tein

li·po·sar·co·ma
pl li·po·sar·co·mas
or li·po·sar·co·ma·ta

li·po·sol·u·bil·i·ty
pl li·po·sol·u·bil·i·ties

li·po·sol·u·ble

li·po·so·mal

li·po·some

li·po·thy·mia

li·po·thy·mic

li·po·tro·pic
also li·po·tro·phic

li·po·tro·pin

li·po·tro·pism

li·po·vac·cine

li·pox·i·dase

li·pox·y·gen·ase

Lippes loop

li·pu·ria

liq·ue·fac·tion

liq·uid
liq·uid·am·bar
li·quor
li·quor am·nii
li·quor fol·li·cu·li
Lis·sau·er's tract
lis·sen·ce·phal·ic
lis·sen·ceph·a·ly
 pl lis·sen·ceph·a·lies
Lis·ter bag
 also Lys·ter bag
lis·ter·el·la
 Lis·ter·el·la
lis·te·ria
lis·te·ri·al
lis·te·ric
lis·te·ri·o·sis
 also lis·ter·el·lo·sis
 pl lis·te·ri·o·ses
 also lis·ter·el·lo·ses
li·ter
 also li·tre
li·tharge
li·the·mia
li·the·mic
li·thi·a·sis
 pl li·thi·a·ses
lith·i·um
lith·o·cho·lic
lith·o·gen·e·sis
 pl lith·o·gen·e·ses
lith·o·gen·ic
lith·ol·a·paxy
 pl lith·ol·a·pax·ies
lith·o·pe·di·on
lith·o·tome

li·thot·o·my
 pl li·thot·o·mies
lith·o·trip·sy
 pl lith·o·trip·sies
lith·o·trip·tor
 or lith·o·trip·ter
lith·o·trite
li·thot·ri·ty
 pl li·thot·ri·ties
li·thu·ria
lit·mus
li·tre
 var of liter
lit·ter
Lit·tle League el·bow
Lit·tle's dis·ease
lit·to·ral cell
Lit·tré's gland
li·ve·do
li·ve·do re·tic·u·lar·is
liv·er
liv·er mor·tis
liv·e·tin
liv·id
li·vid·i·ty
 pl li·vid·i·ties
lix·iv·i·ate
 lix·iv·i·at·ed
 lix·iv·i·at·ing
lix·iv·i·a·tion
lix·iv·i·um
 pl lix·iv·ia
 or lix·iv·i·ums
Loa

lo·a·i·a·sis
 or lo·i·a·sis
 pl lo·a·i·a·ses
 or lo·i·a·ses

loa loa
lo·bar
lo·bate
 also lo·bat·ed
lo·ba·tion
lobe
lo·bec·to·my
 pl lo·bec·to·mies
lo·be·lia
lo·be·line
lo·bi
 pl of lobus
lo·bo·pod
lo·bo·po·di·um
 pl lo·bo·po·dia
 or lo·bo·po·di·ums
lo·bot·o·mize
 lo·bot·o·mized
 lo·bot·o·miz·ing
lo·bot·o·my
 pl lo·bot·o·mies
lob·ster claw
lob·u·lar
lob·u·lat·ed
lob·u·la·tion
lob·ule
lob·u·lus
 pl lob·u·li
lo·bus
 pl lo·bi
lo·cal
lo·cal·iza·tion

lo·cal·ize
  lo·cal·ized
  lo·cal·iz·ing
lo·chia
  pl lo·chia
lo·chi·al
lo·ci
  pl of locus
Locke's so·lu·tion
  also Locke so·lu·tion
lock·jaw
lo·co
  pl lo·cos
  or lo·coes
lo·co·ism
lo·co·mo·tion
lo·co·mo·tive
lo·co·mo·tor
lo·co·mo·to·ry
lo·co·weed
loc·u·lar
loc·u·lat·ed
loc·u·la·tion
loc·u·lus
  pl loc·u·li
lo·cum-te·nen·cy
  pl lo·cum-te·nen·cies
lo·cum te·nens
  pl lo·cum te·nen·tes
lo·cus
  pl lo·ci
lo·cus coe·ru·le·us
  also lo·cus ce·ru·le·us
  pl lo·ci coe·ru·lei
  also lo·ci ce·ru·lei
Loef·fler's syn·drome

log·o·pe·dia
log·o·pe·dic
log·o·pe·dics
log·o·pe·dist
log·or·rhea
log·or·rhe·ic
log·o·ther·a·py
  pl log·o·ther·a·pies
lo·i·a·sis
  var of loaiasis
lo·mus·tine
lon·gev·i·ty
  pl lon·gev·i·ties
lon·gis·si·mus
  pl lon·gis·si·mi
lon·gis·si·mus cap·i·tis
lon·gis·si·mus cer·vi·cis
lon·gis·si·mus dor·si
lon·gis·si·mus thor·a·cis
lon·gi·tu·di·na·lis lin·guae
long·sight·ed
lon·gus
  pl lon·gi
lon·gus cap·i·tis
loop of Hen·le
loph·o·dont
Lo·phoph·o·ra
lo·phoph·o·rine
lo·phot·ri·chous
  or lo·phot·ri·chate
lor·az·e·pam
lor·do·sis

lor·dot·ic
lo·ri·ca
  pl lo·ri·cae
lo·tion
Lou Geh·rig's dis·ease
loupe
loup·ing ill
louse
  pl lice
louse-borne
lou·si·cid·al
lou·si·cide
lous·i·ness
lousy
  lous·i·er
  lous·i·est
lov·age
Lox·os·ce·les
lox·os·ce·lism
loz·enge
L-phase
lubb-dupp
  also lub-dup
  or lub-dub
lu·can·thone
lu·cid
lu·cid·i·ty
  pl lu·cid·i·ties
lu·cif·er·ase
lu·cif·er·in
Lu·cil·ia
lüc·ken·schä·del
Lud·wig's an·gi·na
Lu·er sy·ringe
lu·es
  pl lu·es

lymphadenopathic

lu·et·ic
lu·et·i·cal·ly
lu·e·tin
Lu·gol's so·lu·tion
lum·ba·go
lum·bar
lum·bar·i·za·tion
lum·bo·dor·sal
lum·bo·sa·cral
lum·bri·cal
lum·bri·ca·lis
  pl lum·bri·ca·les
lu·men
  pl lu·mi·na
  or lu·mens
lu·mi·chrome
lu·mi·fla·vin
lu·mi·nal
  also lu·me·nal
lu·mi·nesce
  lu·mi·nesced
  lu·mi·nesc·ing
lu·mi·nes·cence
lu·mi·nes·cent
lu·mi·nif·er·ous
lu·mi·nos·i·ty
  pl lu·mi·nos·i·ties
lu·mi·nous
lu·mi·rho·dop·sin
lu·mis·ter·ol
lump·ec·to·my
  pl lump·ec·to·mies
lu·na·cy
  pl lu·na·cies
lu·nar
lu·nate
lu·na·tic

lung·er
lung·worm
lu·nu·la
  pl lu·nu·lae
lu·nule
lu·pine
  also lu·pin
lu·pi·no·sis
  pl lu·pi·no·ses
lu·poid
lu·pu·lin
lu·pu·lon
  also lu·pu·lone
lu·pus
lu·pus er·y·the·ma·
  to·sus
lu·pus ne·phri·tis
lu·pus per·nio
lu·pus vul·gar·is
Lusch·ka's gland
lu·te·al
lu·tein
lu·tein·iza·tion
lu·tein·ize
  lu·tein·ized
  lu·tein·iz·ing
lu·te·ol·y·sis
  pl lu·te·ol·y·ses
lu·teo·lyt·ic
lu·te·o·ma
  pl lu·te·o·mas
  or lu·te·o·ma·ta
lu·te·o·ma·tous
lu·teo·tro·pic
  or lu·teo·tro·phic
lu·teo·tro·pin
  or lu·teo·tro·phin

lu·te·tium
  also lu·te·cium

lux·ate
  lux·at·ed
  lux·at·ing
lux·a·tion
ly·ase
ly·can·thro·py
  pl ly·can·thro·pies
ly·co·pene
ly·co·pen·emia
Ly·co·per·don
ly·co·po·dine
ly·co·po·di·um
Ly·ell's syn·drome
ly·ing-in
  pl ly·ings-in
  or ly·ing-ins

Lyme dis·ease
Lym·naea
lym·nae·id
Lym·nae·idae
lymph·ad·e·nec·to·
  my
  pl lymph·ad·e·nec·to·
  mies

lymph·ad·e·nit·ic
lymph·ad·e·ni·tis
lym·phad·e·noid
lymph·ad·e·no·ma
  pl lymph·ad·e·no·mas
  or lymph·ad·e·no·ma·
  ta

lymph·ad·e·no·
  path·ic

lymph·ad·e·nop·a·thy
pl lymph·ad·e·nop·a·thies

lymph·ad·e·nop·a·thy-as·so·ci·at·ed vi·rus

lymph·ad·e·no·sis
pl lymph·ad·e·no·ses

lymph·a·gogue

lymph·an·gi·ec·ta·sia

lymph·an·gi·ec·ta·sis
pl lymph·an·gi·ec·ta·ses

lymph·an·gi·ec·tat·ic

lymph·an·gio·en·do·the·li·o·ma
pl lymph·an·gio·en·do·the·li·o·mas
or lymph·an·gio·en·do·the·li·o·ma·ta

lymph·an·gio·gram

lymph·an·gio·graph·ic

lymph·an·gi·og·ra·phy
pl lymph·an·gi·og·ra·phies

lymph·an·gi·o·ma
pl lymph·an·gi·o·mas
or lymph·an·gi·o·ma·ta

lymph·an·gi·om·a·tous

lymph·an·gio·sar·co·ma
pl lymph·an·gio·sar·co·mas
or lymph·an·gio·sar·co·ma·ta

lymph·an·gi·ot·o·my
pl lymph·an·gi·ot·o·mies

lym·phan·gi·tis
pl lym·phan·git·i·des

lym·phan·gi·tis ep·i·zo·ot·i·ca

lym·phat·ic

lym·phat·i·cal·ly

lym·phat·i·co·ve·nous

lym·pha·tism

lymph·ede·ma

lymph·edem·a·tous

lym·pho·blast

lym·pho·blas·tic

lym·pho·blas·toid

lym·pho·blas·to·ma
pl lym·pho·blas·to·mas
or lym·pho·blas·to·ma·ta

lym·pho·blas·to·sis
pl lym·pho·blas·to·ses

lym·pho·cyte

lym·pho·cyt·ic

lym·pho·cy·to·blast

lym·pho·cy·to·gen·e·sis
pl lym·pho·cy·to·gen·e·ses

lym·pho·cy·toid

lym·pho·cy·to·ma
pl lym·pho·cy·to·mas
or lym·pho·cy·to·ma·ta

lym·pho·cy·to·pe·nia

lym·pho·cy·to·pe·nic

lym·pho·cy·to·poi·e·sis
pl lym·pho·cy·to·poi·e·ses

lym·pho·cy·to·poi·et·ic

lym·pho·cy·to·sis
pl lym·pho·cy·to·ses

lym·pho·cy·tot·ic

lym·pho·cy·to·tox·ic

lym·pho·cy·to·tox·ic·i·ty
pl lym·pho·cy·to·tox·ic·i·ties

lym·pho·ep·i·the·li·al

lym·pho·gen·e·sis
pl lym·pho·gen·e·ses

lym·phog·e·nous
also lym·pho·gen·ic

lym·pho·gram

lym·pho·gran·u·lo·
ma
pl lym·pho·gran·u·lo·
mas
or lym·pho·gran·u·lo·
ma·ta

lym·pho·gran·u·lo·
ma in·gui·na·le

lym·pho·gran·u·lo·
ma·to·sis
pl lym·pho·gran·u·lo·
ma·to·ses

lym·pho·gran·u·lo·
mat·ous

lym·pho·gran·u·lo·
ma ve·ne·re·um

lym·pho·graph·ic

lym·phog·ra·phy
pl lym·phog·ra·phies

lym·phoid

lym·phoid·o·cyte

lym·pho·kine

lym·phol·y·sis
pl lym·phol·y·ses

lym·pho·lyt·ic

lym·pho·ma
pl lym·pho·mas
or lym·pho·ma·ta

lym·pho·ma·gen·e·
sis
pl lym·pho·ma·gen·e·
ses

lym·pho·ma·gen·ic

lym·pho·ma·toid

lym·pho·ma·to·sis
pl lym·pho·ma·to·ses

lym·pho·ma·tot·ic

lym·pho·ma·tous

lym·pho·path·ia
ve·ne·re·um

lym·pho·pe·nia

lym·pho·pe·nic

lym·pho·poi·e·sis
pl lym·pho·poi·e·ses

lym·pho·poi·et·ic

lym·pho·pro·lif·er·
a·tive

lym·pho·re·tic·u·
lar

lym·pho·re·tic·u·lo·
sis
pl lym·pho·re·tic·u·
lo·ses

lym·phor·rhage

lym·pho·sar·co·ma
pl lym·pho·sar·co·
mas
or lym·pho·sar·co·
ma·ta

lym·pho·sar·co·ma·
tous

lym·pho·scin·tig·
ra·phy
pl lym·pho·scin·tig·
ra·phies

lym·pho·tox·ic

lym·pho·tox·in

lymph·uria

lyn·es·tre·nol

Ly·on hy·poth·e·sis

lyo·phile
also lyo·phil

lyo·phil·ic

ly·oph·i·li·za·tion

ly·oph·i·lize

ly·oph·i·lized

ly·oph·i·liz·ing

ly·oph·i·liz·er

lyo·pho·bic

lyo·sorp·tion

lyo·tro·pic

ly·ot·ro·py
pl ly·ot·ro·pies

ly·ra

ly·sate

lyse
lysed
lys·ing

Ly·sen·ko·ism

ly·ser·gic

ly·ser·gide

ly·sim·e·ter

ly·si·met·ric

ly·sim·e·try
pl ly·sim·e·tries

ly·sin

ly·sine

ly·sis
pl ly·ses

ly·so·ceph·a·lin

ly·so·gen

ly·so·gen·e·sis
pl ly·so·gen·e·ses

ly·so·gen·ic

ly·so·ge·nic·i·ty
pl ly·so·ge·nic·i·ties

ly·sog·e·ni·za·tion

ly·sog·e·nize

ly·sog·e·nized

ly·sog·e·niz·ing

ly·sog·e·ny
pl ly·sog·e·nies
ly·so·lec·i·thin
ly·so·phos·pha·tide
ly·so·phos·pha·ti·
dyl·cho·line
ly·so·som·al
ly·so·some
ly·so·staph·in
ly·so·zyme
lys·sa
lys·sic
Lys·ter bag
var of Lister bag
lyt·ic
ly·ti·cal·ly
Lyt·ta
lyx·o·fla·vin
lyx·ose

M

Ma·ca·ca
ma·caque
Mac·Con·key's
agar
or Mac·Con·key agar
mac·er·ate
mac·er·at·ed
mac·er·at·ing
mac·er·a·tion
mac·er·a·tive
Mach num·ber
Ma·chu·po vi·rus
mack·er·el shark
Mac·leod's syn·
drome

mac·ra·can·tho·
rhyn·chi·a·sis
pl mac·ra·can·tho·
rhyn·chi·a·ses
*Mac·ra·can·tho·
rhyn·chus*
mac·ro
mac·ro·ag·gre·gate
mac·ro·ag·gre·gat·
ed
mac·ro·anal·y·sis
pl mac·ro·anal·y·ses
Mac·rob·del·la
mac·ro·bi·ot·ics
mac·ro·blast
mac·ro·ceph·a·lous
or mac·ro·ce·phal·ic
mac·ro·ceph·a·lus
pl mac·ro·ceph·a·li
mac·ro·ceph·a·ly
pl mac·ro·ceph·a·lies
mac·ro·co·nid·i·
um
pl mac·ro·co·nid·ia
mac·ro·cra·ni·al
mac·ro·cyst
mac·ro·cyte
mac·ro·cyt·ic
mac·ro·cy·to·sis
pl mac·ro·cy·to·ses
mac·ro·dont
mac·ro·fau·na
mac·ro·fau·nal
mac·ro·flo·ra
mac·ro·flo·ral
mac·ro·ga·mete

mac·ro·ga·me·to·
cyte
mac·ro·gen·i·to·so·
mia
mac·ro·gen·i·to·so·
mia pre·cox
mac·ro·glia
mac·ro·gli·al
mac·ro·glob·u·lin
mac·ro·glob·u·lin·
emia
mac·ro·glob·u·lin·
emic
mac·ro·glos·sia
mac·ro·lec·i·thal
mac·ro·lide
mac·ro·ma·nia
mac·ro·ma·ni·a·cal
mac·ro·mas·tia
mac·ro·mere
mac·ro·meth·od
mac·ro·mo·lec·u·
lar
mac·ro·mol·e·cule
mac·ro·mu·tant
mac·ro·mu·ta·tion
mac·ro·nod·u·lar
mac·ro·nor·mo·
blast
mac·ro·nor·mo·
blas·tic
mac·ro·nu·cle·ar
mac·ro·nu·cle·us
pl mac·ro·nu·clei
also mac·ro·nu·cle·us·
es
mac·ro·nu·tri·ent

mac·ro·os·mat·ic
var of macrosmatic

mac·ro·phage

mac·ro·phag·ic

mac·ro·pol·y·cyte

mac·rop·sia

mac·rop·sy
pl mac·rop·sies

mac·rop·tic

mac·ro·scop·ic

mac·ro·scop·i·cal·ly

mac·ro·sec·tion

mac·ros·mat·ic
also mac·ro·os·mat·ic

mac·ro·so·mia

mac·ro·so·mic

mac·ro·splanch·nic

mac·ro·spore

mac·ro·struc·tur·al

mac·ro·struc·ture

mac·ro·tome

mac·u·la
pl mac·u·lae
also mac·u·las

mac·u·la acu·sti·ca
pl mac·u·lae acu·sti·cae

mac·u·la den·sa

mac·u·la lu·tea
pl mac·u·lae lu·te·ae

mac·u·lar

mac·u·la sac·cu·li

mac·u·la·tion

mac·u·la utri·cu·li

mac·ule

mac·u·lo·pap·u·lar

mac·u·lo·pap·ule

mad·a·ro·sis
pl mad·a·ro·ses

mad·a·rot·ic

Mad·dox rod

mad·ness

Ma·du·ra foot

mad·u·ro·my·co·sis
pl mad·u·ro·my·co·ses

mad·u·ro·my·cot·ic

maf·e·nide

ma·gen·stras·se

ma·gen·ta

mag·got

mag·ic bul·let

ma·gis·tral

mag·ma

mag·ne·sia

mag·ne·sium

mag·net·ic

mag·net·i·cal·ly

mag·ne·tism

mag·ne·ti·za·tion

mag·ne·to·car·dio·gram

mag·ne·to·car·dio·graph

mag·ne·to·car·dio·graph·ic

mag·ne·to·car·di·og·ra·phy
pl mag·ne·to·car·di·og·ra·phies

mag·ne·to·en·ceph·a·lo·gram

mag·ne·to·en·ceph·a·log·ra·phy
pl mag·ne·to·en·ceph·a·log·ra·phies

mag·ne·to·graph

mag·ne·tom·e·ter

mag·ne·to·met·ric

mag·ne·tom·e·try
pl mag·ne·tom·e·tries

mag·ne·ton

mag·ne·to·tac·tic

mag·ne·tron

mag·ni·fi·ca·tion

mag·ni·fy
mag·ni·fied
mag·ni·fy·ing

mag·ni·tude

mag·no·cel·lu·lar

ma·huang

maid·en·hair

maid·en·head

main·te·nance

ma·jor·med·i·cal

mal·ab·sorp·tion

mal·ab·sorp·tive

ma·la·cia

ma·lac·ic

mal·a·co·pla·kia
also mal·a·ko·pla·kia

mal·a·cot·ic

mal·ad·ap·ta·tion

mal·adap·tive

mal·a·die de Ro·ger

mal·ad·just·ed

mal·ad·jus·tive

mal·ad·just·ment

mal·ad·min·is·tra·
tion
mal·a·dy
  pl mal·a·dies
mal·aise
mal·aligned
mal·align·ment
ma·lar
ma·lar·ia
ma·lar·i·ae ma·lar·
ia
ma·lar·ial
ma·lar·i·o·log·i·cal
ma·lar·i·ol·o·gist
ma·lar·i·ol·o·gy
  pl ma·lar·i·ol·o·gies
ma·lar·i·o·met·ric
ma·lar·i·om·e·try
  pl ma·lar·i·om·e·tries
ma·lar·io·ther·a·py
  pl ma·lar·io·ther·a·
    pies
ma·lar·i·ous
mal·as·sim·i·la·
tion
ma·late
mal·a·thi·on
mal de ca·de·ras
mal del pin·to
mal de mer
mal·de·vel·op·
ment
male
ma·le·ate
ma·le·ic
mal·for·ma·tion
mal·formed

mal·func·tion
ma·lic
ma·lig·nan·cy
  pl ma·lig·nan·cies
ma·lig·nant
ma·lin·ger
  ma·lin·gered
  ma·lin·ger·ing
ma·lin·ger·er
mal·le·in
mal·le·in·i·za·tion
mal·le·o·lar
mal·le·o·lus
  pl mal·le·o·li
Mal·leo·my·ces
mal·let fin·ger
mal·le·us
  pl mal·lei
Mal·loph·a·ga
Mal·lo·ry's tri·ple
stain
mal·nour·ished
mal·nu·tri·tion
mal·nu·tri·tion·al
mal·oc·clu·ded
mal·oc·clu·sion
mal·o·nate
ma·lo·nic
mal·o·nyl
mal·o·nyl CoA
mal·o·nyl·urea
Mal·pi·ghi·an body
Mal·pi·ghi·an cor·
pus·cle
Mal·pi·ghi·an lay·
er

Mal·pi·ghi·an pyr·
a·mid
mal·posed
mal·po·si·tion
mal·prac·tice
  mal·prac·ticed
  mal·prac·tic·ing
mal·pre·sen·ta·tion
mal·ro·ta·ted
mal·ro·ta·tion
Mal·ta fe·ver
malt·ase
Mal·thu·sian
Mal·thu·sian·ism
malt·ose
mal·union
mal·unit·ed
mam·ba
mam·e·lon
mam·il·la·ry
  var of mammillary
mam·il·lat·ed
  var of mammillated
mam·il·la·tion
  var of mammillation
mam·il·li·form
  var of mammilliform
mam·il·lo·tha·lam·
ic tract
  var of mammillotha-
  lamic tract
mam·ma
  pl mam·mae
mam·mal
Mam·ma·lia
mam·ma·li·an
mam·mal·o·gist

mantle

mam·mal·o·gy
pl mam·mal·o·gies

mam·ma·plas·ty
pl mam·ma·plas·ties

mam·ma·ry
pl mam·ma·ries

mam·mate

mam·mec·to·my
pl mam·mec·to·mies

mam·mif·er·ous

mam·mi·form

mam·mil·la·ry
or mam·il·la·ry

mam·mil·lat·ed
or mam·il·lat·ed

mam·mil·la·tion
or mam·il·la·tion

mam·mil·li·form
or ma·mil·li·form

mam·mil·lo·tha·
lam·ic tract
or ma·mil·lo·tha·lam·
ic tract

mam·mi·tis
pl mam·mit·i·des

mam·mo·gen

mam·mo·gen·ic

mam·mo·gen·i·cal·
ly

mam·mo·gram

mam·mo·graph

mam·mo·graph·ic

mam·mog·ra·phy
pl mam·mog·ra·phies

mam·mo·plas·ty
pl mam·mo·plas·ties

mam·mo·tro·pic
or mam·mo·tro·phic

mam·mo·tro·pin
also mam·mo·tro·
phin

man·a·ca

man·age
man·aged
man·ag·ing

man·age·ment

man·ci·nism

man·del·ate

man·del·ic

man·de·lo·ni·trile

man·di·ble

man·dib·u·la
pl man·dib·u·lae

man·dib·u·lar

man·di·bu·lo·fa·
cial

man·drake

man·drel
also man·dril

man·drin

ma·neu·ver

man·ga·nese

man·gan·ic

man·ga·nous

mange

man·gy
also man·gey
man·gi·er
man·gi·est

ma·nia

ma·ni·ac

ma·ni·a·cal

man·ic

man·i·cal·ly

man·ic-de·pres·
sion

man·ic-de·pres·
sive

man·i·fes·ta·tion

man·i·fest con·tent

man·i·kin

Ma·nila hemp

ma·nip·u·late
ma·nip·u·lat·ed
ma·nip·u·lat·ing

ma·nip·u·la·tion

ma·nip·u·la·tive

man·kind

man·na

man·nan

man·ner·ism

man·ni·tol

man·no·hep·tu·
lose

man·no·nic

man·nose

man·nos·i·do·sis
pl man·nos·i·do·ses

man·nu·ron·ic

ma·nom·e·ter

mano·met·ric

mano·met·ri·cal·ly

ma·nom·e·try
pl ma·nom·e·tries

man·op·to·scope

man·slaugh·ter

Man·son·el·la

Man·so·nia

Man·son's dis·ease

man·tle

Man·toux test
man·u·al
man·u·al·ist
ma·nu·bri·al
ma·nu·bri·um
  pl ma·nu·bria
  also ma·nu·bri·ums
ma·nu·bri·um ster·
  ni
ma·nus
  pl ma·nus
many·plies
ma·ran·ta
ma·ran·tic
ma·ras·ma
ma·ras·mic
ma·ras·mus
mar·ble·iza·tion
Mar·burg dis·ease
Mar·burg vi·rus
marc
Mar·ek's dis·ease
Ma·rey's law
Mar·fan's syn·
  drome
  or Mar·fan syn·drome

mar·gar·ic
mar·ga·rine
Mar·gar·o·pus
mar·gin·at·ed
mar·gin·a·tion
Ma·rie-Strüm·pell
  dis·ease
  also Ma·rie-Strüm·
  pell's dis·ease

mar·i·jua·na
  also mar·i·hua·na

mark·er
mar·mo·rat·ed
mar·mo·ra·tion
mar·mot
Mar·o·teaux-La·my
  syn·drome
mar·row
Mar·seilles fe·ver
marsh·mal·low
Marsh test
mar·su·pi·al·iza·
  tion
mar·su·pi·al·ize
  mar·su·pi·al·ized
  mar·su·pi·al·iz·
  ing
Mar·ti·not·ti cell
  or Mar·ti·not·ti's cell

Mar·ti·us yel·low
mas·cu·line
mas·cu·lin·i·ty
  pl mas·cu·lin·i·ties
mas·cu·lin·iza·tion
mas·cu·lin·ize
  mas·cu·lin·ized
  mas·cu·lin·iz·ing
mas·cu·lin·ovo·
  blas·to·ma
  pl mas·cu·lin·ovo·
    blas·to·mas
  or mas·cu·lin·ovo·
    blas·to·ma·ta

ma·ser
mas·och·ism
mas·och·ist
mas·och·is·tic
mas·och·is·ti·cal·ly

mas·sage
  mas·saged
  mas·sag·ing
mas·sa in·ter·me·
  dia
mas·se·ter
mas·se·ter·ic
mas·seur
mas·seuse
mas·si·cot
mas·so·ther·a·pist
mas·so·ther·a·py
  pl mas·so·ther·a·pies
mas·tal·gia
mas·tec·to·mee
mas·tec·to·my
  pl mas·tec·to·mies
mas·tic
mas·ti·cate
  mas·ti·cat·ed
  mas·ti·cat·ing
mas·ti·ca·tion
mas·ti·ca·to·ry
  pl mas·ti·ca·to·ries
Mas·ti·goph·ora
mas·ti·goph·o·ran
mas·tit·ic
mas·ti·tis
  pl mas·tit·i·des
mas·to·cyte
mas·to·cy·to·ma
  pl mas·to·cy·to·mas
  or mas·to·cy·to·ma·ta
mas·to·cy·to·sis
  pl mas·to·cy·to·ses
mas·to·dyn·ia
mas·toid

mas·toid·ec·to·my
pl mas·toid·ec·to·mies

mas·toid·itis
pl mas·toid·it·i·des

mas·toid·ot·o·my
pl mas·toid·ot·o·mies

mas·to·mys
pl mas·to·mys

mas·top·a·thy
pl mas·top·a·thies

mas·tot·o·my
pl mas·tot·o·mies

mas·tur·bate
mas·tur·bat·ed
mas·tur·bat·ing

mas·tur·ba·tion
mas·tur·ba·tor
mas·tur·ba·to·ry

mat
or matt
or matte

mate
mat·ed
mat·ing

ma·té
or ma·te

ma·te·ria al·ba
ma·te·ria med·i·ca
ma·ter·nal
ma·ter·ni·ty
pl ma·ter·ni·ties

ma·ti·co
mat·ing
ma·tri·cal
mat·ri·car·ia
pl mat·ri·car·ia
or mat·ri·car·ias

ma·tri·cide
mat·ri·cli·nous
ma·trix
pl ma·tri·ces
or ma·trix·es

mat·ro·cli·nal
mat·ro·clin·ic
mat·ro·cli·nous
mat·ro·cli·ny
pl mat·ro·cli·nies

mat·ter
mat·tery
mat·tress su·ture
mat·u·rate
mat·u·rat·ed
mat·u·rat·ing

mat·u·ra·tion
mat·u·ra·tion·al
ma·tur·a·tive
ma·ture
ma·tur·er
ma·tur·est

ma·ture
ma·tured
ma·tur·ing

ma·tu·ri·ty
pl ma·tu·ri·ties

ma·tu·ri·ty-on·set
di·a·be·tes

Mau·rer's dots
max·il·la
pl max·il·lae
or max·il·las

max·il·lary
pl max·il·lar·ies

max·il·lec·to·my
pl max·il·lec·to·mies

max·il·lo·al·ve·o·
lar

max·il·lo·fa·cial
max·il·lo·tur·bi·nal
max·i·mal
max·i·mum
pl max·i·ma
or max·i·mums

may·ap·ple
May-Grün·wald
stain

may·hem
may·tan·sine
ma·zin·dol
ma·zo·pla·sia
Maz·zi·ni test
M band
Mc·Ar·dle's dis·
ease

Mc·Bur·ney's point
mea·dow mush·
room

mea·sle
mea·sles
mea·sly
mea·sli·er
mea·sli·est

mea·sur·able
mea·sur·ably
mea·sure
mea·sured
mea·sur·ing

mea·sure·ment
me·a·tal
me·ato·plas·ty
pl me·ato·plas·ties

me·a·tot·o·my
  pl me·a·tot·o·mies

me·atus
  pl me·atus·es
  or me·atus

me·ben·da·zole

me·bu·ta·mate

mec·a·myl·a·mine

Mec·ca bal·sam

me·chan·i·cal

me·chan·ics

mech·a·nism

mech·a·nis·tic

mech·a·no·chem·i·cal

mech·a·no·chem·is·try
  pl mech·a·no·chem·is·tries

mech·a·no·re·cep·tion

mech·a·no·re·cep·tive

mech·a·no·re·cep·tor

mech·a·no·sen·so·ry

mech·a·no·ther·a·pist

mech·a·no·ther·a·py
  pl mech·a·no·ther·a·pies

mech·lor·eth·amine

Me·cis·to·cir·rus

Meck·el's car·ti·lage

Meck·el's cave

Meck·el's di·ver·tic·u·lum

Meck·el's gan·gli·on

mec·li·zine

mec·lo·fe·nam·ic

me·con·ic

mec·o·nin
  also mec·o·nine

me·co·ni·um

me·cro·li·ter

me·daz·e·pam

med·e·vac
  also med·i·vac
  noun

med·e·vac
  verb

  med·e·vacked

  med·e·vack·ing

me·dia
  pl me·di·ae

me·dia
  pl of me·di·um

me·di·ad

me·di·al

me·di·an

me·di·as·ti·nal

me·di·as·ti·ni·tis
  pl me·di·as·ti·nit·i·des

me·di·as·ti·no·peri·car·di·tis
  pl me·di·as·ti·no·peri·car·dit·i·des

me·di·as·ti·nos·co·py
  pl me·di·as·ti·nos·co·pies

me·di·as·ti·not·o·my
  pl me·di·as·ti·not·o·mies

me·di·as·ti·num
  pl me·di·as·ti·na

me·di·ate

  me·di·at·ed

  me·di·at·ing

me·di·a·tion

me·di·a·tion·al

me·di·a·tor

me·di·a·to·ry

med·ic

med·i·ca·ble

med·ic·aid

med·i·cal

me·di·ca·ment

med·i·ca·men·tous

med·i·cant

medi·care

med·i·cate

  med·i·cat·ed

  med·i·cat·ing

med·i·ca·tion

me·dic·i·nal

med·i·cine

med·i·co
  pl med·i·cos

med·i·co·le·gal

Me·di·na worm

me·dio·car·pal

me·dio·lat·er·al

melanization

me·di·o·ne·cro·sis
  pl me·di·o·ne·cro·ses

Med·i·ter·ra·nean
  fe·ver

me·di·um
  pl me·di·ums
  or me·dia

med·i·vac
  var of medevac

med·ro·ges·tone

me·droxy·pro·ges·
  ter·one

me·dul·la
  pl me·dul·las
  or me·dul·lae

me·dul·la ob·lon·
  ga·ta
  pl me·dul·la ob·lon·
    ga·tas
  or me·dul·lae ob·lon·
    ga·tae

med·ul·lary

med·ul·lat·ed

med·ul·la·tion

med·ul·lec·to·my
  pl med·ul·lec·to·mies

me·dul·lin

me·dul·lo·blast

me·dul·lo·blas·to·
  ma
  pl me·dul·lo·blas·to·
    mas
  also me·dul·lo·blas·to·
    ma·ta

me·dul·lo·blas·to·
  ma·tous

mef·e·nam·ic

mega·co·lon

mega·cu·rie

mega·cy·cle

mega·dont

mega·don·ty
  pl mega·don·ties

mega·dose

mega·dos·ing

mega·du·o·de·num
  pl mega·du·o·de·na
  or mega·du·o·de·
    nums

mega·esoph·a·gus
  pl mega·esoph·a·gi

mega·hertz

mega·kary·o·blast

mega·kary·o·cyte

mega·kary·o·cyt·ic

mega·lec·i·thal

meg·a·lo·blast

meg·a·lo·blas·tic

meg·a·lo·ceph·a·ly
  pl meg·a·lo·ceph·a·
    lies

meg·a·lo·cor·nea

meg·a·lo·cyte

meg·a·lo·cyt·ic

meg·a·lo·ma·nia

meg·a·lo·ma·ni·ac

meg·a·lo·ma·ni·a·
  cal
  also meg·a·lo·man·ic

mega·mol·e·cule

mega·rad

mega·spore

mega·spor·ic

mega·unit

mega·vi·ta·min

mega·volt

mega·volt·age

mega·watt

me·ges·trol

meg·lu·mine

meg·ohm

me·grim

Meh·lis' gland

mei·bo·mian gland

mei·bo·mi·a·ni·tis

meio·cyte

mei·o·sis
  pl mei·o·ses

meio·stoma·tous

meio·stome

mei·ot·ic

mei·ot·i·cal·ly

Meiss·ner's cor·
  pus·cle

Mek·er burn·er

mel

mel·a·leu·ca

mel·a·mine

mel·an·cho·lia

mel·an·cho·li·ac

mel·an·chol·ic

mel·an·cho·lious

mel·an·choly
  pl mel·an·chol·ies

mel·ane·mia

Me·la·nia

me·lan·ic

mel·a·nif·er·ous

mel·a·nin

mel·a·nism

mel·a·nis·tic

mel·a·ni·za·tion

mel·a·nize
  mel·a·nized
  mel·a·niz·ing
me·la·no
me·la·no·blast
me·la·no·blas·tic
me·la·no·blas·to·
  ma
  pl me·la·no·blas·to·
    mas
  or me·la·no·blas·to·
    ma·ta
mel·a·no·car·ci·no·
  ma
  pl mel·a·no·car·ci·no·
    mas
  or mel·a·no·car·ci·no·
    ma·ta
me·la·no·cyte
me·la·no·cyte-stim·
  u·lat·ing hor·
  mone
me·la·no·cyt·ic
me·la·no·cy·to·ma
  pl me·la·no·cy·to·mas
  or me·la·no·cy·to·ma·
    ta
mel·a·no·der·ma
mel·a·no·der·mic
me·la·no·gen
me·la·no·gen·e·sis
  pl me·la·no·gen·e·ses
me·la·no·ge·net·ic
me·la·no·gen·ic
mel·a·noid
mel·a·no·ma
  pl mel·a·no·mas
  also mel·a·no·ma·ta

mel·a·no·ma·to·sis
  pl mel·a·no·ma·to·ses
me·la·no·phage
me·la·no·phore
me·la·no·phore-
  stim·u·lat·ing
  hor·mone
me·la·no·phor·ic
me·la·no·pla·kia
me·la·no·sar·co·ma
  pl me·la·no·sar·co·
    mas
  or me·la·no·sar·co·
    ma·ta
mel·a·no·sis
  pl mel·a·no·ses
mel·a·no·sis co·li
me·la·no·som·al
me·la·no·some
mel·a·not·ic
me·la·no·tro·pic
  also me·la·no·tro·phic
me·la·no·tro·pin
mel·an·uria
mel·an·uric
me·lar·so·prol
me·las·ma
me·las·mic
me·la·to·nin
me·le·na
mel·en·ges·trol
me·lez·i·tose
mel·i·bi·ose
mel·i·oi·do·sis
  pl mel·i·oi·do·ses
me·lis·sa
me·lis·sic

mel·i·ten·sis
mel·i·tose
me·lit·tin
mel·i·tu·ria
  or mel·li·tu·ria
melo·ma·nia
melo·ma·ni·ac
mel·on-seed body
Me·loph·a·gus
mel·o·plas·ty
  pl mel·o·plas·ties
melo·rhe·os·to·sis
  pl melo·rhe·os·to·ses
  or melo·rhe·os·to·sis·
    es
mel·pha·lan
mem·ber
mem·bra·na
  pl mem·bra·nae
mem·bra·na·ceous
mem·bra·nal
mem·brane
mem·braned
mem·bra·nel·lar
mem·bra·nelle
  also mem·bra·nel·la
  pl mem·bra·nelles
  also mem·bra·nel·lae
mem·bra·nol·o·gist
mem·bra·nol·o·gy
  pl mem·bra·nol·o·gies
mem·bra·no·pro·
  lif·er·a·tive
mem·bra·nous
mem·o·ry
  pl mem·o·ries
men·ac·me

men·a·di·one
men·a·quin·one
men·ar·che
men·ar·che·al
  or men·ar·chal
  also men·ar·chi·al

men·a·zon
men·de·le·vi·um
Men·de·lian
Men·de·lian·ism
Men·de·lian·ist
Men·del·ism
Men·del·ist
men·del·ize
  men·del·ized
  men·del·iz·ing
Men·del's law
men·go·vi·rus
Mé·nière's dis·ease
men·in·ge·al
me·nin·ges
  pl of meninx

me·nin·gi·o·ma
  pl me·nin·gi·o·mas
  or me·nin·gi·o·ma·ta

men·in·gism
men·in·gis·mus
  pl men·in·gis·mi

men·in·git·ic
men·in·gi·tis
  pl men·in·git·i·des

me·nin·go·cele
  also me·nin·go·coele

me·nin·go·coc·cal
  also me·nin·go·coc·cic

me·nin·go·coc·ce·mia
me·nin·go·coc·cus
  pl me·nin·go·coc·ci

me·nin·go·en·ceph·a·lit·ic
me·nin·go·en·ceph·a·li·tis
  pl me·nin·go·en·ceph·a·lit·i·des

me·nin·go·en·ceph·a·lo·cele
me·nin·go·en·ceph·a·lo·my·eli·tis
  pl me·nin·go·en·ceph·a·lo·my·elit·i·des

me·nin·go·my·elo·cele
me·nin·go·pneu·mo·nit·is
  pl me·nin·go·pneu·mo·nit·i·des

me·nin·go·vas·cu·lar
me·ninx
  pl me·nin·ges

me·nis·cal
men·is·cec·to·my
  pl men·is·cec·to·mies

me·nis·co·cy·to·sis
  pl me·nis·co·cy·to·ses

me·nis·cus
  pl me·nis·ci
  also me·nis·cus·es

meno·met·ror·rha·gia

meno·paus·al
meno·pause
men·or·rha·gia
men·or·rhag·ic
men·ses
men·strua
  pl of menstruum

men·stru·al
men·stru·ate
  men·stru·at·ed
  men·stru·at·ing
men·stru·a·tion
men·stru·um
  pl men·stru·ums
  or men·strua

men·tal
men·ta·lis
  pl men·ta·les

men·tal·ism
men·tal·is·tic
men·tal·i·ty
  pl men·tal·i·ties

men·ta·tion
Men·tha
men·thol
men·tho·lat·ed
men·thyl
men·ti·cide
men·ton
men·tum
  pl men·ta

mep·a·zine
me·pen·zo·late
me·per·i·dine
me·phen·e·sin
meph·en·ox·a·lone
me·phen·ter·mine

me·phen·y·to·in
mepho·bar·bi·tal
me·piv·a·caine
mep·ro·bam·ate
me·ral·gia
me·ral·gia par·es·
thet·i·ca
mer·al·lu·ride
mer·bro·min
mer·cap·tal
mer·cap·tan
mer·cap·tide
mer·cap·to
mer·cap·to·eth·a·
nol
mer·cap·tom·er·in
mer·cap·to·pu·rine
mer·cap·tu·ric
Mer·cier's bar
mer·cu·mat·i·lin
mer·cu·ri·al
mer·cu·ri·al·ism
mer·cu·ric
mer·cu·ro·phyl·
line
mer·cu·rous
mer·cu·ry
    pl mer·cu·ries
mer·cu·ry-va·por
lamp
mer·eth·ox·yl·line
me·rid·i·an
me·rid·i·o·nal
me·ris·tic
me·ris·ti·cal·ly
Mer·kel's disk
mero·blas·tic

mero·blas·ti·cal·ly
mero·crine
mer·o·gon·ic
me·rog·o·ny
    pl me·rog·o·nies
mero·my·o·sin
mero·zo·ite
mero·zy·gote
mer·sal·yl
me·sad
    also me·si·ad
me·sal
    var of mesial
mes·an·gi·al
mes·an·gi·um
    pl mes·an·gia
mes·aor·ti·tis
    pl mes·aor·tit·i·des
mes·ar·ter·i·tis
    pl mes·ar·ter·it·i·des
me·sat·i·pel·lic
mes·ax·on
mes·cal
mes·ca·line
mes·ec·to·derm
mes·ec·to·der·mal
    or mes·ec·to·der·mic
mes·en·ce·phal·ic
mes·en·ceph·a·lon
mes·en·chy·ma
mes·en·chy·mal
mes·en·chyme
mes·en·chy·mo·ma
    pl mes·en·chy·mo·
    mas
    or mes·en·chy·mo·
    ma·ta

mes·en·do·derm
    or mes·en·to·derm
mes·en·ter·ic
mes·en·teri·o·lum
    pl mes·en·teri·o·la
mes·en·ter·i·tis
mes·en·ter·on
    pl mes·en·tera
mes·en·tery
    pl mes·en·ter·ies
mesh·work
me·si·ad
    var of mesad
me·si·al
    also me·sal
me·sio·buc·cal
me·sio·clu·sion
    also me·si·oc·clu·sion
me·sio·dis·tal
me·sio·lin·gual
mes·mer·ism
mes·mer·ist
mes·mer·iza·tion
mes·mer·ize
    mes·mer·ized
    mes·mer·iz·ing
me·so·ap·pen·di·
ce·al
me·so·ap·pen·dix
    pl me·so·ap·pen·dix·
    es
    or me·so·ap·pen·di·
    ces
me·so·bili·ru·bin
me·so·blast
me·so·blas·tic
me·so·car·dia

me·so·car·di·um
me·so·ce·cum
pl me·so·ce·ca

me·so·ce·phal·ic
me·so·ceph·a·ly
pl me·so·ceph·a·lies

Me·so·ces·toi·des
me·so·ces·toid·id
me·so·chon·dri·um
pl me·so·chon·dria

me·so·cne·mic
me·so·coele
also me·so·coel

me·so·co·lon
meso·conch
also me·so·chon·chic

me·so·con·chy
pl me·so·con·chies

me·so·cra·nic
also me·so·cra·ni·al

me·so·cra·ny
pl me·so·cra·nies

me·so·derm
me·so·der·mal
also me·so·der·mic

me·so·dont
me·so·don·ty
pl me·so·don·ties

me·so·duo·de·num
pl me·so·duo·de·na
or me·so·duo·de·
nums

me·so·e·soph·a·gus
me·so·gas·ter
me·so·gas·tric
me·so·gas·tri·um
pl me·so·gas·tria

me·so·gna·thion
me·sog·na·thous
also me·sog·nath·ic

me·sog·na·thy
pl me·sog·na·thies

me·so·ino·si·tol
me·so·lec·i·thal
me·so·mere
me·so·mer·ic
me·som·er·ism
me·so·me·tri·al
or me·so·me·tric

me·so·me·tri·um
pl me·so·me·tria

me·so·morph
me·so·mor·phic
also me·so·mor·phous

me·so·mor·phism
me·so·mor·phy
pl me·so·mor·phies

me·son
me·so·neph·ric
me·so·ne·phro·ma
pl me·so·ne·phro·mas
or me·so·ne·phro·ma·
ta

me·so·neph·ros
pl me·so·neph·roi

me·so·on·to·morph
me·so·phile
also me·so·phil

me·so·phil·ic
me·soph·ry·on
pl me·soph·rya

me·so·pic
me·so·por·phy·rin
me·so·pro·so·pic

me·so·pros·o·py
pl me·so·pros·o·pies

me·sor·chi·um
pl me·sor·chia

me·so·rec·tum
pl me·so·rec·tums
or me·so·rec·ta

mes·orid·a·zine
me·sor·rhine
also me·sor·rhin·ic

me·sor·rhi·ny
pl me·sor·rhi·nies

me·so·sal·pinx
pl me·so·sal·pin·ges

me·so·sig·moid
me·so·some
me·so·staph·y·line
me·so·ster·num
pl me·so·ster·na

me·so·tar·sal
me·so·the·li·al
me·so·the·li·o·ma
pl me·so·the·li·o·mas
or me·so·the·li·o·ma·
ta

me·so·the·li·um
pl me·so·the·lia

me·so·thor·i·um
mes·ovar·i·um
pl mes·ovar·ia

mes·ox·a·lyl·urea
Me·so·zoa
me·so·zo·an
mes·sen·ger RNA
mes·tra·nol
me·su·ran·ic

me·su·rany
  pl me·su·ran·ies

me·tab·a·sis
  pl me·tab·a·ses

meta·bi·o·sis
  pl meta·bi·o·ses

meta·bi·ot·ic

meta·bi·sul·fite

met·a·bol·ic

met·a·bol·i·cal·ly

me·tab·o·lim·e·ter

me·tab·o·lism

me·tab·o·lite

me·tab·o·liz·abil·i·ty
  pl me·tab·o·liz·abil·i·ties

me·tab·o·liz·able

me·tab·o·lize
  me·tab·o·lized
  me·tab·o·liz·ing

me·tab·o·liz·er

meta·car·pal

meta·car·po·pha·lan·ge·al

meta·car·pus

meta·cen·tric

meta·cer·car·ia
  pl meta·cer·car·i·ae

meta·cer·car·i·al

meta·ces·tode

meta·chro·ma·sia

meta·chro·ma·sy
  also meta·chro·ma·cy
  pl meta·chro·ma·sies
  also meta·chro·ma·cies

meta·chro·mat·ic

meta·chro·mat·i·cal·ly

meta·chro·ma·tin

meta·chro·ma·tin·ic

meta·chro·ma·tism

me·tach·ro·nous

meta·cone

meta·co·nid

meta·con·trast

meta·co·nule

meta·cre·sol

meta·cryp·to·zo·ite

meta·cy·clic

meta·gen·e·sis
  pl meta·gen·e·ses

meta·ge·net·ic

Meta·gon·i·mus

meta·ken·trin

me·tal·lo·en·zyme

met·al·loid

me·tal·lo·por·phy·rin

me·tal·lo·pro·tein

me·tal·lo·thio·ne·in

meta·mer

meta·mere

meta·mer·ic

meta·mer·i·cal·ly

me·tam·er·ism

meta·mor·phose
  meta·mor·phosed
  meta·mor·phos·ing

meta·mor·pho·sis
  pl meta·mor·pho·ses

meta·my·elo·cyte

meta·neph·ric

meta·neph·rine

meta·neph·ro·gen·ic

meta·neph·ros
  pl meta·neph·roi

meta·phase

meta·phos·pho·ric

me·taph·y·se·al
  also me·taph·y·si·al

me·taph·y·sis
  pl me·taph·y·ses

meta·pla·sia

meta·plas·tic

meta·pro·tein

meta·pro·ter·e·nol

meta·psy·cho·log·i·cal

meta·psy·chol·o·gy
  pl meta·psy·chol·o·gies

meta·ram·i·nol

meta·rho·dop·sin

met·ar·te·ri·ole

meta·sta·bil·i·ty
  pl meta·sta·bil·i·ties

meta·sta·ble

me·tas·ta·sis
  pl me·tas·ta·ses

me·tas·ta·si·za·tion

me·tas·ta·size
  me·tas·ta·sized
  me·tas·ta·siz·ing

met·a·sta·tic

met·a·stat·i·cal·ly
meta·stron·gyle
meta·stron·gy·lid
Meta·stron·gyl·i·dae
Meta·stron·gy·lus
meta·tar·sal
meta·tar·sal·gia
meta·tar·sec·to·my
 pl meta·tar·sec·to·mies
meta·tar·so·pha·lan·ge·al
meta·tar·sus
meta·thal·a·mus
 pl meta·thal·a·mi
meta·tro·phic
met·ax·a·lone
meta·zoa
meta·zo·an
met·en·ce·phal·ic
met·en·ceph·a·lon
Met·en·keph·a·lin
me·te·or·ism
me·ter
met·es·trus
metha·cho·line
meth·ac·ry·late
metha·cy·cline
meth·a·done
 also meth·a·don
meth·am·phet·amine
meth·an·dro·sten·o·lone
meth·ane

meth·ane·sul·fo·nate
me·than·o·gen
me·than·o·gen·e·sis
 pl me·than·o·gen·e·ses
me·than·o·gen·ic
meth·a·nol
meth·a·no·lic
meth·a·nol·y·sis
 pl meth·a·nol·y·ses
meth·an·the·line
meth·a·pyr·i·lene
meth·aqua·lone
meth·ar·bi·tal
meth·a·zol·amide
met·hem·al·bu·min
met·he·mo·glo·bin
met·he·mo·glo·bi·ne·mia
met·he·mo·glo·bin·uria
me·the·na·mine
meth·i·cil·lin
me·thi·ma·zole
meth·io·dal
me·thi·o·nine
me·thi·o·nyl
meth·is·a·zone
me·thix·ene
meth·o·car·ba·mol
meth·od
meth·o·hex·i·tal
me·tho·ni·um
meth·o·trex·ate

meth·o·tri·mep·ra·zine
me·thox·amine
me·thox·sa·len
me·thoxy·flu·rane
8-meth·oxy·psor·a·len
meth·sco·pol·amine
meth·sux·i·mide
meth·y·clo·thi·azide
meth·yl
meth·yl·al
meth·yl·ase
meth·yl·ate
 meth·yl·at·ed
 meth·yl·at·ing
meth·yl·ation
meth·yl·ben·zene
meth·yl·ben·ze·tho·ni·um
meth·yl·cel·lu·lose
meth·yl·cho·lan·threne
meth·yl·cyt·o·sine
meth·yl·di·hy·dro·mor·phi·none
meth·yl·do·pa
meth·yl·er·go·no·vine
meth·yl·glu·ca·mine
meth·yl·gly·ox·al
me·thyl·ic
meth·yl·ma·lon·ic

meth·yl·mer·cu·ry
   pl meth·yl·mer·cu·ries

meth·yl·para·ben

meth·yl·phe·ni·date

meth·yl·pred·nis·o·lone

meth·yl·ros·an·i·line

meth·yl·tes·tos·ter·one

meth·yl·thio·ura·cil

meth·yl·trans·fer·ase

meth·yl·ty·ro·sine

meth·y·pry·lon

meth·y·ser·gide

me·ti·amide

met·myo·glo·bin

met·o·clo·pra·mide

me·to·la·zone

me·top·ic

me·to·pi·on

met·o·pism

Me·to·pi·um

met·o·pon

met·o·pro·lol

me·tra
   pl me·trae

me·tra·term

me·tri·al

met·ric
   or met·ri·cal

met·ri·cal·ly

met·rio·cra·nic

met·rio·cra·ny
   pl met·rio·cra·nies

me·tri·tis

me·triz·a·mide

met·ri·zo·ate

met·ro·ni·da·zole

me·tror·rha·gia

me·tror·rhag·ic

me·tu·re·depa

me·tyr·a·pone

me·val·o·nate

mev·a·lon·ic

me·ze·re·on

me·ze·re·um

mho
   pl mhos

Mi·a·neh fe·ver

mi·an·ser·in

mi·as·ma
   pl mi·as·mas
   also mi·as·ma·ta

mi·as·mal

mi·as·mat·ic

mi·as·mic

mice
   pl of mouse

mi·cel·la
   pl mi·cel·lae

mi·cel·lar

mi·celle

Mi·chae·lis con·stant

Mi·chel clip

mi·con·a·zole

mi·cra
   pl of micron

mi·cren·ceph·a·ly
   pl mi·cren·ceph·a·lies

mi·cro

mi·cro·ab·scess

mi·cro·ad·e·no·ma
   pl mi·cro·ad·e·no·mas
   or mi·cro·ad·e·no·ma·ta

mi·cro·aero·phile

mi·cro·aero·phil·ic

mi·cro·aero·phil·i·cal·ly

mi·cro·ag·gre·gate

mi·cro·anal·y·sis
   pl mi·cro·anal·y·ses

mi·cro·an·a·lyt·ic
   or mi·cro·an·a·lyt·i·cal

mi·cro·ana·tom·i·cal

mi·cro·anat·o·mist

mi·cro·anat·o·my
   pl mi·cro·anat·o·mies

mi·cro·an·eu·rysm

mi·cro·an·eu·rys·mal

mi·cro·an·gio·graph·ic

mi·cro·an·gi·og·ra·phy
   pl mi·cro·an·gi·og·ra·phies

mi·cro·an·gio·path·ic

microembolus

mi·cro·an·gi·op·a·
thy
pl mi·cro·an·gi·op·a·
thies

mi·cro·bac·te·ri·
um
pl mi·cro·bac·te·ria

mi·cro·bal·ance

mi·crobe

mi·cro·beam

mi·cro·bi·al

mi·cro·bic

mi·cro·bi·ci·dal

mi·cro·bi·cide

mi·cro·bi·o·log·i·
cal
also mi·cro·bi·o·log·ic

mi·cro·bi·ol·o·gist

mi·cro·bi·ol·o·gy
pl mi·cro·bi·ol·o·gies

mi·cro·bi·o·ta

mi·cro·bi·ot·ic

mi·cro·blast

mi·cro·body
pl mi·cro·bod·ies

mi·cro·bu·rette
or mi·cro·bu·ret

mi·cro·cal·o·rim·e·
ter

mi·cro·ca·lo·ri·
met·ric

mi·cro·cal·o·rim·e·
try
pl mi·cro·cal·o·rim·e·
tries

mi·cro·cap·sule

mi·cro·ce·phal·ic

mi·cro·ceph·a·lus
pl mi·cro·ceph·a·li

mi·cro·ceph·a·ly
pl mi·cro·ceph·a·lies

mi·cro·chem·i·cal

mi·cro·chem·is·try
pl mi·cro·chem·is·
tries

mi·cro·cin·e·mat·o·
graph·ic

mi·cro·cin·e·ma·
tog·ra·phy
pl mi·cro·cin·e·ma·
tog·ra·phies

mi·cro·cir·cu·la·
tion

mi·cro·cir·cu·la·to·
ry

Mi·cro·coc·ca·ce·ae

mi·cro·coc·cal

mi·cro·coc·cus
pl mi·cro·coc·ci

mi·cro·co·lo·nial

mi·cro·col·o·ny
pl mi·cro·col·o·nies

mi·cro·co·nid·i·al

mi·cro·co·nid·i·um
pl mi·cro·co·nid·ia

mi·cro·cor·nea

mi·cro·cou·lomb

mi·cro·crys·tal

mi·cro·crys·tal·line

mi·cro·crys·tal·lin·
i·ty
pl mi·cro·crys·tal·lin·
i·ties

mi·cro·cul·tur·al

mi·cro·cul·ture

mi·cro·cu·rie

mi·cro·cyst

mi·cro·cys·tic

mi·cro·cyte

mi·cro·cy·the·mia

mi·cro·cy·the·mic

mi·cro·cyt·ic

mi·cro·cy·to·sis
pl mi·cro·cy·to·ses

mi·cro·cy·to·tox·ic·
i·ty

mi·cro·de·ter·mi·
na·tion

mi·cro·dis·sect·ed

mi·cro·dis·sec·tion

mi·cro·dose

mi·cro·do·sim·e·try
pl mi·cro·do·sim·e·
tries

mi·cro·drop

mi·cro·drop·let

mi·cro·elec·trode

mi·cro·elec·tro·
pho·re·sis
pl mi·cro·elec·tro·
pho·re·ses

mi·cro·elec·tro·
pho·ret·ic

mi·cro·elec·tro·
pho·ret·i·cal·ly

mi·cro·el·e·ment

mi·cro·em·bo·lus
pl mi·cro·em·bo·li

mi·cro·en·cap·su·late

mi·cro·en·cap·su·lat·ed

mi·cro·en·cap·su·lat·ing

mi·cro·en·cap·su·la·tion

mi·cro·en·vi·ron·ment

mi·cro·en·vi·ron·men·tal

mi·cro·evo·lu·tion

mi·cro·evo·lu·tion·ary

mi·cro·far·ad

mi·cro·fau·na

mi·cro·fau·nal

mi·cro·fi·bril

mi·cro·fi·bril·lar

mi·cro·fil·a·ment

mi·cro·fil·a·men·tous

mi·cro·fil·a·re·mia

mi·cro·fi·lar·ia
  pl mi·cro·fi·lar·i·ae

mi·cro·fi·lar·i·al

mi·cro·flo·ra

mi·cro·flo·ral

mi·cro·flu·o·rom·e·ter

mi·cro·flu·o·ro·met·ric

mi·cro·flu·o·rom·e·try
  pl mi·cro·flu·o·rom·e·tries

mi·cro·ga·mete

mi·cro·ga·me·to·cyte

mi·crog·lia

mi·crog·li·al

β_2-mi·cro·glob·u·lin

mi·cro·gna·thia

mi·cro·gram

mi·cro·graph

mi·crog·ra·phy
  pl mi·crog·ra·phies

mi·cro·gy·ria

mi·cro·gy·ric

mi·cro·hab·i·tat

mi·cro·he·mat·o·crit

mi·cro·het·ero·ge·ne·ity
  pl mi·cro·het·ero·ge·ne·ities

mi·crohm

mi·cro·in·cin·er·a·tion

mi·cro·in·farct

mi·cro·in·ject

mi·cro·in·jec·tion

mi·cro·in·va·sion

mi·cro·in·va·sive

mi·cro·ion·to·pho·re·sis
  pl mi·cro·ion·to·pho·re·ses

mi·cro·ion·to·pho·ret·ic

mi·cro·ion·to·pho·ret·i·cal·ly

mi·cro·li·ter

mi·cro·lith

mi·cro·li·thi·a·sis
  pl mi·cro·li·thi·a·ses

mi·cro·ma·nip·u·late

mi·cro·ma·nip·u·lat·ed

mi·cro·ma·nip·u·lat·ing

mi·cro·ma·nip·u·la·tion

mi·cro·ma·nip·u·la·tor

mi·cro·ma·nom·e·ter

mi·cro·mas·tia

mi·cro·me·lia

mi·cro·me·lic

mi·cro·mer·al
  or mi·cro·mer·ic

mi·cro·mere

mi·cro·me·tas·ta·sis
  pl mi·cro·me·tas·ta·ses

mi·cro·met·a·stat·ic

mi·crom·e·ter
  measuring instrument

mi·cro·me·ter
  unit of length

mi·cro·meth·od

mi·cro·met·ric

mi·crom·e·try
  pl mi·crom·e·tries

mi·cro·mi·cro·cu·rie

mi·cro·mi·cron

mi·cro·mil·li·me·ter

mi·cro·mo·lar

mi·cro·mole

mi·cro·mo·lec·u·lar

mi·cro·mol·e·cule

mi·cro·mono·spo·ra
   pl mi·cro·mono·spo·rae

mi·cro·mor·pho·log·ic
   or mi·cro·mor·pho·log·i·cal

mi·cro·mor·phol·o·gy
   pl mi·cro·mor·phol·o·gies

mi·cron
   pl mi·crons
   also mi·cra

mi·cro·nee·dle

mi·cron·iza·tion

mi·cron·ize
   mi·cron·ized
   mi·cron·iz·ing

mi·cro·nod·u·lar

mi·cro·nu·cle·ar

mi·cro·nu·cle·us

mi·cro·nu·tri·ent

mi·cro·nych·ia

mi·cro·or·gan·ic

mi·cro·or·gan·ism

mi·cro·or·gan·is·mal

mi·cro·par·a·site

mi·cro·par·a·sit·ic

mi·cro·pe·nis
   pl mi·cro·pe·nes
   or mi·cro·pe·nis·es

mi·cro·per·fused

mi·cro·per·fu·sion

mi·cro·phage

mi·croph·a·gous

mi·croph·a·gy
   pl mi·croph·a·gies

mi·cro·pha·kia

mi·cro·phal·lus

mi·cro·phone

mi·cro·phon·ic

mi·cro·pho·to·graph

mi·cro·pho·tog·ra·pher

mi·cro·pho·to·graph·ic

mi·cro·pho·tog·ra·phy
   pl mi·cro·pho·tog·ra·phies

mi·cro·pho·tom·e·ter

mi·cro·pho·to·met·ric

mi·cro·pho·to·met·ri·cal·ly

mi·cro·pho·tom·e·try
   pl mi·cro·pho·tom·e·tries

mi·croph·thal·mia

mi·croph·thal·mic

mi·croph·thal·mus
   or mi·croph·thal·mos
   pl mi·croph·thal·mi
   or mi·croph·thal·moi

mi·cro·phys·i·o·log·i·cal

mi·cro·phys·i·ol·o·gist

mi·cro·phys·i·ol·o·gy
   pl mi·cro·phys·i·ol·o·gies

mi·cro·phyte

mi·cro·phyt·ic

mi·cro·pi·no·cy·to·sis
   pl mi·cro·pi·no·cy·to·ses

mi·cro·pi·no·cy·tot·ic

mi·cro·pi·pette
   or mi·cro·pi·pet
   noun

mi·cro·pi·pette
   verb
   mi·cro·pi·pet·ted
   mi·cro·pi·pet·ting

mi·cro·pop·u·la·tion

mi·cro·probe

mi·crop·sia

mi·crop·sy
   pl mi·crop·sies

mi·crop·tic

mi·cro·punc·ture

mi·cro·py·lar
mi·cro·pyle
mi·cro·ra·dio·graph
mi·cro·ra·dio·graph·ic
mi·cro·ra·di·og·ra·phy
pl mi·cro·ra·di·og·ra·phies
mi·cro·res·pi·rom·e·ter
mi·cro·res·pi·rom·e·try
pl mi·cro·res·pi·rom·e·tries
mi·cro·scis·sors
mi·cro·scope
mi·cro·scop·ic
or mi·cro·scop·i·cal
mi·cros·co·pist
mi·cros·co·py
pl mi·cros·co·pies
mi·cro·sec·ond
mi·cro·sec·tion
mi·cro·slide
mi·cros·mat·ic
mi·cro·som·al
mi·cro·some
mi·cro·spec·tro·graph
mi·cro·spec·tro·graph·ic
mi·cro·spec·trog·ra·phy
pl mi·cro·spec·trog·ra·phies

mi·cro·spec·tro·pho·tom·e·ter
mi·cro·spec·tro·pho·to·met·ric
mi·cro·spec·tro·pho·tom·e·try
pl mi·cro·spec·tro·pho·tom·e·tries
mi·cro·spec·tro·scope
mi·cro·spec·tro·scop·ic
mi·cro·spec·tros·co·py
pl mi·cro·spec·tros·co·pies
mi·cro·sphe·ro·cy·to·sis
pl mi·cro·sphe·ro·cy·to·ses
mi·cro·spore
Mi·cro·spo·rid·ia
mi·cro·spo·rid·i·an
Mi·cros·po·ron
mi·cro·spo·ro·sis
pl mi·cro·spo·ro·ses
mi·cros·po·rum
pl mi·cros·po·ra
mi·cro·sto·mia
mi·cro·struc·tur·al
mi·cro·struc·ture
mi·cro·sur·gery
pl mi·cro·sur·ger·ies
mi·cro·sur·gi·cal
mi·cro·sy·ringe
mi·cro·tech·nique
also mi·cro·tech·nic

mi·cro·tia
mi·cro·ti·ter
mi·cro·ti·tra·tion
mi·cro·tome
mi·cro·tomed
mi·cro·tom·ing
mi·crot·o·my
pl mi·crot·o·mies
mi·cro·trau·ma
mi·cro·tu·bu·lar
mi·cro·tu·bule
Mi·cro·tus
mi·cro·unit
mi·cro·vas·cu·lar
mi·cro·vas·cu·la·ture
mi·cro·ves·i·cle
mi·cro·ves·sel
mi·cro·vil·lar
mi·cro·vil·lous
mi·cro·vil·lus
pl mi·cro·vil·li
mi·cro·volt
mi·cro·watt
mi·cro·wave
mi·cro·zoa
mi·cro·zo·an
mi·crur·gi·cal
also mi·crur·gic
mi·crur·gy
pl mi·crur·gies
Mi·cru·rus
mic·tion
mic·tu·rate
mic·tu·rat·ed
mic·tu·rat·ing
mic·tu·ri·tion

mic·tu·ri·tion·al
mid·ax·il·lary
mid·brain
mid·car·pal
mid·cla·vic·u·lar
mid·dle-aged
mid·for·ceps
midge
midg·et
midg·et·ism
mid·gut
mid·life
mid·line
mid·riff
mid·sag·it·tal
mid·sec·tion
mid·stream
mid·tar·sal
mid·tri·mes·ter
mid·wife
mid·wife·ry
  pl mid·wife·ries
mi·graine
mi·grain·eur
mi·grain·ous
mi·grate
  mi·grat·ed
  mi·grat·ing
mi·gra·tion
mi·gra·to·ry
Mi·ku·licz cell
Mi·ku·licz re·sec·
  tion
Mi·ku·licz's dis·
  ease
mil·dew
mil·i·ar·ia

mil·i·ar·ia crys·tal·
  li·na
mil·i·ar·i·al
mil·i·ary
mi·lieu
  pl mi·lieus
  or mi·lieux
mi·lieu in·te·ri·eur
mil·i·um
  pl mil·ia
milk·er's nod·ules
milk·i·ness
Milk·man's syn·
  drome
milky
  milk·i·er
  milk·i·est
Mil·ler-Ab·bott
  tube
mil·li·am·me·ter
mil·li·am·pere
mil·li·bar
mil·li·cu·rie
mil·li·equiv·a·lent
mil·li·gram
mil·li·gram-hour
mil·li·li·ter
mil·li·me·ter
mil·li·mi·cron
mil·li·mol·ar
mil·li·mo·lar·i·ty
  pl mil·li·mo·lar·i·ties
mil·li·mole
mil·li·nor·mal
mil·li·os·mol
  or mil·li·os·mole
mil·li·os·mo·lal

mil·li·os·mo·lal·i·ty
  pl mil·li·os·mo·lal·i·
  ties

mil·li·os·mo·lar
mil·li·pede
mil·li·rad
mil·li·rem
mil·li·roent·gen
mil·li·sec·ond
mil·li·unit
mil·li·volt
Mil·lon's re·agent
  or Mil·lon re·agent

Mil·roy's dis·ease
mi·met·ic
mim·ic
  mim·icked
  mim·ick·ing
mim·ic·ry
  pl mim·ic·ries

Min·a·mata dis·
  ease
mind-set
min·er·al
min·er·al·iza·tion
min·er·al·ize
  min·er·al·ized
  min·er·al·iz·ing
min·er·al·o·cor·ti·
  coid
min·er's asth·ma
min·er's con·
  sump·tion
min·er's phthi·sis

mini·lap·a·rot·o·
my
pl mini·lap·a·rot·o·
mies
min·im
min·i·mal
min·i·mum
pl min·i·ma
or min·i·mums
mini·pill
Min·ne·so·ta Mul·
ti·pha·sic Per·
son·al·i·ty In·
ven·to·ry
min·o·cy·cline
mi·nom·e·ter
min·ox·i·dil
min·ute
mio·lec·i·thal
mi·o·sis
also my·o·sis
pl mi·o·ses
also my·o·ses
mi·ot·ic
also my·ot·ic
mi·ra·cid·i·al
mi·ra·cid·i·um
pl mi·ra·cid·ia
mir·a·cil D
mir·a·cle drug
mi·rex
mis·car·riage
mis·car·ry
mis·car·ried
mis·car·ry·ing
mis·ce·ge·na·tion
mis·ci·bil·i·ty
pl mis·ci·bil·i·ties

mis·ci·ble
mis·di·ag·nose
mis·di·ag·nosed
mis·di·ag·nos·
ing
mis·di·ag·no·sis
pl mis·di·ag·no·ses
mi·sog·y·nist
mi·sog·y·nis·tic
mi·sog·y·ny
pl mi·sog·y·nies
miso·ne·ism
miso·pe·dia
mi·so·pho·bia
var of my·so·pho·bia
mis·sense
mis·tle·toe
mith·ra·my·cin
mith·ri·da·tism
mi·ti·cid·al
mi·ti·cide
mit·i·gate
mit·i·gat·ed
mit·i·gat·ing
mit·i·ga·tion
mi·tis
mi·to·chon·dri·al
mi·to·chon·dri·on
pl mi·to·chon·dria
mi·to·gen
mi·to·gen·e·sis
pl mi·to·gen·e·ses
mi·to·ge·net·ic
mi·to·gen·ic
mi·to·ge·nic·i·ty
pl mi·to·ge·nic·i·ties
mi·to·my·cin

mi·to·sis
pl mi·to·ses
mi·to·spore
mi·tot·ic
mi·tot·i·cal·ly
mi·tral
mit·tel·schmerz
mixo·sco·pia
mixo·scop·ic
mix·os·co·py
pl mix·os·co·pies
mix·ture
Mi·ya·ga·wa·nel·la
M line
M-mode
mne·me
mne·mic
mo·bile
mo·bil·i·ty
pl mo·bil·i·ties
mo·bi·liz·able
mo·bi·li·za·tion
mo·bi·lize
mo·bi·lized
mo·bi·liz·ing
Mö·bius syn·
drome
moc·ca·sin
mo·dal·i·ty
pl mo·dal·i·ties
mod·el
mod·er·ate
mod·er·at·ed
mod·er·at·ing
mod·er·a·tion
mod·i·fi·ca·tion
mod·i·fi·er

mod·i·fy
  mod·i·fied
  mod·i·fy·ing
mo·di·o·lar
mo·di·o·lus
  pl mo·di·o·li

mod·u·late
  mod·u·lat·ed
  mod·u·lat·ing
mod·u·la·tion
mod·u·la·tor
mod·u·la·to·ry
mod·u·lus
  pl mod·u·li

Mohs' scale
Mohs' tech·nique
moi·ety
  pl moi·eties

mol
  var of mole

mol·al
mo·lal·i·ty
  pl mo·lal·i·ties

mol·ar
mo·lar·i·form
mo·lar·i·ty
  pl mo·lar·i·ties

mold
  also mould

moldy
  also mouldy
  mold·i·er
    also mould·i·er
  mold·i·est
    also mould·i·est

mole
  bodily spot or an
    abnormal growth
mole
  also mol
    chemical amount
mo·lec·u·lar
mo·lec·u·lar·i·ty
  pl mo·lec·u·lar·i·ties
mol·e·cule
mo·li·men
  pl mo·lim·i·na
mol·in·done
Mo·lisch test
Moll's gland
Mol·lus·ca
mol·lus·can
  also mol·lus·kan
    adjective
mol·lus·ci·cid·al
  also mol·lus·ca·cid·al
mol·lus·ci·cide
  also mol·lus·ca·cide
mol·lus·cous
mol·lus·cum
  pl mol·lus·ca
mol·lus·cum con·
  ta·gi·o·sum
  pl mol·lus·ca con·ta·
    gi·o·sa
mol·lusk
  or mol·lusc
    noun

Mo·lo·ney test
molt
  also moult
mo·lyb·date
mo·lyb·de·num

mo·lyb·dic
mo·lyb·dous
mo·nad
mon·am·ine
  var of monoamine
mo·nar·da
mon·ar·tic·u·lar
  var of monoarticular
mon·as·ter
mon·atom·ic
mon·au·ral
Möncke·berg's
  scle·ro·sis
mo·nen·sin
mon·es·trous
mon·gol
mon·go·lian
mon·gol·ism
mon·gol·oid
mo·nie·zia
mo·nil·e·thrix
  pl mon·i·let·ri·ches

mo·nil·ia
  pl mo·nil·ias
  or mo·nil·ia
  also mo·nil·i·ae
    fungus
mo·nil·ia
  pl mo·nil·ias
    fungus infection
Mo·nil·i·a·ce·ae
Mo·nil·i·al
Mo·nil·i·a·les
mo·nil·i·a·sis
  pl mo·ni·li·a·ses
mo·nil·i·form
Mo·nil·i·for·mis

mo·nil·iid
mon·i·tor
  mon·i·tored
  mon·i·tor·ing
monks·hood
mono
mono·ac·e·tin
mono·ac·id
mono·am·ide
mono·am·ine
  also mon·am·ine
mono·am·in·er·gic
mono·ar·tic·u·lar
  or mon·ar·tic·u·lar

mono·ba·sic
mono·ben·zone
mono·blast
mono·bro·min·a·
  tion
mono·car·box·yl·ic
mono·chlo·ro·ace·
  tic
  also mono·chlor·ace·
    tic

mono·chord
mono·cho·ri·on·ic
  also mono·cho·ri·al

mono·chro·ma·cy
  also mono·chro·ma·sy
  pl mono·chro·ma·cies
  also mono·chro·ma·
    sies

mono·chro·mat
mono·chro·mat·ic
mono·chro·mat·ic·
  i·ty
  pl mono·chro·ma·tic·
    i·ties

mono·chro·ma·
  tism
mono·chro·ma·tor
mono·clin·ic
mono·clo·nal
mono·cro·ta·line
mono·crot·ic
mon·oc·u·lar
mono·cyte
mono·cyt·ic
mono·cyt·oid
mono·cy·to·pe·nia
mono·cy·to·sis
  pl mono·cy·to·ses

mono·dis·perse
mono·es·ter
mono·eth·a·nol·
  amine
mono·fac·to·ri·al
mono·fil·a·ment
mono·func·tion·al
mo·nog·a·mist
mo·nog·a·mous
  also mono·gam·ic

mo·nog·a·my
mono·gas·tric
Mono·ge·nea
mono·ge·ne·an
mono·ge·net·ic
mono·gen·ic
mono·gen·i·cal·ly
mono·glyc·er·ide
mono·go·nad·ic
mo·nog·o·ny
  pl mo·nog·o·nies

mono·graph
mono·hy·brid

mono·hy·drate
mono·hy·drat·ed
mono·hy·dric
mono·hy·droxy
mono·ide·ism
mono·ide·is·tic
mono·iodo·ty·ro·
  sine
mono·kary·on
mono·kary·ot·ic
mono·lay·er
mono·ma·nia
mono·ma·ni·ac
  noun

mono·ma·ni·a·cal
  also mono·ma·ni·ac
    adjective

mono·me·lic
mono·mer
mo·no·mer·ic
mono·mo·lec·u·lar
mono·mor·phic
mono·mor·phism
mono·neu·ri·tis
  pl mono·neu·rit·i·des
  or mono·neu·ri·tis·es

mono·neu·ri·tis
  mul·ti·plex
mono·nu·cle·ar
mono·nu·cle·at·ed
  also mono·nu·cle·ate

mono·nu·cle·o·sis
mono·nu·cle·o·tide
mono·ox·y·gen·ase
mono·pha·sic
mono·phos·phate
mono·phy·let·ic

morphogenesis

mono·phy·ly
  pl mono·phy·lies

mono·ple·gia

mono·ple·gic

mono·ploid

mono·po·lar

mono·po·lar·i·ty
  pl mono·po·lar·i·ties

mon·or·chid

mon·or·chid·ism
  also mon·or·chism

mono·rhi·nic

mono·sac·cha·ride

mono·so·di·um glu·ta·mate

mono·some

mono·so·mic

mono·so·my
  pl mono·so·mies

mono·spe·cif·ic

mono·spec·i·fic·i·ty
  pl mono·spec·i·fic·i·ties

mono·sper·mic

mono·sper·my
  pl mono·sper·mies

mon·os·tot·ic

mono·sub·sti·tut·ed

mono·sub·sti·tu·tion

mono·symp·tom·at·ic

mono·syn·ap·tic

mono·syn·ap·ti·cal·ly

mo·not·o·cous

Mono·trem·a·ta

mono·treme

mo·not·ri·chous

mono·typ·ic

mono·un·sat·u·rat·ed

mono·va·lent

mon·ovu·lar

mo·nox·e·nous

mon·ox·ide

mono·zo·ot·ic

mono·zy·gos·i·ty
  pl mono·zy·gos·i·ties

mono·zy·gote

mono·zy·got·ic

mono·zy·gous

mons
  pl mon·tes

mons pu·bis
  pl mon·tes pu·bis

mon·ster

mon·stros·i·ty
  pl mon·stros·i·ties

mon·strous

mons ve·ne·ris
  pl mon·tes ve·ne·ris

Mon·teg·gia frac·ture
  or Mon·teg·gia's frac·ture

Mon·te·zu·ma's re·venge

Mont·gom·ery's gland

mon·tic·u·lus

Moon's mo·lar
  or Moon mo·lar

Mor·ax·el·la

mor·bid

mor·bid·i·ty
  pl mor·bid·i·ties

mor·bif·ic

mor·bil·li

mor·bil·li·form

mor·bus
  pl mor·bi

mor·bus cox·ae se·nil·is

mor·cel·la·tion

mor·dant

morgue

mor·i·bund

morn·ing-af·ter pill

mo·ron

mo·ron·ic

mo·ron·ism

mo·ron·i·ty
  pl mo·ron·i·ties

Moro re·flex

mor·phal·lax·is
  pl mor·phal·lax·es

mor·phea
  pl mor·phe·ae

mor·phia

mor·phine

mor·phin·ism

mor·phin·ist

mor·phin·iza·tion

mor·phin·ized

mor·pho·dif·fer·en·ti·a·tion

mor·pho·gen·e·sis
  pl mor·pho·gen·e·ses

mor·pho·ge·net·ic
mor·pho·ge·net·i·
  cal·ly
mor·pho·gen·ic
mor·pho·log·i·cal
  also mor·pho·log·ic
mor·phol·o·gist
mor·phol·o·gy
  pl mor·phol·o·gies
mor·pho·met·rics
mor·phom·e·try
  pl mor·phom·e·tries
Mor·quio's dis·ease
mor·rhu·ate
mor·rhu·ic
mor·tal
mor·tal·i·ty
  pl mor·tal·i·ties

mor·tar
mor·ti·cian
mor·ti·fi·ca·tion
mor·ti·fy
  mor·ti·fied
  mor·ti·fy·ing
Mor·ton's toe
mor·tu·ary
  pl mor·tu·ar·ies

mor·u·la
  pl mor·u·lae

mor·u·lar
mor·u·la·tion
mo·sa·ic
mo·sa·i·cal·ly
mo·sa·icism
mos·qui·to
  pl mos·qui·toes
  also mos·qui·tos

mossy fi·ber
mo·tile
mo·til·i·ty
  pl mo·til·i·ties
mo·ti·vate
  mo·ti·vat·ed
  mo·ti·vat·ing
mo·ti·va·tion
mo·ti·va·tion·al
mo·ti·va·tive
mo·tive
mo·to·neu·ron
mo·to·neu·ro·nal
mo·tor
mo·tor·ic
mo·tor·i·cal·ly
mo·to·ri·um
  pl mo·to·ria

mot·tled enam·el
mou·lage
mould
  var of mold
mouldy
  var of moldy
moult
  var of molt
mount
moun·tant
moun·te·bank
mouse
  pl mice

mouse·pox
mouth
  pl mouths
mouth breath·er
mouth·part
mouth-to-mouth

mouth·wash
moxa
mox·i·bus·tion
mu
  pl mu

mu·cate
mu·cic
mu·ci·car·mine
mu·cif·er·ous
mu·ci·fi·ca·tion
mu·ci·gen
mu·ci·lage
mu·ci·lag·i·nous
mu·cin
mu·cin·o·gen
mu·ci·no·lyt·ic
mu·ci·no·sis
  pl mu·ci·no·ses

mu·ci·nous
mu·co·buc·cal
mu·co·cele
mu·co·cil·i·ary
mu·co·cu·ta·ne·ous
mu·co·epi·der·
  moid
mu·co·gin·gi·val
mu·coid
mu·coi·tin·sul·fu·
  ric
mu·co·lyt·ic
mu·co·pep·tide
mu·co·peri·os·te·al
mu·co·peri·os·te·
  um
mu·co·poly·sac·
  cha·ride

mu·co·poly·sac·
cha·ri·do·sis
pl mu·co·poly·sac·
cha·ri·do·ses

mu·co·pro·tein

mu·co·pu·ru·lent

mu·co·pus

mu·cor

Mu·co·ra·ce·ae

mu·co·ra·ceous

Mu·co·ra·les

mu·cor·my·co·sis
pl mu·cor·my·co·ses

mu·cor·my·cot·ic

mu·co·sa
pl mu·co·sae
or mu·co·sas

mu·co·sal

mu·co·se·rous

mu·co·si·tis

mu·co·stat·ic

mu·cous
adjective (see mucus)

mu·co·vis·ci·do·sis
pl mu·co·vis·ci·do·ses

Mu·cu·na

mu·cus
noun (see mucous)

Mules op·er·a·tion

mull·er

Mül·ler cell
also Mül·ler's cell

mül·le·ri·an
also muel·le·ri·an

Mül·le·ri·an duct
also Muel·le·ri·an
duct

Mül·ler's mus·cle

mult·an·gu·lar

mul·ti·an·gu·lar

mul·ti·cel·lu·lar

mul·ti·cel·lu·lar·i·
ty
pl mul·ti·cel·lu·lar·i·
ties

mul·ti·cen·ter

mul·ti·cen·tric

mul·ti·cen·tri·cal·
ly

mul·ti·cen·tric·i·ty
pl mul·ti·cen·tric·i·
ties

mul·ti·ceps

mul·ti·chain

mul·ti·clo·nal

mul·ti·cys·tic

mul·ti·den·tate

mul·ti·dose

mul·ti·en·zyme

mul·ti·fac·to·ri·al
or mul·ti·fac·tor

mul·ti·fac·to·ri·al·i·
ty
pl mul·ti·fac·to·ri·al·
i·ties

mul·tif·i·dus
pl mul·tif·i·di

mul·ti·fo·cal

mul·ti·form

mul·ti·for·mi·ty
pl mul·ti·for·mi·ties

mul·ti·gen·ic

mul·ti·grav·i·da

mul·ti·han·di·
capped

mul·ti·hos·pi·
tal

mul·ti·lay·er
noun

mul·ti·lay·ered
or mul·ti·lay·er
adjective

mul·ti·lobed

mul·ti·loc·u·lar

mul·ti·mam·mate

mul·ti·mo·dal

mul·ti·nod·u·lar

mul·ti·nu·cle·ate
or mul·ti·nu·cle·at·ed

mul·ti·or·gas·mic

mul·tip·a·ra

mul·ti·par·i·ty
pl mul·ti·par·i·ties

mul·tip·a·rous

mul·ti·ple

mul·ti·plic·i·ty
pl mul·ti·plic·i·ties

mul·ti·po·lar

mul·ti·po·lar·i·ty
pl mul·ti·po·lar·i·
ties

mul·tip·o·tent

mul·ti·po·ten·tial

mul·ti·re·sis·tance

mul·ti·re·sis·tant

mul·ti·spe·cial·ty
pl mul·ti·spe·cial·
ties

mul·ti·syn·ap·tic

mul·ti·sys·tem
also mul·ti·sys·te·mic

mul·ti·va·lent

mul·ti·vi·ta·min

mum·mi·fi·ca·tion

mum·mi·fy
mum·mi·fied
mum·mi·fy·
ing

mumps

Mun·chau·sen syn·
drome
or Mun·chau·sen's
syn·drome

mu·ral

mu·ram·ic

mu·ram·i·dase

mu·rein

mu·rex·ide

mu·ri·ate

mu·ri·at·ic

mu·rid

Mu·ri·dae

mu·rine

mur·mur

mur·ri·na

Mus

Mus·ca

mus·cae vo·li·tan·
tes

mus·ca·rine

mus·ca·rin·ic

mus·cid

Mus·ci·dae

mus·cle

mus·cu·lar

mus·cu·la·ris

mus·cu·la·ris ex·
ter·na

mus·cu·la·ris mu·
co·sae
also mus·cu·la·ris mu·
co·sa

mus·cu·lar·i·ty
pl mus·cu·lar·i·ties

mus·cu·la·ture

mus·cu·li pec·ti·
na·ti

mus·cu·lo·cu·ta·ne·
ous

mus·cu·lo·fas·cial

mus·cu·lo·fi·brous

mus·cu·lo·mem·
bra·nous

mus·cu·lo·phren·ic

mus·cu·lo·skel·e·
tal

mus·cu·lo·spi·ral

mus·cu·lo·ten·di·
nous

mus·cu·lo·tro·pic

mus·cu·lus
pl mus·cu·li

mush·room

mu·si·co·gen·ic

mus·tard

mu·ta·bil·i·ty
pl mu·ta·bil·i·ties

mu·ta·ble

mu·ta·fa·cient

mu·ta·gen

mu·ta·gen·e·sis
pl mu·ta·gen·e·ses

mu·ta·gen·ic

mu·ta·gen·i·cal·ly

mu·ta·ge·nic·i·ty
pl mu·ta·ge·nic·i·ties

mu·ta·gen·ize
mu·ta·gen·ized
mu·ta·gen·iz·ing

mu·tant

mu·ta·ro·tase

mu·ta·ro·tate
mu·ta·ro·tat·ed
mu·ta·ro·tat·ing

mu·ta·ro·ta·tion

mu·tase

mu·tate
mu·tat·ed
mu·tat·ing

mu·ta·tion

mu·ta·tion·al

mu·ta·tive

mu·ta·tor

mute
mut·er
mut·est

mu·ti·late
mu·ti·lat·ed
mu·ti·lat·ing

mu·ti·la·tion

mut·ism

mu·ton

mu·tu·al·ism

mu·tu·al·ist

mu·tu·al·is·tic

my·al·gia

my·al·gic

my·an·e·sin

my·as·the·nia

my·as·the·nia gra·
vis
my·as·then·ic
my·ce·li·al
my·ce·li·oid
my·ce·li·um
  pl my·ce·lia
my·ce·tis·mus
  pl my·ce·tis·mi
my·ce·to·ma
  pl my·ce·to·mas
  or my·ce·to·ma·ta
my·ce·to·ma·tous
My·co·bac·te·ri·a·
ce·ae
my·co·bac·te·ri·al
my·co·bac·te·ri·o·
sis
  pl my·co·bac·te·ri·o·
  ses
my·co·bac·te·ri·um
  pl my·co·bac·te·ria
my·co·bac·tin
my·co·cide
my·col·ic
my·co·log·i·cal
my·col·o·gist
my·col·o·gy
  pl my·col·o·gies
my·co·my·cin
my·co·phe·no·lic
my·co·plas·ma
  pl my·co·plas·mas
  or my·co·plas·ma·ta
my·co·plas·mal
My·co·plas·ma·ta·
ce·ae

my·co·sis
  pl my·co·ses
my·co·sis fun·goi·
des
my·co·stat
my·co·stat·ic
my·cos·ter·ol
my·cot·ic
my·co·tox·i·co·sis
  pl my·co·tox·i·co·ses
my·co·tox·in
my·dri·a·sis
  pl my·dri·a·ses
myd·ri·at·ic
my·ec·to·my
  pl my·ec·to·mies
my·el·en·ce·phal·ic
my·el·en·ceph·a·
lon
my·elin
my·elin·at·ed
my·e·li·na·tion
my·elin·ic
my·e·lin·iza·tion
my·eli·nol·y·sis
  pl my·eli·nol·y·ses
my·elit·ic
my·eli·tis
  pl my·elit·i·des
my·elo·blast
my·elo·blas·tic
my·elo·blas·to·ma
  pl my·elo·blas·to·mas
  or my·elo·blas·to·ma·
  ta
my·elo·cele
  form of spina bifida

my·elo·coele
  central spinal canal
my·elo·cyte
my·elo·cyt·ic
my·elo·dys·pla·sia
my·elo·dys·plas·tic
my·elo·fi·bro·sis
  pl my·elo·fi·bro·ses
my·elo·fi·brot·ic
my·elog·e·nous
  also my·elo·gen·ic
my·elo·gram
my·elo·graph·ic
my·elo·graph·i·cal·
ly
my·elog·ra·phy
  pl my·elog·ra·phies
my·eloid
my·elo·ma
  pl my·elo·mas
  or my·elo·ma·ta
my·elo·ma·to·sis
  pl my·elo·ma·to·ses
my·elo·ma·tous
my·elo·me·nin·go·
cele
my·elo·mono·cyte
my·elo·mono·cyt·ic
my·elo·path·ic
my·elop·a·thy
  pl my·elop·a·thies
my·elo·per·ox·i·
dase
my·elo·phthi·sic
my·elo·plax
my·elo·poi·e·sis
  pl my·elo·poi·e·ses

my·elo·poi·et·ic
my·elo·pro·lif·er·a·tive
my·elo·ra·dic·u·li·tis
my·elo·scle·ro·sis
  pl my·elo·scle·ro·ses
my·elo·sis
  pl my·elo·ses
my·elo·sup·pres·sion
my·elo·sup·pres·sive
my·elot·o·my
  pl my·elot·o·mies
my·elo·tox·ic
my·elo·tox·ic·i·ty
  pl my·elo·tox·ic·i·ties
my·en·ter·ic
my·en·ter·on
my·ia·sis
  pl my·ia·ses
my·lo·hy·oid
my·lo·hy·oi·de·us
  pl my·lo·hy·oi·dei
myo·blast
myo·blas·to·ma
  pl myo·blas·to·mas
  or myo·blas·to·ma·ta
myo·car·di·al
myo·car·dio·graph
myo·car·dio·graph·ic
myo·car·di·op·a·thy
  pl myo·car·di·op·a·thies

myo·car·di·tis
myo·car·di·um
  pl myo·car·dia
myo·car·do·sis
  pl myo·car·do·ses
myo·clo·nia
myo·clon·ic
myo·oc·lo·nus
myo·coele
  or myo·coel
myo·com·ma
  pl myo·com·ma·ta
  also myo·com·mas
myo·cyte
myo·elas·tic
myo·elec·tric
  also myo·elec·tri·cal
myo·epi·the·li·al
myo·epi·the·lium
  pl myo·epi·the·lia
myo·fas·cial
myo·fi·bril
myo·fi·bril·lar
myo·fi·bro·ma
  pl myo·fi·bro·mas
  also myo·fi·bro·ma·ta
myo·fil·a·ment
myo·ge·lo·sis
my·o·gen
myo·gen·e·sis
  pl myo·gen·e·ses
myo·gen·ic
  also my·og·e·nous
myo·ge·nic·i·ty
  pl myo·ge·nic·i·ties
myo·glo·bin
myo·glo·bin·uria

myo·graph
myo·graph·ic
myo·graph·i·cal·ly
my·og·ra·phy
  pl my·og·ra·phies
myo·he·ma·tin
myo·he·mo·glo·bin
my·oid
myo·ino·si·tol
myo·ki·nase
my·o·log·ic
  or my·o·log·i·cal
my·ol·o·gy
  pl my·ol·o·gies
my·o·ma
  pl my·o·mas
  or my·o·ma·ta
my·o·ma·tous
myo·mec·to·my
  pl myo·mec·to·mies
myo·me·tri·al
myo·me·tri·tis
myo·me·tri·um
my·o·neme
myo·neu·ral
myo·path·ic
my·op·a·thy
  pl my·op·a·thies
my·ope
myo·peri·car·di·tis
  pl myo·peri·car·dit·i·des
my·o·pia
my·o·pic
my·o·pi·cal·ly
myo·re·lax·ant

myo·sar·co·ma
  pl myo·sar·co·mas
  or myo·sar·co·ma·ta

myo·sep·tum
  pl myo·sep·ta

my·o·sin

my·o·sis
  var of miosis

myo·si·tis

myo·si·tis os·sif·i·cans

myo·tat·ic

my·ot·ic
  var of miotic

myo·to·mal

myo·tome

my·ot·o·my
  pl my·ot·o·mies

myo·to·nia

myo·to·nia con·gen·i·ta

myo·ton·ic

my·ot·o·nus

myo·trop·ic

myo·tube

myr·i·cyl

myr·in·ga

myr·in·gi·tis

my·rin·go·plas·ty
  pl my·rin·go·plas·ties

myr·in·got·o·my
  pl myr·in·got·o·mies

myr·io·pod
  also myr·ia·pod

Myr·i·op·o·da

my·ris·tate

my·ris·tic

my·ro·sin

myrrh

my·so·phil·ia

my·so·pho·bia
  or mi·so·pho·bia

my·so·pho·bic

my·ta·cism

mytho·ma·nia

mytho·ma·ni·ac

myx·ede·ma

myx·ede·ma·tous

myxo·fi·bro·sar·co·ma
  pl myxo·fi·bro·sar·co·mas
  or myxo·fi·bro·sar·co·ma·ta

myx·oid

myx·o·ma
  pl myx·o·mas
  or myx·o·ma·ta

myx·o·ma·to·sis
  pl myx·o·ma·to·ses

myx·o·ma·tous

myxo·my·cete

Myxo·my·ce·tes

myxo·my·ce·tous

Myxo·phy·ce·ae

myxo·sar·co·ma
  pl myxo·sar·co·mas
  or myxo·sar·co·ma·ta

myxo·sar·co·ma·tous

Myxo·spo·rid·ia

myxo·spo·rid·i·an

myxo·vi·ral

myxo·vi·rus

N

na·bo·thi·an

na·do·lol

naf·cil·lin

naf·ox·i·dine

na·ga·na
  also n'ga·na

Na·ga sore

Nai·ro·bi dis·ease

na·ive
  or na·ïve

na·iv·er
  or na·ïv·er

na·iv·est
  or na·ïv·est

Na·ja

na·li·dix·ic

na·lor·phine

nal·ox·one

nal·trex·one

nan·dro·lone

na·nism

nano·ce·phal·ic

nano·cu·rie

nano·gram

nano·li·ter

nano·me·ter

nano·mo·lar

nano·mole

nano·sec·ond

na·no·so·mia

na·phaz·o·line

naph·tha·lene

naph·tha·lene·sul·fon·ic

naph·tha·len·ic

naph·thol
naph·tho·qui·none
  also naph·tha·qui·none

naph·thyl·amine
na·pi·form
nap·ra·path
na·prap·a·thy
  pl na·prap·a·thies

na·prox·en
nap·syl·ate
nar·ce·ine
nar·cism
nar·cis·sism
nar·cis·sist
nar·cis·sis·tic
nar·cis·sis·ti·cal·ly
nar·cis·tic
nar·co·anal·y·sis
  pl nar·co·anal·y·ses

nar·co·di·ag·no·sis
  pl nar·co·di·ag·no·ses

nar·co·hyp·no·sis
  pl nar·co·hyp·no·ses

nar·co·lep·sy
  pl nar·co·lep·sies

nar·co·lep·tic
nar·cose
nar·co·sis
  pl nar·co·ses

nar·co·sug·ges·tion
nar·co·syn·the·sis
  pl nar·co·syn·the·ses

nar·co·ther·a·py
  pl nar·co·ther·a·pies

nar·cot·ic
nar·cot·i·cism

nar·co·tine
nar·co·tism
nar·co·ti·za·tion
nar·co·tize
  nar·co·tized
  nar·co·tiz·ing
nar·co·tol·ine
na·ris
  pl na·res

nar·row-an·gle
  glau·co·ma
nar·row-spec·trum
na·sal
na·sa·lis
na·scent
na·si·on
Na·smyth's mem·
  brane
na·so·bas·i·lar
na·so·cil·i·ary
na·so·fron·tal
na·so·gas·tric
na·so·la·bi·al
na·so·lac·ri·mal
  also na·so·lach·ry·mal

na·so·max·il·lary
na·so·pal·a·tine
na·so·pha·ryn·geal
na·so·phar·yn·gi·tis
  pl na·so·phar·yn·git·i·
  des

na·so·pha·ryn·go·
  scope
na·so·pha·ryn·go·
  scop·ic

na·so·phar·yn·gos·
  co·py
  pl na·so·phar·yn·gos·
  co·pies

na·so·phar·ynx
  pl na·so·pha·ryn·ges
  also na·so·phar·ynx·
  es

na·so·spi·na·le
na·so·tra·che·al
na·tal
na·tal·i·ty
  pl na·tal·i·ties

Na·tal sore
na·tes
Na·tion·al For·mu·
  lary
na·tri·um
na·tri·ure·sis
  also na·tru·re·sis

na·tri·uret·ic
nat·u·ral
na·tu·ro·path
  also na·ture·o·path

na·tu·ro·path·ic
  also na·ture·o·path·ic

na·tu·rop·a·thy
  also na·ture·op·a·thy
  pl na·tu·rop·a·thies
  also na·ture·op·a·thies

nau·path·ia
nau·sea
nau·se·ant
nau·se·ate
  nau·se·at·ed
  nau·se·at·ing
nau·seous
na·vel

na·vic·u·lar
near·sight·ed
ne·ben·kern
neb·u·la
  pl neb·u·las
  or neb·u·lae

neb·u·li·za·tion
neb·u·lize
  neb·u·lized
  neb·u·liz·ing
neb·u·liz·er
Ne·ca·tor
ne·ca·to·ri·a·sis
  pl ne·ca·to·ri·a·ses

nec·ro
nec·ro·bac·il·lo·sis
  pl nec·ro·bac·il·lo·ses
nec·ro·bi·o·sis
  pl nec·ro·bi·o·ses

nec·ro·bi·o·sis li·
  poid·i·ca
nec·ro·bi·ot·ic
nec·ro·phile
  also nec·ro·phil

nec·ro·phil·ia
nec·ro·phil·i·ac
nec·ro·phil·ic
nec·roph·i·lism
nec·roph·i·ly
  pl nec·roph·i·lies

nec·rop·sy
  pl nec·rop·sies

nec·rop·sy
  nec·rop·sied
  nec·rop·sy·ing

nec·rose
  nec·rosed
  nec·ros·ing
nec·ro·sin
ne·cro·sis
  pl ne·cro·ses
nec·ro·sper·mia
ne·crot·ic
nec·ro·tiz·ing
nec·ro·tox·in
ne·en·ceph·a·lon
neg·a·tive
neg·a·tiv·ism
neg·a·tiv·ist·ic
Ne·gri body
Neis·se·ria
Neis·ser·i·a·ce·ae
neis·se·ri·an
  or neis·se·ri·al
nem·a·thel·minth
Nem·a·thel·min·
  thes
ne·mat·ic
ne·ma·to·cid·al
  also ne·ma·ti·cid·al
ne·ma·to·cide
  also ne·ma·ti·cide
  or nem·a·cide
ne·ma·to·cyst
Nem·a·to·da
nem·a·tode
nem·a·to·di·a·sis
  pl nem·a·to·di·a·ses
nem·a·to·di·ri·a·sis
  pl nem·a·to·di·ri·a·
  ses
Nem·a·to·di·rus

nem·a·to·log·i·cal
nem·a·tol·o·gist
nem·a·tol·o·gy
  pl nem·a·tol·o·gies

Nem·a·to·mor·pha
nem·bu·tal·ized
nem·ic
neo·ars·phen·a·
  mine
neo·blas·tic
neo·cer·e·bel·lar
neo·cer·e·bel·lum
  pl neo·cer·e·bel·lums
  or neo·cer·e·bel·la

neo·cin·cho·phen
neo·cor·tex
  pl neo·cor·ti·ces
  or neo·cor·tex·es

neo·cor·ti·cal
neo-Dar·win·ian
neo-Dar·win·ism
neo-Dar·win·ist
neo·dym·i·um
neo·for·ma·tion
neo·for·ma·tive
neo-Freud·ian
neo·hes·per·i·din
  di·hy·dro·chal·
  cone
ne·ol·o·gism
neo·morph
neo·my·cin
ne·on
neo·na·tal
ne·o·nate
neo·na·tol·o·gist

neo·na·tol·o·gy
  pl neo·na·tol·o·gies

neo·pal·li·al
neo·pal·li·um
  pl neo·pal·lia

neo·pho·bia
neo·pho·bic
ne·o·pine
neo·pla·sia
neo·plasm
neo·plas·tic
neo·plas·ti·cal·ly
neo·sal·var·san
neo·sti·bo·san
neo·stig·mine
neo·stri·a·tal
neo·stri·a·tum
  pl neo·stri·a·tums
  or neo·stri·a·ta

neo·thal·a·mus
  pl neo·thal·a·mi

neo·vas·cu·lar
neo·vas·cu·lar·i·ty
  pl neo·vas·cu·lar·i·
    ties

neo·vas·cu·lar·iza·
  tion
nep·e·ta·lac·tone
neph·e·lom·e·ter
neph·e·lo·met·ric
neph·e·lom·e·try
  pl neph·e·lom·e·tries

ne·phrec·to·mize
  ne·phrec·to·
    mized
  ne·phrec·to·miz·
    ing

ne·phrec·to·my
  pl ne·phrec·to·mies

neph·ric
ne·phrid·i·al
ne·phrid·i·um
  pl ne·phrid·ia

ne·phrit·ic
ne·phri·tis
  pl ne·phrit·i·des

neph·ri·to·gen·ic
neph·ro·cal·ci·no·
  sis
  pl neph·ro·cal·ci·no·
    ses

neph·ro·coel
  or neph·ro·coele

neph·ro·gen·e·sis
  pl neph·ro·gen·e·ses

neph·ro·gen·ic
neph·ro·gram
ne·phrog·ra·phy
  pl ne·phrog·ra·phies

neph·ro·li·thi·a·sis
  pl neph·ro·li·thi·a·ses

neph·ro·li·thot·o·
  my
  pl neph·ro·li·thot·o·
    mies

ne·phrol·o·gist
ne·phrol·o·gy
  pl ne·phrol·o·gies

ne·phro·ma
  pl ne·phro·mas
  also ne·phro·ma·ta

neph·ro·mere
neph·ron
neph·ro·path·ic

ne·phrop·a·thy
  pl ne·phrop·a·thies

neph·ro·pexy
  pl neph·ro·pex·ies

neph·rop·to·sis
  pl neph·rop·to·ses

ne·phror·rha·phy
  pl ne·phror·rha·phies

neph·ro·scle·ro·sis
  pl neph·ro·scle·ro·ses

neph·ro·scle·ro·tic
ne·phro·sis
  pl ne·phro·ses

ne·phros·to·gram
ne·phros·to·ma
  pl neph·ro·sto·ma·ta

neph·ro·stome
ne·phros·to·my
  pl ne·phros·to·mies

ne·phrot·ic
neph·ro·tome
neph·ro·to·mo·
  gram
neph·ro·to·mo·
  graph·ic
neph·ro·to·mog·ra·
  phy
  pl neph·ro·to·mog·ra·
    phies

ne·phrot·o·my
  pl ne·phrot·o·mies

neph·ro·tox·ic
neph·ro·tox·ic·i·ty
  pl neph·ro·tox·i·ci·
    ties

neph·ro·tox·in
nep·tu·ni·um

Nernst equa·tion
nerve of Her·ing
nerve of Lan·ci·si
nerve of Wris·berg
ner·vi ner·vo·rum
ner·von
  or ner·vone

ner·von·ic
ner·vous
ner·vus
  pl ner·vi
ner·vus er·i·gens
  pl ner·vi er·i·gen·tes
ner·vus in·ter·me·
  di·us
ner·vus ra·di·a·lis
  pl ner·vi ra·di·a·les
ner·vus ter·mi·na·
  lis
  pl ner·vi ter·mi·na·les
ness·ler·iza·tion
ness·ler·ize
  ness·ler·ized
  ness·ler·iz·ing
Ness·ler's re·agent
neth·a·lide
net·tle
net·work
neu·ral
neu·ral·gia
neu·ral·gic
neu·ral·gi·form
neur·amin·ic
neur·amin·i·dase
neur·aprax·ia
neur·as·the·nia
neur·as·then·ic

neur·ax·is
  pl neur·ax·es
neur·ax·on
  also neur·ax·one
neur·rec·to·my
  pl neur·rec·to·mies
neur·en·ter·ic
neur·rer·gic
neu·ri·lem·ma
neu·ri·lem·mal
neu·ri·lem·mo·ma
  or neu·ri·le·mo·ma
  or neu·ro·lem·mo·ma
  pl neu·ri·lem·mo·mas
  or neu·ri·lem·mo·ma·
    ta
  or neu·ri·le·mo·mas
  or neu·ri·le·mo·ma·ta
  or neu·ro·lem·mo·
    mas
  or neu·ro·lem·mo·
    ma·ta
neu·ril·i·ty
  pl neu·ril·i·ties
neu·rine
neu·ri·no·ma
  pl neu·ri·no·mas
  or neu·ri·no·ma·ta
neu·rite
neu·rit·ic
neu·ri·tis
  pl neu·rit·i·des
  or neu·ri·tis·es
neu·ro·ac·tive
neu·ro·ana·tom·i·
  cal
  also neu·ro·ana·tom·
    ic
neu·ro·anat·o·mist

neu·ro·anat·o·my
  pl neu·ro·anat·o·mies
neu·ro·be·hav·ior·
  al
neu·ro·bi·o·log·i·
  cal
neu·ro·bi·ol·o·gist
neu·ro·bi·ol·o·gy
  pl neu·ro·bi·ol·o·gies
neu·ro·bio·tac·tic
  or neu·ro·bio·tac·ti·
    cal
neu·ro·bio·tax·is
  pl neu·ro·bio·tax·es
neu·ro·blast
neu·ro·blas·tic
neu·ro·blas·to·ma
  pl neu·ro·blas·to·mas
  or neu·ro·blas·to·ma·
    ta
neu·ro·blas·to·mal
neu·ro·cen·tral
neu·ro·cen·trum
  pl neu·ro·cen·trums
  or neu·ro·cen·tra
neu·ro·chem·i·cal
neu·ro·chem·ist
neu·ro·chem·is·try
  pl neu·ro·chem·is·
    tries
neu·ro·cir·cu·la·to·
  ry
neu·ro·cra·ni·al
neu·ro·cra·ni·um
  pl neu·ro·cra·ni·ums
  or neu·ro·cra·nia
neu·ro·cu·ta·ne·
  ous

neu·ro·cyte
neu·ro·cy·to·ma
  pl neu·ro·cy·to·mas
  or neu·ro·cy·to·ma·ta

neu·ro·der·ma·tit·
  ic
neu·ro·der·ma·ti·
  tis
  pl neu·ro·der·ma·ti·
    tis·es
  or neu·ro·der·ma·tit·
    i·des

neu·ro·der·ma·to·
  sis
  pl neu·ro·der·ma·to·
    ses

neu·ro·de·vel·op·
  ment
neu·ro·de·vel·op·
  ment·al
neu·ro·di·ag·nos·
  tic
neu·ro·dy·nam·ics
neu·ro·ec·to·derm
neu·ro·ec·to·der·
  mal
neu·ro·ef·fec·tor
neu·ro·elec·tric
  also neu·ro·elec·tri·
    cal

neu·ro·elec·tric·i·ty
  pl neu·ro·elec·tric·i·
    ties

neu·ro·em·bry·o·
  log·ic
  or neu·ro·em·bry·o·
    log·i·cal

neu·ro·em·bry·ol·o·
  gist
neu·ro·em·bry·ol·o·
  gy
  pl neu·ro·em·bry·ol·
    o·gies

neu·ro·en·do·crine
neu·ro·en·do·cri·
  no·log·i·cal
  also neu·ro·en·do·cri·
    no·log·ic

neu·ro·en·do·cri·
  nol·o·gist
neu·ro·en·do·cri·
  nol·o·gy
  pl neu·ro·en·do·cri·
    nol·o·gies

neu·ro·ep·i·the·li·
  al
neu·ro·epi·the·li·
  um
  pl neu·ro·epi·the·lia

neu·ro·fi·bril
neu·ro·fi·bril·la
  pl neu·ro·fi·bril·lae

neu·ro·fi·bril·lary
  also neu·ro·fi·bril·lar

neu·ro·fi·bro·ma
  pl neu·ro·fi·bro·mas
  also neu·ro·fi·bro·ma·
    ta

neu·ro·fi·bro·ma·
  to·sis
  pl neu·ro·fi·bro·ma·
    to·ses

neu·ro·fil·a·ment
neu·ro·fil·a·men·
  tous

neu·ro·gen
neu·ro·gen·e·sis
  pl neu·ro·gen·e·ses

neu·ro·ge·net·ic
neu·ro·gen·ic
  also neu·rog·e·nous

neu·ro·gen·i·cal·ly
neu·ro·glan·du·lar
neu·ro·glia
neu·ro·gli·al
neu·ro·gram
neu·ro·gram·mic
neu·ro·his·to·log·i·
  cal
  also neu·ro·his·to·log·
    ic

neu·ro·his·tol·o·
  gist
neu·ro·his·tol·o·gy
  pl neu·ro·his·tol·o·
    gies

neu·ro·hor·mon·al
neu·ro·hor·mone
neu·ro·hu·mor
neu·ro·hu·mor·al
neu·ro·hy·po·phy·
  se·al
  or neu·ro·hy·po·phy·
    si·al

neu·ro·hy·poph·y·
  sis
neu·ro·im·mu·nol·
  o·gy
  pl neu·ro·im·mu·nol·
    o·gies

neu·ro·ker·a·tin
neu·ro·kyme

neu·ro·lept·an·al·
ge·sia
or neu·ro·lep·to·an·
al·ge·sia

neu·ro·lept·an·al·
ge·sic

neu·ro·lep·tic

neu·ro·lin·guis·tics

neu·ro·log·i·cal
or neu·ro·log·ic

neu·rol·o·gist

neu·rol·o·gy
pl neu·rol·o·gies

neu·ro·lym·pho·
ma·to·sis

neu·ro·lyt·ic

neu·ro·ma
pl neu·ro·mas
or neu·ro·ma·ta

neu·ro·mere

neu·ro·met·rics

neu·ro·mi·me·sis
pl neu·ro·mi·me·ses

neu·ro·mi·met·ic

neu·ro·mod·u·la·
tor

neu·ro·mod·u·la·to·
ry

neu·ro·mo·tor

neu·ro·mus·cu·lar

neu·ro·my·al

neu·ro·my·op·a·thy
pl neu·ro·my·op·a·
thies

neu·ro·my·o·si·tis

neu·ron
also neu·rone

neu·ro·nal
also neu·ron·ic

neu·ro·neu·ro·nal

neu·ro·ne·vus
pl neu·ro·ne·vi

neu·ron·i·tis

neu·ro·nog·ra·phy
pl neu·ro·nog·ra·
phies

neu·ro·no·pha·gia

neu·ro·noph·a·gy
pl neu·ro·noph·a·gies

neu·ro·oph·thal·
mo·log·ic
or neu·ro·oph·thal·
mo·log·i·cal

neu·ro·oph·thal·
mol·o·gy
pl neu·ro·oph·thal·
mol·o·gies

neu·ro·oto·log·ic
or neu·ro·oto·log·i·cal

neu·ro·otol·o·gy
pl neu·ro·otol·o·gies

neu·ro·par·a·lyt·ic

neu·ro·path

neu·ro·path·ic

neu·ro·path·i·cal·ly

neu·ro·patho·gen·
e·sis
pl neu·ro·patho·gen·e·
ses

neu·ro·path·o·log·
ic
or neu·ro·path·o·log·
i·cal

neu·ro·pa·thol·o·
gist

neu·ro·pa·thol·o·gy
pl neu·ro·pa·thol·o·
gies

neu·rop·a·thy
pl neu·rop·a·thies

neu·ro·pep·tide

neu·ro·phar·ma·co·
log·i·cal
also neu·ro·phar·ma·
co·log·ic

neu·ro·phar·ma·
col·o·gist

neu·ro·phar·ma·
col·o·gy
pl neu·ro·phar·ma·
col·o·gies

neu·ro·phil·ic

neu·ro·phy·sin

neu·ro·phys·i·o·log·
i·cal
also neu·ro·phys·i·o·
log·ic

neu·ro·phys·i·ol·o·
gist

neu·ro·phys·i·ol·o·
gy
pl neu·ro·phys·i·ol·o·
gies

neu·ro·pil
also neu·ro·pile

neu·ro·pi·lar

neu·ro·plasm

neu·ro·plas·mat·ic
or neu·ro·plas·mic

neu·ro·ple·gic

neu·ro·pore

neu·ro·psy·chi·at·
ric

neu·ro·psy·chi·at·
ri·cal·ly
neu·ro·psy·chi·a·
trist
neu·ro·psy·chi·a·
try
  pl neu·ro·psy·chi·a·
  tries
neu·ro·psy·chic
  also neu·ro·psy·chi·
  cal
neu·ro·psy·cho·log·
i·cal
neu·ro·psy·chol·o·
gist
neu·ro·psy·chol·o·
gy
  pl neu·ro·psy·chol·o·
  gies
neu·ro·psy·cho·
phar·ma·col·o·gy
  pl neu·ro·psy·cho·
  phar·ma·col·o·gies
neu·ro·ra·dio·log·i·
cal
  also neu·ro·ra·dio·log·
  ic
neu·ro·ra·di·ol·o·
gist
neu·ro·ra·di·ol·o·gy
  pl neu·ro·ra·di·ol·o·
  gies
neu·ro·ret·i·ni·tis
  pl neu·ro·ret·i·nit·i·
  des
neu·ror·rha·phy
  pl neu·ror·rha·phies
neu·ro·sci·ence

neu·ro·sci·en·tist
neu·ro·se·cre·tion
neu·ro·se·cre·to·ry
neu·ro·sen·so·ry
neu·ro·sis
  pl neu·ro·ses
neu·ro·some
neu·ros·po·ra
neu·ro·stim·u·la·
tor
neu·ro·sur·geon
neu·ro·sur·gery
  pl neu·ro·sur·ger·ies
neu·ro·sur·gi·cal
neu·ro·syph·i·lis
neu·ro·syph·i·lit·ic
neu·ro·ten·di·nous
neu·rot·ic
neu·rot·i·cal·ly
neu·rot·i·cism
neu·ro·to·gen·ic
neu·ro·tox·ic
neu·ro·tox·ic·i·ty
  pl neu·ro·tox·ic·i·ties
neu·ro·tox·i·co·log·
i·cal
neu·ro·tox·i·col·o·
gist
neu·ro·tox·i·col·o·
gy
  pl neu·ro·tox·i·col·o·
  gies
neu·ro·tox·in
neu·ro·trans·mis·
sion
neu·ro·trans·mit·
ter

neu·ro·trope
neu·ro·troph·ic
neu·ro·trop·ic
neu·rot·ro·pism
neu·ro·tu·bule
neu·ro·vac·cine
neu·ro·vac·cin·ia
neu·ro·vas·cu·lar
neu·ro·veg·e·ta·tive
neu·ro·vir·u·lence
neu·ro·vir·u·lent
neu·ro·vis·cer·al
neu·ru·la
  pl neu·ru·lae
  or neu·ru·las
neu·ru·lar
neu·ru·la·tion
neu·ter
neu·tral
neu·tral·iza·tion
neu·tro·clu·sion
neu·tron
neu·tro·pe·nia
neu·tro·pe·nic
neu·tro·phil
  or neu·tro·phil·ic
  also neu·tro·phile
  adjective
neu·tro·phil
  also neu·tro·phile
  noun
neu·tro·phil·ia
ne·vo·car·ci·no·ma
  pl ne·vo·car·ci·no·
  mas
  or ne·vo·car·ci·no·
  ma·ta
ne·void

ne·vus
   pl ne·vi

ne·vus flam·me·us

new·born
   pl new·born
   or new·borns

New·cas·tle dis·ease

new·ton

New·ton's rings

nex·us
   pl nex·us·es
   or nex·us

n'ga·na
   var of nagana

ni·a·cin

ni·a·cin·amide

ni·al·amide

nick·el

nick·ing

Ni·co·ti·ana

nic·o·tin·amide

nic·o·tin·ate

nic·o·tine

nic·o·tin·ic

nic·o·tin·ism

ni·dal

ni·da·tion

ni·dus
   pl ni·di
   or ni·dus·es

Nie·mann-Pick dis·ease

ni·fed·i·pine

ni·fur·ox·ime

night-blind

night blind·ness

night·mare

night·shade

ni·gral

ni·gro·stri·a·tal

nik·eth·amide

Nile blue

nin·hy·drin

ni·o·bi·um

nip·per

nip·ple

Nip·po·stron·gy·lus

Ni·pride

ni·sin

Nissel sub·stance

Nissl bod·ies

ni·ter

ni·trate
   ni·trat·ed
   ni·trat·ing

ni·tra·tion

ni·tric

ni·trid·a·tion

ni·tride

ni·tri·fi·ca·tion

ni·tri·fy·ing

ni·trile

ni·trite

ni·tri·toid

ni·tro·ben·zene

ni·tro·cel·lu·lose

ni·tro·fu·ran

ni·tro·fu·ran·to·in

ni·tro·fu·ra·zone

ni·tro·gen

ni·tro·ge·nase

ni·trog·e·nous

ni·tro·glyc·er·in
   or ni·tro·glyc·er·ine

ni·tro·hy·dro·chlo·ric

ni·tro·mer·sol

ni·trom·e·ter

ni·tro·prus·side

ni·tro·sa·mine
   also ni·tro·so·amine

ni·tro·sate
   ni·tro·sat·ed
   ni·tro·sat·ing

ni·tro·sa·tion

ni·tro·so·di·meth·yl·amine

ni·tro·so·gua·ni·dine

ni·tro·so·urea

ni·tro·syl

ni·trous

no·bel·i·um

no·car·dia

no·car·di·al

no·car·di·o·sis
   pl no·car·di·o·ses

no·ci·cep·tive

no·ci·cep·tor

no·ci·fen·sor

no·ci·per·cep·tion

noc·tu·ria

noc·tur·nal

noc·u·ous

nod·al

node of Ran·vier

no·dose

no·dos·i·ty
   pl no·dos·i·ties

nod·u·lar
nod·u·lar·i·ty
  pl nod·u·lar·i·ties
nod·u·la·tion
nod·ule
nod·u·lus
  pl nod·u·li
no·et·ic
no·ma
no·men·cla·tur·al
no·men·cla·ture
No·mi·na An·a·
  tom·i·ca
no·mo·gram
no·mo·graph
no·mo·graph·ic
no·mog·ra·phy
  pl no·mog·ra·phies

non·ab·sorb·able
non·ac·id
non·ad·dict·ing
non·al·le·lic
non·al·ler·gen·ic
non·al·ler·gic
non·an·ti·gen·ic
non·aque·ous
non·as·so·cia·tive
non·bac·te·ri·al
non·bar·bi·tu·rate
non·car·cin·o·gen
non·car·ci·no·gen·
  ic
non·cel·lu·lar
non·chro·mo·som·
  al
non·com·mu·ni·ca·
  ble

non·com·pet·i·tive
non com·pos men·
  tis
non·con·duc·tor
non·cor·o·nary
non·de·form·ing
non·di·a·bet·ic
non·di·a·lyz·able
non·di·rec·tive
non·dis·junc·tion
non·di·vid·ing
non·elas·tic
non·elec·tro·lyte
non·en·zy·mat·ic
  or non·en·zy·mic
  also non·en·zyme
non·en·zy·mat·i·
  cal·ly
non·fa·tal
non·fe·brile
non·gono·coc·cal
non·gran·u·lar
non·heme
non·in·va·sive
non·ke·tot·ic
non·ma·lig·nant
non·med·ul·lat·ed
non·mo·tile
non·my·elin·at·ed
non·nar·cot·ic
non·neo·plas·tic
non·nu·cle·at·ed
non·nu·tri·tive
non·ob·struc·tive
non·of·fi·cial
non·ol·fac·to·ry
non·opaque

non·or·gas·mic
non·par·ous
non·pa·ter·ni·ty
  pl non·pa·ter·ni·ties
non·patho·gen·ic
non·phy·si·cian
non·preg·nant
non·pre·scrip·tion
non·pro·duc·tive
non·pro·pri·etary
non·pro·tein
non·psy·chi·at·ric
non·re·ac·tive
non·re·duc·ing
non·re·duc·tion
non·rheu·ma·toid
non·se·cre·tor
non·self
non·spe·cif·ic
non·spe·cif·i·cal·ly
non·ste·roi·dal
  also non·ste·roid

non·stri·at·ed
non·sur·gi·cal
non·tast·er
non·tox·ic
non·union
non·vas·cu·lar
non·vec·tor
non·vi·a·ble
nor·adren·a·line
  also nor·adren·a·lin
nor·ad·ren·er·gic
nor·epi·neph·rine
nor·eth·in·drone
nor·ethyn·o·drel
nor·ges·trel

nor·leu·cine

nor·mal·i·ty
  pl nor·mal·i·ties

nor·mal·iza·tion

nor·mal·ize
  nor·mal·ized
  nor·mal·iz·ing

nor·mer·gic

nor·meta·neph·
  rine

nor·mo·blast

nor·mo·blas·tic

nor·mo·cal·ce·mia

nor·mo·cal·ce·mic

nor·mo·chro·mia

nor·mo·chro·mic

nor·mo·cyte

nor·mo·cyt·ic

nor·mo·gly·ce·mia

nor·mo·gly·ce·mic

nor·mo·ten·sive

nor·mo·ther·mia

nor·mo·ther·mic

nor·mo·ton·ic

nor·mo·vol·emia

nor·mo·vol·emic

nor·trip·ty·line

nor·va·line

nose·bleed

nose·piece

nos·o·co·mi·al

no·so·log·i·cal
  or no·so·log·ic

no·sol·o·gist

no·sol·o·gy
  pl no·sol·o·gies

Nos·o·psyl·lus

nos·tril

nos·trum

no·ti·fi·able

no·ti·fi·ca·tion

no·ti·fy
  no·ti·fied
  no·ti·fy·ing

no·to·chord

no·to·chord·al

No·to·ed·res

no·to·ed·ric

nour·ish

nour·ish·ment

no·vo·bi·o·cin

no·vo·caine

noxa
  pl nox·ae

nox·ious

nu·bile

nu·bil·i·ty
  pl nu·bil·i·ties

nu·chal

nu·cle·ar

nu·cle·ase

nu·cle·ate
  nu·cle·at·ed
  nu·cle·at·ing

nu·cle·a·tion

nu·clei
  pl of nucleus

nu·cle·ic

nu·cle·in

nu·cleo·cap·sid

nu·cleo·cy·to·plas·
  mic

nu·cleo·his·tone

nu·cle·oid

nu·cle·o·lar

nu·cle·o·lo·ne·ma
  also nu·cle·o·lo·neme
  pl nu·cle·o·lo·ne·mas
  or nu·cle·o·lo·ne·ma·
    ta
  also nu·cle·o·lo·
    nemes

nu·cle·o·lus
  pl nu·cle·o·li

nu·cle·on

nu·cle·on·ic

nu·cleo·phile

nu·cleo·phil·ic

nu·cleo·phi·lic·i·ty
  pl nu·cleo·phi·lic·i·
    ties

nu·cleo·plasm

nu·cleo·plas·mat·ic
  or nu·cleo·plas·mic

nu·cleo·prot·amine

nu·cleo·pro·tein

nu·cle·o·sid·ase

nu·cle·o·side

nu·cleo·so·mal

nu·cleo·some

nu·cle·o·tid·ase

nu·cle·o·tide

nu·cleo·ti·dyl·
  trans·fer·ase

nu·cleo·tox·ic

nu·cle·us
  pl nu·clei
  also nu·cle·us·es

nu·cle·us ac·cum·
  bens

nu·cle·us am·big·u·
  us

nu·cle·us cu·ne·a·tus

nu·cle·us dor·sa·lis
  pl nu·clei dor·sa·les

nu·cle·us grac·i·lis

nu·cle·us pul·po·sus
  pl nu·clei pul·po·si

nu·clide

nu·clid·ic

nul·li·grav·i·da

nul·lip·a·ra
  pl nul·lip·a·ras
  also nul·lip·a·rae

nul·lip·a·rous

nul·li·so·mic

nu·mer·i·cal

num·mu·lar

nurse
  nursed
  nurs·ing

nurse-anes·the·tist

nurse-mid·wife
  pl nurse-mid·wives

nurse-mid·wife·ry
  pl nurse-mid·wife·ries

nurse-prac·ti·tion·er

nurs·ery
  pl nurs·er·ies

nurse's aide

nurs·ling

nur·tur·ance

nur·tur·ant

nut·gall

nu·tri·ent

nu·tri·lite

nu·tri·ment

nu·tri·tion

nu·tri·tion·al

nu·tri·tion·ist

nu·tri·tious

nu·tri·tive

nux vom·i·ca
  pl nux vom·i·ca

nyc·ta·lope

nyc·ta·lo·pia

nyc·to·pho·bia

nyc·tu·ria

ny·lon

nymph

nym·phae

nymph·al

nym·pho
  pl nym·phos

nym·pho·ma·nia

nym·pho·ma·ni·ac
  noun

nym·pho·ma·ni·ac
  or nym·pho·ma·ni·a·cal
  adjective

nys·tag·mo·graph·ic

nys·tag·mog·ra·phy
  pl nys·tag·mog·ra·phies

nys·tag·moid

nys·tag·mus

nys·ta·tin

O

O an·ti·gen

oat-cell

obe·li·on
  pl obe·lia

obese

obe·si·ty
  pl obe·si·ties

obex

ob·jec·tive

ob·li·gate

oblig·a·to·ri·ly

oblig·a·to·ry

oblique

obliq·ui·ty
  pl obliq·ui·ties

ob·li·quus
  pl ob·li·qui

ob·li·quus ex·ter·nus

ob·li·quus ex·ter·nus ab·dom·i·nis

ob·li·quus in·ter·nus

ob·li·quus in·ter·nus ab·dom·i·nis

oblit·er·ate
  oblit·er·at·ed
  oblit·er·at·ing

oblit·er·a·tion

oblit·er·a·tive

ob·nub·i·la·tion

ob·ses·sion

ob·ses·sion·al

ob·ses·sive

ob·stet·ric
   or ob·stet·ri·cal
ob·ste·tri·cian
ob·stet·rics
ob·sti·na·cy
   pl ob·sti·na·cies
ob·sti·nate
ob·sti·pa·tion
ob·struct
ob·struc·tion
ob·struc·tive
ob·tund
ob·tun·da·tion
ob·tund·ent
ob·tu·ra·tion
ob·tu·ra·tor
ob·tu·ra·tor ex·ter·
   nus
ob·tu·ra·tor in·ter·
   nus
oc·cip·i·tal
oc·cip·i·ta·lis
oc·cip·i·to·fron·ta·
   lis
oc·ci·put
   pl oc·ci·puts
   or oc·cip·i·ta
oc·clude
   oc·clud·ed
   oc·clud·ing
oc·clu·sal
oc·clu·sion
oc·clu·sive
oc·cult
ocel·lar
ocel·lus
   pl ocel·li

och·lo·pho·bia
ochro·no·sis
   pl ochro·no·ses
ochro·not·ic
oc·ta·dec·a·no·ic
oc·ta·meth·yl·py·
   ro·phos·phor·a·
   mide
oc·ta·no·ic
oc·ta·pep·tide
oc·ta·va·lent
oc·to·pa·mine
oc·tose
oc·u·lar
oc·u·lar·ist
oc·u·list
oc·u·lo·cu·ta·ne·
   ous
oc·u·lo·gy·ral
oc·u·lo·gy·ric
oc·u·lo·mo·tor
oc·u·lus
   pl oc·u·li
OD
   OD'd
     or ODed
   OD'·ing
   OD's
odon·tal·gia
odon·tal·gic
odon·ti·tis
   pl odon·tit·i·des
odon·to·blast
odon·to·blas·tic
odon·to·cele
odon·to·clast

odon·to·gen·e·sis
   pl odon·to·gen·e·ses
odon·to·gen·ic
odon·toid
odon·to·log·i·cal
odon·tol·o·gist
odon·tol·o·gy
   pl odon·tol·o·gies
odon·to·ma
   pl odon·to·mas
   also odon·to·ma·ta
odon·tome
odon·tot·o·my
   pl odon·tot·o·mies
odor·ant
odor·if·er·ous
odor·ous
odyno·pha·gia
oe·di·pal
Oe·di·pus
oe·soph·a·go·sto·
   mi·a·sis
   pl oe·soph·a·go·sto·
   mi·a·ses
Oe·soph·a·gos·to·
   mum
oes·tri·a·sis
   pl oes·tri·a·ses
oes·trid
Oes·tri·dae
Oes·trus
of·fi·cial
of·fi·ci·nal
ohm
ohm·ic
oid·ium
   pl oid·ia

oint·ment

olea
pl of oleum

ole·ag·i·nous

ole·an·der

ole·an·do·my·cin

ole·an·drin

ole·ate

olec·ra·non

ole·ic

ole·in

ole·o·phil·ic

ole·o·pho·bic

oleo·res·in

oleo·res·in·ous

oleo·tho·rax
pl oleo·tho·rax·es
or oleo·tho·ra·ces

oleo·vi·ta·min

ole·um
pl olea

ol·fac·tion

ol·fac·tom·e·ter

ol·fac·to·met·ric

ol·fac·to·ry

ol·fac·ty
pl ol·fac·ties

ol·i·ge·mia

ol·i·ge·mic

oli·go·chro·me·mia

oli·go·cy·the·mia

oli·go·cy·the·mic

oli·go·den·dro·cyte

oli·go·den·drog·lia

oli·go·den·drog·li·al

oli·go·den·dro·gli·o·ma
pl oli·go·den·dro·gli·o·mas
or oli·go·den·dro·gli·o·ma·ta

oli·go·dy·nam·ic

oli·go·hy·dram·ni·os

oli·go·lec·i·thal

oli·go·men·or·rhea

oligo·mer

oligo·mer·ic

oligo·mer·iza·tion

oli·go·my·cin

oli·go·nu·cle·o·tide

oli·go·phre·nia

oli·go·phren·ic

oli·go·sac·cha·ride

oli·go·sper·mia

ol·i·gu·ria

ol·i·gur·ic

ol·i·vary

ol·ive

ol·i·vo·cer·e·bel·lar

ol·i·vo·spi·nal

olo·li·u·qui

oma·sal

oma·si·tis

oma·sum
pl oma·sa

omen·tal

omen·tal

omen·tec·to·my
pl omen·tec·to·mies

omen·to·pexy
pl omen·to·pex·ies

omen·to·plas·ty
pl omen·to·plas·ties

omen·tor·rha·phy
pl omen·tor·rha·phies

omen·tum
pl omen·ta
or omen·tums

om·niv·o·rous

omo·hy·oid

om·pha·lec·to·my
pl om·pha·lec·to·mies

om·phal·ic

om·phal·i·tis
pl om·pha·lit·i·des

om·pha·lo·cele

om·pha·lo·mes·en·ter·ic

onan·ism

onan·ist

onan·is·tic

On·cho·cer·ca

on·cho·cer·cal

on·cho·cer·ci·a·sis
pl on·cho·cer·ci·a·ses

on·cho·cer·co·ma

on·cho·cer·co·sis
pl on·cho·cer·co·ses

on·cho·sphere
var of oncosphere

on·co·cyte

on·co·cy·to·ma
pl on·co·cy·to·mas
or on·co·cy·to·ma·ta

on·co·fe·tal

on·co·gene

on·co·gen·e·sis
pl on·co·gen·e·ses

on·co·gen·ic
  also on·cog·e·nous

on·co·gen·i·cal·ly
on·co·ge·nic·i·ty
  pl on·co·ge·nic·i·ties

on·co·log·i·cal
  also on·co·log·ic

on·col·o·gist
on·col·o·gy
  pl on·col·o·gies

on·col·y·sis
  pl on·col·y·ses

on·co·lyt·ic
on·co·lyt·i·cal·ly
On·co·me·la·nia
on·com·e·ter
on·co·met·ric
on·cor·na·vi·rus
on·co·sphere
  also on·cho·sphere

on·cot·ic
oni·um
on·lay
on·o·mato·ma·nia
on·set
on·to·gen·e·sis
  pl on·to·gen·e·ses

on·to·ge·net·ic
on·to·ge·net·i·cal·ly
on·to·gen·ic
on·to·gen·i·cal·ly
on·tog·e·ny
  pl on·tog·e·nies

on·ych·a·tro·phia
on·ych·aux·is
  pl on·ych·aux·es

on·ych·ec·to·my
  pl on·ych·ec·to·mies

onych·ia
on·y·cho·gry·po·sis
  pl on·y·cho·gry·po·ses

on·y·cho·het·ero·to·pia
on·y·chol·y·sis
  pl on·y·chol·y·ses

on·y·cho·ma·de·sis
  pl on·y·cho·ma·de·ses

on·y·cho·my·co·sis
  pl on·y·cho·my·co·ses

on·y·choph·a·gy
  pl on·y·choph·a·gies

on·y·chor·rhex·is
  pl on·y·chor·rhex·es

on·y·cho·schiz·ia
on·y·cho·sis
  pl on·y·cho·ses

onyx·is
oo·cy·e·sis
  pl oo·cy·e·ses

oo·cyst
oo·cyte
oog·a·mous
oog·a·my
  pl oog·a·mies

oo·gen·e·sis
  pl oo·gen·e·ses

oo·ge·net·ic
oo·go·ni·al
oo·go·ni·um
oo·ki·nete
oo·lem·ma

oo·pho·rec·to·mize
oo·pho·rec·to·mized
oo·pho·rec·to·miz·ing
oo·pho·rec·to·my
  pl oo·pho·rec·to·mies

oo·pho·ri·tis
oo·plasm
oo·plas·mic
oo·spore
oo·tid
oo·type
opac·i·fi·ca·tion
opac·i·fy
  opac·i·fied
  opac·i·fy·ing
opac·i·ty
  pl opac·i·ties

opaque
open
  opened
  open·ing
open-heart
open·ing
op·er·a·bil·i·ty
  pl op·er·a·bil·i·ties

op·er·a·ble
op·er·ant
op·er·ate
  op·er·at·ed
  op·er·at·ing
op·er·a·tion
op·er·a·tive
op·er·a·tor
op·er·a·to·ry
  pl op·er·a·to·ries

oper·cu·lum
pl oper·cu·la
also oper·cu·lums

op·er·on

oph·thal·mia

oph·thal·mia neo·
na·to·rum

oph·thal·mic

oph·thal·mo·dy·na·
mom·e·try
pl oph·thal·mo·dy·na·
mom·e·tries

oph·thal·mo·graph

oph·thal·mo·log·ic
or oph·thal·mo·log·i·
cal

oph·thal·mol·o·gist

oph·thal·mol·o·gy
pl oph·thal·mol·o·gies

oph·thal·mom·e·
ter

oph·thal·mom·e·
try
pl oph·thal·mom·e·
tries

oph·thal·mo·plas·
tic

oph·thal·mo·ple·
gia

oph·thal·mo·ple·
gic

oph·thal·mo·scope

oph·thal·mo·scop·
ic

oph·thal·mo·scop·i·
cal·ly

oph·thal·mos·co·py
pl oph·thal·mos·co·
pies

oph·thal·mo·trope

oph·thal·mo·tro·
pom·e·ter

opi·ate

opin·ion

opi·oid

opis·the·nar

opis·thi·on
pl opis·thia
or opis·thi·ons

opis·tho·cra·ni·on

opis·thor·chi·a·sis

Opis·thor·chi·idae

Op·is·thor·chis

opis·tho·ton·ic

op·is·thot·o·nos

op·is·thot·o·nus

opi·um

opo·ther·a·py
pl opo·ther·a·pies

op·po·nens
pl op·po·nen·tes
or op·po·nens

op·po·nens dig·i·ti
min·i·mi

op·po·nens pol·li·
cis

op·po·nent

op·por·tun·ist

op·por·tu·nist·ic

op·pos·abil·i·ty
pl op·pos·abil·i·ties

op·pos·able

op·pose

op·posed

op·pos·ing

op·sin

op·son·ic

op·so·nin

op·son·iza·tion

op·son·ize

op·son·ized

op·son·iz·ing

op·so·no·cy·to·pha·
gic

op·tic

op·ti·cal

op·ti·cian

op·ti·cian·ry
pl op·ti·cian·ries

op·tics

op·ti·mal

op·ti·mal·i·ty
pl op·ti·mal·i·ties

op·ti·mism

op·ti·mist

op·ti·mis·tic

op·ti·mum
pl op·ti·ma
also op·ti·mums

op·to·gram

op·to·ki·net·ic

op·tom·e·ter

op·to·met·ric

op·tom·e·trist

op·tom·e·try
pl op·tom·e·tries

op·to·phone

op·to·type

ora
  pl of os

orad

orae ser·ra·tae
  pl of ora serrata

oral
  of the mouth (see
  aural)

ora·le

oral·ism

oral·ist

oral·i·ty
  pl oral·i·ties

ora ser·ra·ta
  pl orae ser·ra·tae

or·bic·u·lar

or·bi·cu·lar·is
  pl or·bi·cu·la·res

or·bi·cu·lar·is oc·u·li
  pl or·bi·cu·la·res oc·u·li

or·bi·cu·lar·is oris
  pl or·bi·cu·la·res oris

or·bit

or·bit·al

or·bi·ta·le
  pl or·bi·ta·lia

or·bi·to·sphe·noid

or·bi·tot·o·my
  pl or·bi·tot·o·mies

or·ce·in

or·chi·dec·to·my
  pl or·chi·dec·to·mies

or·chi·do·pexy
  pl or·chi·do·pex·ies

or·chi·ec·to·my
  also or·chec·to·my
  pl or·chi·ec·to·mies
  also or·chec·to·mies

or·chil
  var of archil

or·chi·o·pexy
  pl or·chi·o·pex·ies

or·chit·ic

or·chi·tis

or·cin

or·cin·ol

or·der

or·der·ly
  pl or·der·lies

or·gan

or·gan·elle

or·gan·ic

or·gan·i·cal·ly

or·gan·i·cism

or·gan·i·cist

or·gan·i·cis·tic

or·ga·nic·i·ty
  pl or·ga·nic·i·ties

or·gan·ism

or·gan·is·mic
  also or·gan·is·mal

or·gan·is·mi·cal·ly

or·ga·ni·za·tion

or·ga·nize
  or·ga·nized
  or·ga·niz·ing

or·ga·niz·er

or·gano·chlo·rine

or·gan of Cor·ti

or·gan of Ja·cob·son

or·gan of Ro·sen·mül·ler

or·gan·o·gen·e·sis
  pl or·gan·o·gen·e·ses

or·gan·o·ge·net·ic

or·ga·nog·e·ny
  pl or·ga·nog·e·nies

or·gan·oid

or·gan·o·lep·tic

or·gan·o·lep·ti·cal·ly

or·gan·ol·o·gy
  pl or·gan·ol·o·gies

or·gano·mer·cu·ri·al

or·gano·mer·cu·ry

or·gano·me·tal·lic

or·gano·phos·phate

or·gano·phos·pho·rus

or·gano·sol

or·gano·ther·a·py
  pl or·gano·ther·a·pies

or·gan·o·tro·phic

or·gan·o·trop·ic

or·gan·o·trop·i·cal·ly

or·gasm

or·gas·mic
  also or·gas·tic

ori·en·ta·tion

ori·ent·ed

or·i·fice

or·i·fi·cial

or·i·gin

Or·mond's dis·ease

or·ni·thine

Or·ni·thod·o·ros
or·ni·tho·sis
pl or·ni·tho·ses

oro·an·tral
oro·fa·cial
oro·na·sal
oro·pha·ryn·geal
oro·phar·ynx
pl oro·pha·ryn·ges
also oro·phar·ynx·es

oro·so·mu·coid
oro·tate
orot·ic
oro·tra·che·al
Oro·ya fe·ver
or·phen·a·drine
or·the·sis
pl or·the·ses

or·tho
or·tho·bo·ric
or·tho·chro·mat·ic
or·tho·cre·sol
or·tho·di·a·gram
or·tho·di·a·graph·ic
or·tho·di·ag·ra·phy
pl or·tho·di·ag·ra·phies

orth·odon·tia
orth·odon·tic
orth·odon·tics
or·tho·don·tist
or·tho·drom·ic
or·tho·drom·i·cal·ly
or·tho·gen·e·sis
pl or·tho·gen·e·ses

or·tho·ge·net·ic
or·thog·na·thism
or·thog·na·thous
also or·thog·nath·ic
or·thog·na·thy
pl or·thog·na·thies

or·thog·o·nal
or·tho·grade
or·tho·kera·tol·o·gist
or·tho·kera·tol·o·gy
pl or·tho·kera·tol·o·gies

or·tho·mo·lec·u·lar
or·tho·pe·dic
or·tho·pe·di·cal·ly
or·tho·pe·dics
or·tho·pe·dist
or·tho·pho·ria
or·tho·phos·phate
or·tho·phos·pho·ric
or·thop·nea
or·thop·ne·ic
or·tho·psy·chi·at·ric
or·tho·psy·chi·a·trist
or·tho·psy·chi·a·try
pl or·tho·psy·chi·a·tries

or·thop·tic
or·thop·tics
or·thop·tist
or·tho·scope
or·tho·sis
pl or·tho·ses

or·tho·stat·ic

or·tho·stat·ism
or·thot·ics
or·thot·ist
or·tho·top·ic
or·tho·top·i·cal·ly
or·tho·vol·tage
ory·ze·nin
os
pl os·sa
bone

os
pl ora
orifice

os cal·cis
pl os·sa cal·cis

os·cil·late
os·cil·lat·ed
os·cil·lat·ing
os·cil·la·tion
os·cil·la·tor
os·cil·la·to·ry
os·cil·lo·gram
os·cil·lo·graph
os·cil·lo·graph·ic
os·cil·lo·graph·i·cal·ly
os·cil·log·ra·phy
pl os·cil·log·ra·phies

os·cil·lom·e·ter
os·cil·lo·met·ric
os·cil·lom·e·try
pl os·cil·lom·e·tries

os·cil·lo·scope
os·cil·lo·scop·ic
os·cil·lo·scop·i·cal·ly

os·cox·ae
 pl os·sa cox·ae

Os·good-Schlat·
 ter's dis·ease
os·mate
os·mic
os·mio·phil·ic
os·mi·oph·i·ly
 pl os·mi·oph·i·lies
os·mi·um
os·mol
 or os·mole
os·mo·lal
os·mo·lal·i·ty
 pl os·mo·lal·i·ties
os·mo·lar
os·mo·lar·i·ty
 pl os·mo·lar·i·ties
os·mom·e·ter
os·mo·met·ric
os·mom·e·try
 pl os·mom·e·tries
os·mo·phil·ic
 also os·mo·phile
os·mo·re·cep·tor
os·mo·reg·u·la·tion
os·mo·reg·u·la·to·
 ry
os·mo·scope
os·mo·sis
 pl os·mo·ses
os·mot·ic
os·mot·i·cal·ly
os·sa
 pl of os
os·sa cal·cis
 pl of os cal·cis

os·sa cox·ae
 pl of os cox·ae

os·se·in
os·se·let
os·se·ous
os·si·cle
os·sic·u·lar
os·si·cu·lec·to·my
 pl os·si·cu·lec·to·mies

os·si·cu·lot·o·my
 pl os·si·cu·lot·o·mies

os·sif·ic
os·si·fi·ca·tion
os·si·fi·ca·to·ry
os·si·fy
 os·si·fied
 os·si·fy·ing
os·te·al
os·tec·to·my
 pl os·tec·to·mies

os·te·it·ic
os·te·itis
 pl os·te·it·i·des

os·te·itis de·for·
 mans
os·te·itis fi·bro·sa
os·te·itis fi·bro·sa
 cys·ti·ca
os·te·itis fi·bro·sa
 cys·ti·ca gen·er·
 al·is·ta
os·teo·ar·thrit·ic
os·teo·ar·thri·tis
 pl os·teo·ar·thrit·i·des

os·teo·ar·throp·a·
 thy
 pl os·teo·ar·throp·a·
 thies

os·teo·ar·tic·u·lar
os·teo·blast
os·teo·blas·tic
os·teo·chon·dri·tis
os·teo·chon·dri·tis
 dis·se·cans
os·teo·chon·dro·ma
 pl os·teo·chon·dro·
 mas
 or os·teo·chon·dro·
 ma·ta

os·teo·chon·dro·sis
 pl os·teo·chon·dro·ses

os·teo·chon·drot·ic
os·te·oc·la·sis
 pl os·te·oc·la·ses

os·teo·clast
os·teo·clas·tic
os·teo·clas·to·ma
 pl os·teo·clas·to·mas
 or os·teo·clas·to·ma·ta

os·teo·cra·ni·um
 pl os·teo·cra·ni·ums
 or os·teo·cra·nia

os·teo·cyte
os·teo·den·tin
os·teo·dys·tro·phia
 de·for·mans
os·teo·dys·tro·phia
 fi·bro·sa
os·teo·dys·tro·phic
os·teo·dys·tro·phy
 pl os·teo·dys·tro·phies

os·teo·fi·bro·sis
pl os·teo·fi·bro·ses

os·teo·gen·e·sis
pl os·teo·gen·e·ses

os·teo·gen·e·sis im·per·fec·ta

os·teo·gen·ic
also os·teo·ge·net·ic

os·te·og·e·nous

os·te·oid

os·teo·lath·y·rism

os·te·o·log·i·cal

os·te·ol·o·gist

os·te·ol·o·gy
pl os·te·ol·o·gies

os·te·ol·y·sis
pl os·te·ol·y·ses

os·te·o·lyt·ic

os·te·o·ma
pl os·te·o·mas
or os·te·o·ma·ta

os·teo·ma·la·cia

os·teo·ma·la·cic

os·teo·met·ric

os·te·om·e·try
pl os·te·om·e·tries

os·teo·my·elit·ic

os·teo·my·eli·tis
pl os·teo·my·elit·i·des

os·te·on
also os·te·one

os·te·on·al

os·teo·ne·cro·sis
pl os·teo·ne·cro·ses

os·teo·path

os·teo·path·ic

os·teo·path·i·cal·ly

os·te·op·a·thy
pl os·te·op·a·thies

os·teo·peri·os·ti·tis

os·teo·pe·tro·sis
pl os·teo·pe·tro·ses

os·teo·pe·trot·ic

os·teo·phyte

os·teo·phyt·ic

os·teo·plas·tic

os·teo·plas·ty
pl os·teo·plas·ties

os·teo·po·ro·sis
pl os·teo·po·ro·ses

os·teo·po·rot·ic

os·te·op·sath·y·ro·sis
pl os·te·op·sath·y·ro·ses

os·teo·ra·dio·ne·cro·sis
pl os·teo·ra·dio·ne·cro·ses

os·teo·sar·co·ma
pl os·teo·sar·co·mas
or os·teo·sar·co·ma·ta

os·teo·scle·ro·sis
pl os·teo·scle·ro·ses

os·teo·scle·rot·ic

os·teo·syn·the·sis
pl os·teo·syn·the·ses

os·te·o·tome

os·te·ot·o·my
pl os·te·ot·o·mies

Os·ter·ta·gia

os·ti·al

os·ti·tis

os·ti·um
pl os·tia

os·ti·um pri·mum

os·ti·um se·cun·dum

os·to·mate

os·to·my
pl os·to·mies

otal·gia

otic

otit·ic

oti·tis
pl otit·i·des

oti·tis ex·ter·na

oti·tis me·dia

Oto·bi·us

oto·co·nia

oto·cyst

Oto·dec·tes

oto·dec·tic

otog·e·nous

oto·lar·yn·go·log·i·cal

oto·lar·yn·gol·o·gist

oto·lar·yn·gol·o·gy
pl oto·lar·yn·gol·o·gies

oto·lith

oto·lith·ic

oto·log·ic
also oto·log·i·cal

oto·log·i·cal·ly

otol·o·gist

otol·o·gy
pl otol·o·gies

oto·my·co·sis
pl oto·my·co·ses

oto·my·cot·ic
oto·neu·ro·log·i·cal
oto·neu·rol·o·gy
 pl oto·neu·rol·o·gies
oto·plas·ty
 pl oto·plas·ties
oto·rhi·no·lar·yn·
 go·log·i·cal
oto·rhi·no·lar·yn·
 gol·o·gist
oto·rhi·no·lar·yn·
 gol·o·gy
 pl oto·rhi·no·lar·yn·
 gol·o·gies
otor·rhea
oto·scle·ro·sis
 pl oto·scle·ro·ses
oto·scle·rot·ic
oto·scope
oto·scop·ic
otos·co·py
 pl otos·co·pies
oto·tox·ic
oto·tox·ic·i·ty
 pl oto·tox·ic·i·ties
oua·bain
ounce
out·bred
out·breed·ing
out·cross
out·cross·ing
out·growth
out·let
out·pa·tient
out·pock·et·ing
out·pouch·ing

ova
 pl of ovum
ov·al·bu·min
ova·le ma·lar·ia
ovalo·cyte
ovalo·cyt·ic
ovalo·cy·to·sis
 pl ovalo·cy·to·ses
ovar·i·an
 also ovar·i·al
ovari·ec·to·mize
 ovari·ec·to·
 mized
 ovari·ec·to·miz·
 ing
ovari·ec·to·my
 pl ovari·ec·to·mies
ovar·io·hys·ter·ec·
 to·my
 pl ovar·io·hys·ter·ec·
 to·mies
ovar·i·ot·o·my
 pl ovar·i·ot·o·mies
ova·ri·tis
 pl ova·rit·i·des
ova·ry
 pl ova·ries
over·ac·tive
over·ac·tiv·i·ty
 pl over·ac·tiv·i·ties
over·bite
over·breathe
 over·breathed
 over·breath·ing

over·com·pen·sate
over·com·pen·
 sat·ed
over·com·pen·
 sat·ing
over·com·pen·sa·
 tion
over·com·pen·sa·
 to·ry
over·cor·rect
over·cor·rec·tion
over·de·ter·mi·na·
 tion
over·de·ter·mined
over·dig·i·tal·iza·
 tion
over·dis·tend·ed
over·dis·ten·sion
 or over·dis·ten·tion
over·dom·i·nance
over·dom·i·nant
over·dos·age
over·dose
 over·dosed
 over·dos·ing
over·eat
 over·ate
 over·eat·en
 over·eat·ing
over·eat·er
over·ex·ert
over·ex·er·tion
over·ex·pose
 over·ex·posed
 over·ex·pos·
 ing
over·ex·po·sure

over·fa·tigue
over·grow
  over·grew
  over·grown
  over·grow·ing
over·growth
over·hang
over·hy·dra·tion
over·jet
over·med·i·cate
  over·med·i·cat·
    ed
  over·med·i·cat·
    ing
over·med·i·ca·
  tion
over·nu·tri·tion
over·pop·u·lat·ed
over·pop·u·la·tion
over·pre·scribe
  over·pre·scribed
  over·pre·scrib·
    ing
over·pre·scrip·
  tion
over·pro·duce
  over·pro·duced
  over·pro·duc·
    ing
over·pro·duc·tion
over·pro·tect
over·pro·tec·tion
over·pro·tec·tive
over·reach
over·se·da·tion
over·shoot
over·shot

over·stim·u·late
  over·stim·u·lat·
    ed
  over·stim·u·lat·
    ing
over·stim·u·la·tion
over-the-count·er
over·ven·ti·la·tion
over·weight
over·work
ovi·cid·al
ovi·du·cal
ovi·duct
ovi·duc·tal
ovi·gen·e·sis
  pl ovi·gen·e·ses
ovip·a·rous
ovi·pos·it
ovi·po·si·tion
ovi·po·si·tion·al
ovi·pos·i·tor
ovo·cyte
ovo·fla·vin
ovo·gen·e·sis
  pl ovo·gen·e·ses
ovoid
ovo·mu·cin
ovo·mu·coid
ovo·tes·tis
  pl ovo·tes·tes
ovo·vi·tel·lin
ovo·vi·vip·a·rous
ovu·lar
ovu·late
  ovu·lat·ed
  ovu·lat·ing
ovu·la·tion

ovu·la·to·ry
ovule
ovum
  pl ova
Ow·ren's dis·ease
ox·a·cil·lin
ox·a·late
  ox·a·lat·ed
  ox·a·lat·ing
ox·al·ic
ox·a·lo·ac·e·tate
  also ox·al·ac·e·tate
ox·a·lo·ace·tic
  also ox·al·ace·tic
ox·a·lo·sis
ox·a·lo·suc·cin·ic
ox·al·uria
ox·a·lyl·urea
ox·az·e·pam
ox·gall
ox·i·dant
ox·i·dase
ox·i·da·tion
ox·i·da·tion-re·duc·
  tion
ox·i·da·tive
ox·ide
ox·i·diz·able
ox·i·dize
  ox·i·dized
  ox·i·diz·ing
ox·i·do·re·duc·tase
ox·ime
ox·im·e·ter
ox·i·met·ric
ox·im·e·try
  pl ox·im·e·tries

ox·ine
ox·o·ni·um
oxo·phen·ar·sine
oxo·trem·o·rine
ox·pren·o·lol
ox·tri·phyl·line
oxy·cal·o·rim·e·ter
oxy·ce·phal·ic
oxy·ceph·a·ly
  pl oxy·ceph·a·lies
oxy·chro·ma·tin
oxy·co·done
ox·y·gen
ox·y·gen·ase
ox·y·gen·ate
  ox·y·gen·at·ed
  ox·y·gen·at·ing
ox·y·gen·ation
ox·y·gen·ator
ox·y·gen·ic
oxy·he·mo·glo·bin
oxy·he·mo·graph
ox·y·mel
oxy·myo·glo·bin
ox·yn·tic
oxy·phen·bu·ta·
  zone
oxy·phen·cy·cli·
  mine
oxy·phil
oxy·phile
oxy·phil·ic
oxy·quin·o·line
oxy·some
Oxy·spi·ru·ra
oxy·tet·ra·cy·cline

oxy·thi·a·mine
  also oxy·thi·a·min
oxy·to·cic
oxy·to·cin
oxy·uri·a·sis
  pl oxy·uri·a·ses
oxy·uric
oxy·uri·cide
oxy·urid
Oxy·uri·dae
oxy·uris
oze·na
ozo·ke·rite
  also ozo·ce·rite
ozone
ozo·nic
ozon·ide
ozon·iza·tion
ozon·ize
  ozon·ized
  ozon·iz·ing
ozon·iz·er
ozon·ol·y·sis
  pl ozon·ol·y·ses

P

pab·u·lum
pac·chi·o·ni·an
  body
pace·mak·er
pace·mak·ing
pac·er
pa·chom·e·ter
pachy·ce·pha·lia
pachy·ceph·a·ly
  pl pachy·ceph·a·lies

pachy·der·ma·tous
pachy·der·mia
pachy·der·mi·al
pachy·men·in·gi·
  tis
  pl pachy·men·in·git·i·
  des
pachy·me·ninx
  pl pachy·me·nin·ges
pachy·ne·ma
pachy·o·nych·ia
pachy·tene
pac·i·fi·er
Pa·cin·i·an cor·
  pus·cle
  also Pa·ci·ni's cor·
  pus·cle
pae·do·gen·e·sis
  also pe·do·gen·e·sis
  pl pae·do·gen·e·ses
  also pe·do·gen·e·ses
pae·do·ge·net·ic
  also pe·do·ge·net·ic
Pag·et's dis·ease
pa·go·pha·gia
pai·dol·o·gy
  pl pai·dol·o·gies
pain·ful
  pain·ful·ler
  pain·ful·lest
pain·kill·er
pain·kill·ing
paint·er's col·ic
pair-bond
pa·ja·ro·el·lo
pal·a·tal
pal·ate

pal·a·tine

pal·a·to·glos·sal

pal·a·to·glos·sus
pl pal·a·to·glos·si

pal·a·to·max·il·lary

pal·a·to·pha·ryn·geal

pal·a·to·pha·ryn·ge·us

pal·a·to·plas·ty
pl pal·a·to·plas·ties

pal·a·tos·chi·sis
pl pal·a·tos·chi·ses
also pal·a·tos·chi·sis·es

pa·le·en·ceph·a·lon
pl pa·le·en·ceph·a·la

pa·leo·cer·e·bel·lar

pa·leo·cer·e·bel·lum
pl pa·leo·cer·e·bel·lums
or pa·leo·cer·e·bel·la

pa·leo·cor·tex
pl pa·leo·cor·ti·ces
or pa·leo·cor·tex·es

pa·leo·pal·li·um
pl pa·leo·pal·lia
or pa·leo·pal·li·ums

pa·leo·pa·thol·o·gist

pa·leo·pa·thol·o·gy
pl pa·leo·pa·thol·o·gies

pa·leo·stri·a·tum
pl pa·leo·stri·a·ta

pali·la·lia

pal·in·drome

pal·in·dro·mic

pal·in·ge·net·ic

pal·i·sade worm

pal·la·di·um

pall·es·the·sia

pal·li·ate
pal·li·at·ed
pal·li·at·ing

pal·li·a·tion

pal·lia·tive

pal·li·dal

pal·li·do·fu·gal

pal·li·dot·o·my
pl pal·li·dot·o·mies

pal·li·dum

pal·li·um
pl pal·lia
or pal·li·ums

pal·lor

pal·mar

pal·mar·is
pl pal·mar·es

pal·mar·is brev·is

pal·mar·is lon·gus

pal·mi·tate

pal·mit·ic

pal·mi·tin

pal·mit·ole·ic

pal·pa·ble

pal·pate
pal·pat·ed
pal·pat·ing

pal·pa·tion
examination by touch
(see palpitation)

pal·pa·to·ry

pal·pe·bra
pl pal·pe·brae

pal·pe·bral

pal·pi·tate
pal·pi·tat·ed
pal·pi·tat·ing

pal·pi·ta·tion
rapid beating of the heart (see palpation)

pal·sied

pal·sy
pl pal·sies

pal·u·dism

pam·a·quine

pam·o·ate

pam·pin·i·form

pan·a·cea

pan·a·ce·an

pan·ag·glu·ti·na·bil·i·ty
pl pan·ag·glu·ti·na·bil·i·ties

pan·ag·glu·ti·na·ble

pan·ag·glu·ti·na·tion

pan·ar·ter·i·tis

pan·car·di·tis

Pan·coast's tu·mor
or Pan·coast tu·mor

pan·cre·as

pan·cre·atec·to·mized

pan·cre·atec·to·my
pl pan·cre·atec·to·mies

papular

pan·cre·at·ic
pan·cre·at·i·co·du·
o·de·nal
pan·cre·at·i·co·du·
o·de·nec·to·my
  pl pan·cre·at·i·co·du·
  o·de·nec·to·mies

pan·cre·at·i·co·du·
o·de·nos·to·my
  pl pan·cre·at·i·co·du·
  o·de·nos·to·mies

pan·cre·at·i·co·je·
ju·nos·to·my
  pl pan·cre·at·i·co·je·
  ju·nos·to·mies

pan·cre·atin
pan·cre·ati·tis
  pl pan·cre·atit·i·des

pan·cre·a·to·du·o·
de·nec·to·my
  pl pan·cre·a·to·du·o·
  de·nec·to·mies

pan·creo·zy·min
pan·cu·ro·ni·um
pan·cy·to·pe·nia
pan·cy·to·pe·nic
pan·dem·ic
Pan·dy's test
pan·en·ceph·a·li·tis
  pl pan·en·ceph·a·lit·i·
  des

pan·en·do·scope
pan·en·do·scop·ic
pan·en·dos·co·py
  pl pan·en·dos·co·pies

Pa·neth cell
pan·gen·e·sis
  pl pan·gen·e·ses

pan·ge·net·ic
pan·hy·po·pi·tu·ita·
rism
pan·hys·ter·ec·to·
my
  pl pan·hys·ter·ec·to·
  mies

pan·ic
pan·leu·ko·pe·nia
pan·mic·tic
pan·mix·ia
pan·mixy
  pl pan·mix·ies

pan·my·elop·a·thy
  pl pan·my·elop·a·
  thies

pan·my·elo·phthi·
sis
  pl pan·my·elo·phthi·
  ses

pan·nic·u·li·tis
pan·nic·u·lus
  pl pan·nic·u·li

pan·nic·u·lus car·
no·sus
pan·nus
  pl pan·ni

pano·pho·bia
pan·oph·thal·mi·tis
pan·sex·u·al·ism
pan·sex·u·al·i·ty
  pl pan·sex·u·al·i·ties

pan·sper·mia
Pan·stron·gy·lus
pan·sys·tol·ic
pan·te·the·ine
pan·to·graph

pan·to·the·nate
pan·to·then·ic
pan·trop·ic
pa·pa·in
pa·pa·in·ase
Pa·pa·ni·co·laou
  smear
Pa·pa·ver
pa·pav·er·ine
pa·pa·ya
pa·pil·la
  pl pa·pil·lae

pa·pil·la of Va·ter
pap·il·lary
pap·il·late
pap·il·lec·to·my
  pl pap·il·lec·to·mies

pap·il·le·de·ma
pa·pil·li·form
pap·il·li·tis
pap·il·lo·ma
  pl pap·il·lo·mas
  or pap·il·lo·ma·ta

pap·il·lo·ma·to·sis
  pl pap·il·lo·ma·to·ses

pap·il·lo·ma·vi·rus
pap·il·lose
pap·il·los·i·ty
  pl pap·il·los·i·ties

pa·po·va·vi·rus
pap·pa·ta·ci fe·ver
  also pa·pa·ta·ci fe·ver
  or pa·pa·ta·si fe·ver

Pap smear
pap·u·la
  pl pap·u·lae

pap·u·lar

pap·ule
pap·u·lo·ne·crot·ic
pap·u·lo·pus·tu·lar
pap·u·lo·sis
pap·u·lo·ve·sic·u·lar
pap·y·ra·ceous
para
  pl par·as
  or par·ae
para-ami·no·ben·zo·ic
para-ami·no·hip·pu·rate
para-ami·no·hip·pu·ric
para-ami·no·sal·i·cyl·ic
para-an·es·the·sia
para-aor·tic
par·a·ban·ic
para·bas·al
para·ben
para·bi·ont
para·bi·o·sis
  pl para·bi·o·ses
para·bi·ot·ic
para·bi·ot·i·cal·ly
para·blast
para·blas·tic
para·car·mine
para·ca·sein
Par·a·cel·sian
para·cen·te·sis
  pl para·cen·te·ses
para·cen·tral
para·cen·tric

par·ac·et·al·de·hyde
para·cet·a·mol
para·chlo·ro·phe·nol
para·chol·era
para·chord·al
para·co·lic
para·co·lon
para·cone
para·co·nid
par·acu·sic
par·acu·sis
  pl par·acu·ses
para·cys·ti·tis
  pl para·cys·tit·i·des
para·den·tal
para·den·tium
  pl para·den·tia
para·den·to·sis
  pl para·den·to·ses
para·did·y·mis
  pl para·did·y·mi·des
par·a·don·to·sis
  pl par·a·don·to·ses
par·a·dox·i·cal
  also par·a·dox·ic
para·esoph·a·ge·al
par·af·fin
par·af·fin·ic
par·af·fin·o·ma
  pl par·af·fin·o·mas
  or par·af·fin·o·ma·ta
para·fol·lic·u·lar
para·form
para·for·mal·de·hyde

para·fo·vea
  pl para·fo·ve·ae
para·fo·ve·al
para·fuch·sin
para·gan·gli·o·ma
  pl para·gan·gli·o·mas
  or para·gan·gli·o·ma·ta
para·gan·gli·on
  pl para·gan·glia
para·gan·gli·on·ic
par·ag·glu·ti·na·tion
par·a·gon·i·mi·a·sis
  pl par·a·gon·i·mi·a·ses
Par·a·gon·i·mus
para·gram·ma·tism
para·gran·u·lo·ma
  pl para·gran·u·lo·mas
  or para·gran·u·lo·ma·ta
para·graph·ia
para·he·mo·phil·ia
para·hor·mone
para·hy·droxy·ben·zo·ic
para·in·flu·en·za
para·ker·a·to·sis
  pl para·ker·a·to·ses
para·ker·a·tot·ic
par·al·de·hyde
par·al·lax
par·al·lel·om·e·ter
para·lo·gia
pa·ral·y·sis
  pl pa·ral·y·ses

parasitologist

par·a·lyt·ic
par·a·ly·zant
par·a·ly·za·tion
par·a·lyze
  par·a·lyzed
  par·a·lyz·ing
par·a·lyz·er
par·a·mag·net·ic
para·mag·ne·tism
para·mas·toid
par·a·me·cin
par·a·me·cium
  pl par·a·me·cia
  also par·a·me·ciums
para·me·di·an
para·med·ic
para·med·i·cal
para·me·so·neph·
  ric
para·metha·di·one
para·meth·a·sone
para·me·tri·al
para·me·tri·tis
para·me·tri·um
  pl para·me·tria
par·am·ne·sia
Par·a·moe·cium
para·mo·lar
para·mor·phine
par·am·phis·tome
*Par·am·phis·to·
  mum*
par·am·y·loid·osis
  pl par·am·y·loid·oses
para·my·oc·lo·nus
  mul·ti·plex
para·myo·to·nia

para·myxo·vi·rus
para·na·sal
para·neo·plas·tic
para·neph·ric
para·noia
para·noi·ac
  also para·no·ic
para·noid
  also para·noi·dal
para·nor·mal
para·pa·re·sis
  pl para·pa·re·ses
para·pa·ret·ic
para·pe·de·sis
  pl para·pe·de·ses
para·pha·ryn·geal
par·a·pha·sia
par·a·pha·sic
para·phen·yl·ene·
  di·amine
para·phil·ia
para·phil·iac
para·phi·mo·sis
  pl para·phi·mo·ses
para·phre·nia
para·phren·ic
pa·raph·y·se·al
  or par·a·phys·i·al
pa·raph·y·sis
  pl pa·raph·y·ses
para·ple·gia
para·ple·gic
para·prax·ia
para·prax·is
  pl para·prax·es
para·pro·fes·sion·
  al

para·pro·tein
para·pro·tein·emia
para·pso·ri·a·sis
  pl para·pso·ri·a·ses
para·psy·cho·log·i·
  cal
para·psy·chol·o·
  gist
para·psy·chol·o·gy
  pl para·psy·chol·o·
  gies
para·quat
para·rec·tus
para·re·nal
para·ros·an·i·line
para·sa·cral
para·sag·it·tal
Par·as·ca·ris
para·sex·u·al
para·sex·u·al·i·ty
  pl para·sex·u·al·i·ties
par·a·site
par·a·sit·emia
par·a·sit·ic
  also par·a·sit·i·cal
par·a·sit·i·ci·dal
par·a·sit·i·cide
par·a·sit·ism
par·a·sit·iza·tion
par·a·sit·ize
  par·a·sit·ized
  par·a·sit·iz·ing
par·a·sit·oid
Par·a·si·toi·dea
par·a·si·to·log·i·cal
  also par·a·si·to·log·ic
par·a·si·tol·o·gist

par·a·si·tol·o·gy
  pl par·a·si·tol·o·gies

par·a·sit·o·sis
  pl par·a·sit·o·ses

para·spe·cif·ic

para·spi·nal

para·ster·nal

para·sym·pa·thet·ic

para·sym·pa·thet·i·co·mi·met·ic

para·sym·pa·tho·lyt·ic

para·sym·pa·tho·mi·met·ic

para·syn·ap·sis
  pl para·syn·ap·ses

para·syn·ap·tic

para·syph·i·lis

para·syph·i·lit·ic

para·sys·to·le

para·tax·ic

para·tax·is
  pl para·tax·es

para·ten·on

para·thi·on

par·a·thor·mone

para·thy·roid

para·thy·roid·ec·to·mized

para·thy·roid·ec·to·my
  pl para·thy·roid·ec·to·mies

para·thy·ro·pri·val
  or para·thy·ro·priv·ic

para·thy·ro·trop·ic

para·tra·che·al

para·tu·ber·cu·lo·sis
  pl para·tu·ber·cu·lo·ses

para·tu·ber·cu·lous

para·ty·phoid

para·ure·thral

para·vac·cin·ia

para·vag·i·nal

para·ven·tric·u·lar

para·ver·te·bral

par·ax·i·al

par·e·go·ric

pa·ren·chy·ma

pa·ren·chy·mal

par·en·chy·ma·tous

par·en·ter·al

par·er·ga·sia

pa·re·sis
  pl pa·re·ses

par·es·the·sia

par·es·thet·ic

pa·ret·ic

par·fo·cal

par·fo·cal·i·ty
  pl par·fo·cal·i·ties

par·gy·line

par·i·es
  pl pa·ri·etes

pa·ri·etal

pa·ri·e·to·mas·toid

pa·ri·e·to·oc·cip·i·tal

pa·ri·e·to·tem·po·ral

Par·i·naud's oc·u·lo·glan·du·lar syn·drome

Par·i·naud's syn·drome

Par·is green

par·i·ty
  pl par·i·ties

Par·ker's flu·id

par·kin·so·nian

par·kin·son·ism

Par·kin·son's dis·ease

par·odon·tal

pa·rol·able

pa·role
  pa·roled
  pa·rol·ing

par·ol·fac·to·ry

par·o·mo·my·cin

par·o·nych·ia

par·ooph·o·ron

par·os·mia

pa·rot·ic

pa·rot·id

par·o·tit·ic

par·o·ti·tis

par·ous

par·o·var·i·an

par·o·var·i·um

par·ox·ysm

par·ox·ys·mal

pars
  pl par·tes

pars com·pac·ta

pars dis·ta·lis

pars in·ter·me·dia

pars irid·i·ca ret·i·
nae
pars ner·vo·sa
pars tu·ber·a·lis
par·tes
pl of pars
par·the·no·gen·e·
sis
pl par·the·no·gen·e·
ses
par·the·no·ge·net·
ic
also par·the·no·gen·ic
par·the·no·ge·net·i·
cal·ly
par·tial den·ture
par·tial·ism
par·ti·cle
par·tic·u·late
par·tu·ri·ent
par·tu·ri·tion
pa·ru·lis
pl pa·ru·li·des
par·um·bil·i·cal
par·vo
par·vo·cel·lu·lar
also par·vi·cel·lu·lar
par·vo·vi·rus
par·vule
Pas·cal's law
pasque·flow·er
pas·sage
pas·saged
pas·sag·ing
pas·sive
pas·siv·i·ty
pl pas·siv·i·ties

pas·tern
Pas·teur ef·fect
pas·teu·rel·la
pl pas·teu·rel·las
or pas·teu·rel·lae
pas·teu·rel·lo·sis
pl pas·teu·rel·lo·ses
pas·teur·iza·tion
pas·teur·ize
pas·teur·ized
pas·teur·iz·ing
pas·teur·iz·er
pas·tille
also pas·til
past-point
pa·tel·la
pl pa·tel·lae
or pa·tel·las
pa·tel·lar
pat·el·lec·to·my
pl pat·el·lec·to·mies
pa·tel·lo·fem·o·ral
pa·ten·cy
pl pa·ten·cies
pa·tent
pa·tent med·i·cine
pa·ter·ni·ty
path·er·gy
pl path·er·gies
patho·bi·ol·o·gy
pl patho·bi·ol·o·gies
patho·gen
patho·gen·e·sis
pl patho·gen·e·ses
patho·ge·net·ic
patho·gen·ic
pa·tho·gen·i·cal·ly

patho·ge·nic·i·ty
pl patho·ge·nic·i·ties
path·og·nom·ic
pa·tho·gno·mon·ic
patho·log·i·cal
also patho·log·ic
patho·log·i·cal·ly
pa·thol·o·gist
pa·thol·o·gy
pl pa·thol·o·gies
patho·mor·pho·log·
i·cal
or patho·mor·pho·log·
ic
patho·mor·phol·o·
gy
pl patho·mor·phol·o·
gies
patho·phys·i·o·log·
i·cal
also patho·phys·i·o·
log·ic
patho·phys·i·ol·o·
gy
pl patho·phys·i·ol·o·
gies
pa·tho·sis
pl pa·tho·ses
path·way
pa·tient
pat·ro·cli·nous
pat·ro·cli·ny
pl pat·ro·cli·nies
pat·tern·ing
pat·u·lin
pat·u·lous
Paul-Bun·nell test

paunch
pa·vil·ion
Pav·lov·ian
Pav·lov pouch
pav·or noc·tur·nus
pea·nut oil
peck·ing or·der
  also peck or·der
pec·tase
pec·ten
  pl pec·ti·nes
pec·te·no·sis
  pl pec·te·no·ses
  or pec·te·no·sis·es
pec·tic
pec·tin
pec·tin·ase
pec·tin·e·al
pec·tin·es·ter·ase
pec·tin·e·us
  pl pec·tin·ei
pec·tin·ic
pec·tin·i·form
pec·ti·no·lyt·ic
pec·to·lyt·ic
pec·to·ral
pec·to·ra·lis
  pl pec·to·ra·les
pec·to·ril·o·quy
  pl pec·to·ril·o·quies
pec·tose
pec·tus ex·ca·va·
  tum
ped·al
ped·er·ast`
ped·er·as·tic

ped·er·as·ty
  pl ped·er·as·ties
pe·des
  pl of pes
pe·di·at·ric
pe·di·a·tri·cian
pe·di·at·rics
pe·di·a·trist
ped·i·cle
ped·i·cled
pe·dic·u·li·cid·al
pe·dic·u·li·cide
Ped·i·cu·li·dae
Pe·dic·u·loi·des
pe·dic·u·lo·sis
  pl pe·dic·u·lo·ses
pe·dic·u·lo·sis cap·
  i·tis
pe·dic·u·lo·sis cor·
  po·ris
pe·dic·u·lo·sis pu·
  bis
pe·dic·u·lus
  pl pe·dic·u·li
  or pe·dic·u·lus
ped·i·cure
ped·i·gree
Ped·i·lan·thus
pe·do·don·tia
pe·do·don·tics
pe·do·don·tist
pe·do·phile
pe·do·phil·ia
pe·do·phil·i·ac
pe·do·phil·ic
pe·dun·cle
pe·dun·cu·lar

pe·dun·cu·lat·ed
  also pe·dun·cu·late
pe·dun·cu·lot·o·my
  pl pe·dun·cu·lot·o·
  mies
pe·dun·cu·lus ce·
  re·bel·la·ris in·
  fe·ri·or
pe·li·o·sis hep·a·ti·
  tis
pel·la·gra
pel·la·gra·gen·ic
pel·la·grin
pel·la·grous
pel·let
pel·le·tier·ine
pel·li·cle
pel·lic·u·lar
pel·oid
pel·ta·tin
pel·ves
  pl of pelvis
pel·vic
pel·vim·e·ter
pel·vi·met·ric
pel·vim·e·try
  pl pel·vim·e·tries
pel·vio·li·thot·o·my
  pl pel·vio·li·thot·o·
  mies
pel·vis
  pl pel·vis·es
  or pel·ves
pel·vi·scope
pem·o·line
pem·phi·goid

perceived

pem·phi·gus
  pl pem·phi·gus·es
  or pem·phi·gi

pem·phi·gus er·y·
  the·ma·to·sus

pem·phi·gus fo·li·
  a·ce·us

pem·phi·gus vul·
  gar·is

pen·du·lar

pe·nes
  pl of penis

pen·e·trance

pen·e·trate
  pen·e·trat·ed
  pen·e·trat·ing

pen·e·tra·tion

pen·flur·i·dol

pen·i·cil·la·mine

pen·i·cil·lic

pen·i·cil·lin

pen·i·cil·lin·ase

pen·i·cil·li·o·sis
  pl pen·i·cil·li·o·ses

pen·i·cil·li·um
  pl pen·i·cil·lia

pen·i·cil·lo·ic

pen·i·cil·lo·yl·poly·
  ly·sine

pen·i·cil·lus
  pl pen·i·cil·li

pe·nile

pe·nis
  pl pe·nes
  or pe·nis·es

pen·nate

pen·ni·form

pen·ny·roy·al

pen·ny·weight

pe·no·scro·tal

Pen·rose drain

pen·ta·chlo·ro·phe·
  nol

pen·ta·eryth·ri·tol

pen·ta·eryth·ri·tol
  te·tra·ni·trate

pen·ta·gas·trin

pen·tal·o·gy
  pl pen·tal·o·gies

pen·ta·mer

pen·ta·me·tho·ni·
  um

pent·am·i·dine

pen·tane

pen·ta·pep·tide

pen·ta·pip·eride
  meth·yl·sul·fate

pen·ta·ploid

pen·ta·ploi·dy
  pl pen·ta·ploi·dies

pen·ta·quine
  also pen·ta·quin

pen·tas·to·mid

Pen·ta·stom·i·da

pen·ta·tom·ic

pen·ta·va·lent

pen·taz·o·cine

pen·tene

pen·to·bar·bi·tal

pen·to·bar·bi·tone

pen·to·lin·i·um

pen·to·san

pen·tose

pen·to·side

pen·tos·uria

pen·tyl·ene·tet·ra·
  zol

pe·po
  pl pe·pos

pep·per

pep·per·mint

pep·per·minty

pep·sin

pep·sin·o·gen

pep·tic

pep·ti·dase

pep·tide

pep·tid·er·gic

pep·tid·ic

pep·ti·do·gly·can

pep·ti·za·tion

pep·tize
  pep·tized
  pep·tiz·ing

pep·tiz·er

pep·to·coc·cus
  pl pep·to·coc·ci

pep·tone

pep·to·niz·a·tion

pep·to·nize
  pep·to·nized
  pep·to·niz·ing

per·ace·tic

per·ac·id

per·acute

per·bo·rate

per·ceiv·able

per·ceiv·ably

per·ceive
  per·ceived
  per·ceiv·ing

per·ceiv·er
per·cen·tile
per·cept
per·cep·ti·bil·i·ty
  pl per·cep·ti·bil·i·ties
per·cep·ti·ble
per·cep·ti·bly
per·cep·tion
per·cep·tive
per·cep·tiv·i·ty
  pl per·cep·tiv·i·ties
per·cep·tu·al
per·chlo·rate
per·chlo·ric
per·chlo·ride
per·chlo·ro·eth·y·
  lene
  also per·chlor·eth·y·
  lene
per·co·late
  per·co·lat·ed
  per·co·lat·ing
per·co·la·tion
per·co·la·tor
per·co·morph
per·cuss
per·cus·sion
per·cu·ta·ne·ous
per·fec·tion·ism
per·fec·tion·ist
per·fec·tion·is·tic
per·fo·rate
  per·fo·rat·ed
  per·fo·rat·ing
per·fo·ra·tion
per·fo·ra·tor

per·fo·ra·to·ri·um
  pl per·fo·ra·to·ria
per·fus·ate
per·fuse
  per·fused
  per·fus·ing
per·fu·sion
per·hex·i·lene
peri·ad·e·ni·tis
peri·anal
peri·aor·tic
  also peri·aor·tal
peri·api·cal
peri·aq·ue·duc·tal
peri·ar·te·ri·al
peri·ar·te·ri·o·lar
peri·ar·ter·i·tis no·
  do·sa
peri·ar·thri·tis
  pl peri·ar·thrit·i·des
peri·ar·tic·u·lar
peri·bron·chi·al
peri·bron·chi·o·lar
peri·cap·il·lary
peri·car·di·al
peri·car·di·ec·to·
  my
  pl peri·car·di·ec·to·
  mies
peri·car·dio·cen·te·
  sis
  pl peri·car·dio·cen·te·
  ses
peri·car·dio·phren·
  ic

peri·car·di·os·to·
  my
  pl peri·car·di·os·to·
  mies
peri·car·di·ot·o·my
  pl peri·car·di·ot·o·
  mies
peri·car·dit·ic
peri·car·di·tis
  pl peri·car·dit·i·des
peri·car·di·um
  pl peri·car·dia
peri·cary·on
  var of perikaryon
peri·cel·lu·lar
peri·ce·men·ti·tis
peri·cen·tric
peri·chon·dral
peri·chon·dri·al
peri·chon·dri·um
  pl peri·chon·dria
peri·chord
peri·chord·al
peri·co·ro·nal
peri·cor·o·ni·tis
  pl peri·cor·o·ni·tis·i·des
peri·cra·ni·al
peri·cra·ni·um
  pl peri·cra·nia
peri·cyst
peri·cys·tic
peri·cyte
peri·den·tal
peri·derm
peri·du·ral
peri·en·ter·ic
peri·fo·cal

peri·fol·lic·u·lar
peri·gan·gli·on·ic
peri·hep·a·ti·tis
 pl peri·hep·a·tit·i·des

peri·kary·al
peri·kary·on
 also peri·cary·on
 pl peri·karya
 also peri·carya

peri·lymph
peri·lym·phat·ic
pe·rim·e·ter
peri·met·ric
peri·me·tri·um
 pl peri·me·tria

pe·rim·e·try
 pl pe·rim·e·tries

peri·my·si·al
peri·my·si·um
 pl peri·my·sia

per·i·nae·um
 var of perineum

peri·na·tal
peri·na·tol·o·gist
peri·na·tol·o·gy
 pl peri·na·tol·o·gies

per·i·ne·al
 relating to the peri-
 neum (see perito-
 neal, peroneal)

per·i·ne·or·rha·phy
 pl per·i·ne·or·rha·
 phies

peri·neph·ric
peri·ne·phri·tis
 pl peri·ne·phrit·i·des

peri·neph·ri·um
 pl peri·neph·ria

per·i·ne·um
 also per·i·nae·um
 pl per·i·nea
 also per·i·naea
 area of tissue mark-
 ing the pelvic outlet
 (see perineurium,
 peritoneum)

peri·neu·ral
peri·neu·ri·al
peri·neu·ri·um
 pl peri·neu·ria
 nerve sheath of con-
 nective tissue (see
 perineum, perito-
 neum)

peri·nu·cle·ar
pe·ri·od
per·io·date
pe·ri·od·ic
per·iod·ic acid-
 Schiff
pe·ri·od·ic·i·ty
 pl pe·ri·od·ic·i·ties

peri·odon·tal
peri·odon·tia
peri·odon·tics
peri·odon·tist
peri·odon·ti·tis
peri·odon·ti·tis
 sim·plex
peri·odon·tium
 pl peri·odon·tia

peri·odon·to·cla·sia
peri·odon·tol·o·gist
peri·odon·tol·o·gy
 pl peri·odon·tol·o·gies

peri·odon·to·sis
 pl peri·odon·to·ses

peri·onych·i·um
 pl peri·onych·ia

peri·on·yx
peri·op·er·a·tive
peri·or·bit·al
peri·os·te·al
peri·os·te·um
 pl peri·os·tea

peri·os·ti·tis
peri·otic
peri·pha·ryn·geal
pe·riph·er·al
pe·riph·ery
 pl pe·riph·er·ies

peri·phle·bi·tis
 pl peri·phle·bit·i·des

Peri·pla·ne·ta
peri·plas·mic
peri·por·tal
peri·rec·tal
peri·re·nal
peri·scop·ic
peri·sple·ni·tis
pe·ris·so·dac·tyl
Pe·ris·so·dac·tyla
peri·stal·sis
 pl peri·stal·ses

peri·stal·tic
peri·ten·di·ni·tis
peri·the·li·al
peri·the·li·o·ma
 pl peri·the·li·o·mas
 or peri·the·li·o·ma·ta

peri·the·li·um
 pl peri·the·lia

peri·to·ne·al
relating to the peritoneum (see perineal, peroneal)

peri·to·neo·cen·te·sis
pl peri·to·neo·cen·te·ses

peri·to·neo·scope
peri·to·neo·scop·ic
peri·to·ne·os·co·py
pl peri·to·ne·os·co·pies

peri·to·neo·ve·nous
peri·to·ne·um
pl peri·to·ne·ums
or peri·to·nea
membrane lining the abdominal cavity (see perineum, perineurium)

peri·to·ni·tis
peri·to·nize
peri·to·nized
peri·to·niz·ing
peri·ton·sil·lar
peri·tra·che·al
peri·trich·ic
pe·rit·ri·chous
peri·tu·bu·lar
peri·um·bi·li·cal
peri·un·gual
peri·ure·thral
peri·vas·cu·lar
situated around a blood vessel (see perivisceral)

peri·ve·nous
peri·ven·tric·u·lar

peri·vis·cer·al
situated around the viscera (see perivascular)

peri·vi·tel·line
per·i·win·kle
perle
per·lèche
per·man·ga·nate
per·man·gan·ic
per·me·abil·i·ty
pl per·me·abil·i·ties

per·me·able
per·me·ant
per·me·ase
per·me·ate
per·me·at·ed
per·me·at·ing
per·me·ation
per·mis·sive
per·ni·cious
per·nio
pl per·ni·o·nes

pe·ro·ne·al
relating to the fibula (see perineal, peritoneal)

per·o·ne·us
pl per·o·nei

per·o·ne·us brev·is
per·o·ne·us lon·gus
per·o·ne·us ter·ti·us
per·oral
per os
pe·ro·sis
pl pe·ro·ses

pe·rot·ic
per·ox·i·dase
per·ox·i·dat·ic
per·ox·i·da·tion
per·ox·ide
per·ox·i·som·al
per·ox·i·some
per·oxy
per·phen·a·zine
per pri·mam
per rec·tum
per·salt
per·se·cu·tion com·plex
per·se·cu·to·ry
per·sev·er·ate
per·sev·er·at·ed
per·sev·er·at·ing
per·sev·er·a·tion
per·sev·er·a·tive
per·sic
per·sis·tent
per·so·na
pl per·so·nas

per·son·al·i·ty
pl per·son·al·i·ties

per·spi·ra·tion
per·spi·ra·to·ry
per·spire
per·spired
per·spir·ing
per·sua·sion
per·sul·fate
per·sul·fu·ric
per·tus·sal
per·tus·sis
Peru bal·sam

pharmaceutical

Pe·ru·vi·an bal·
sam
per·vap·o·ra·tion
per·ver·sion
per·vert
pes
  pl pe·des
pes an·se·ri·nus
pes ca·vus
pes hip·po·cam·pi
pes·sa·ry
  pl pes·sa·ries
pes·si·mism
pes·si·mis·tic
pes·ti·cide
pes·tif·er·ous
pes·ti·lence
pes·ti·len·tial
pes·tle
pe·te·chia
  pl pe·te·chi·ae
pe·te·chi·al
pe·te·chi·a·tion
peth·i·dine
pe·tit mal
pe·tri dish
pet·ri·fac·tion
pet·ri·fi·ca·tion
pet·ri·fy
  pet·ri·fied
  pet·ri·fy·ing
pe·tris·sage
pet·ro·la·tum
pe·tro·leum
pe·tro·leum ben·
zin
pe·tro·sal

pe·tro·si·tis
pe·tro·tym·pan·ic
pe·trous
pe·trox·o·lin
Pey·er's patch
pey·o·te
  also pey·otl
Pey·ro·nie's dis·
ease
Pfan·nen·stiel's in·
ci·sion
Pfeif·fer·el·la
Pfeif·fer's ba·cil·
lus
phaco·emul·si·fi·
ca·tion
  also phako·emul·si·fi·
ca·tion
phage
phag·e·de·na
  also phag·e·dae·na
phag·e·de·nic
  also phag·e·dae·nic
phago·cyt·able
phago·cyte
  phago·cyt·ed
  phago·cyt·ing
phago·cyt·ic
phago·cy·tize
  phago·cy·tized
  phago·cy·tiz·ing
phago·cy·tos·able
phago·cy·tose
  phago·cy·tosed
  phago·cy·tos·ing
phago·cy·to·sis
  pl phago·cy·to·ses

phago·cy·tot·ic
phago·some
phako·emul·si·fi·
ca·tion
  var of phacoemulsifi-
cation
phal·a·cro·sis
  pl phal·a·cro·ses
pha·lan·ge·al
  relating to the phalanx
  (see pharyngeal)
pha·lan·gec·to·my
  pl pha·lan·gec·to·
mies
pha·lanx
  pl pha·lan·ges
phal·li
  pl of phallus
phal·lic
phal·li·cism
phal·loid
phal·loi·din
  also phal·loi·dine
phal·lus
  pl phal·li
  or phal·lus·es
phan·er·o·gen·ic
phan·er·o·sis
  pl phan·er·o·ses
phan·ero·zo·ite
phan·ero·zo·it·ic
phan·ta·sy
  var of fantasy
phan·tom
  also fan·tom
phar·ma·ceu·ti·cal
  also phar·ma·ceu·tic

phar·ma·ceu·tics

phar·ma·cist

phar·ma·co·dy·nam·ic

phar·ma·co·dy·nam·i·cal·ly

phar·ma·co·dy·nam·ics

phar·ma·co·ge·net·ics

phar·ma·cog·no·sist

phar·ma·cog·nos·tic
or phar·ma·cog·nos·ti·cal

phar·ma·cog·no·sy
pl phar·ma·cog·no·sies

phar·ma·co·ki·net·ics

phar·ma·co·log·i·cal
also phar·ma·co·log·ic

phar·ma·col·o·gist

phar·ma·col·o·gy
pl phar·ma·col·o·gies

phar·ma·co·poe·ia
or phar·ma·co·pe·ia

phar·ma·co·poe·ial
or phar·ma·co·pe·ial

phar·ma·co·ther·a·peu·tic
also phar·ma·co·ther·a·peu·ti·cal

phar·ma·co·ther·a·peu·tics

phar·ma·co·ther·a·py
pl phar·ma·co·ther·a·pies

phar·ma·cy
pl phar·ma·cies

pha·ryn·geal
relating to the pharynx
(see phalangeal*)*

phar·yn·gec·to·my
pl phar·yn·gec·to·mies

phar·yn·gi·tis
pl phar·yn·git·i·des

pha·ryn·go·esoph·a·ge·al

pha·ryn·go·pal·a·tine

pha·ryn·go·pal·a·ti·nus
pl pha·ryn·go·pal·a·ti·ni

pha·ryn·go·plas·ty
pl pha·ryn·go·plas·ties

phar·yn·gos·to·my
pl phar·yn·gos·to·mies

pha·ryn·go·ton·sil·li·tis

pha·ryn·go·tym·pan·ic

phar·ynx
pl pha·ryn·ges
also phar·ynx·es
part of the alimentary canal (see lar·ynx*)*

phase-con·trast

pha·sic

pha·si·cal·ly

phas·mid

Phas·mid·ia

phas·mid·ian

phe·na·caine

phen·ac·e·tin

phen·ace·tu·ric

phen·an·threne

phe·naz·o·cine

phen·a·zone

phen·cy·cli·dine

phen·el·zine

phe·neth·i·cil·lin

phen·eth·yl

phe·net·i·dine
also phe·net·i·din

phen·for·min

phen·in·di·one

phen·ir·amine

phen·met·ra·zine

phe·no·bar·bi·tal

phe·no·bar·bi·tone

phe·no·copy
pl phe·no·cop·ies

phe·nol

phe·no·lase

phe·no·late

phe·no·lat·ed

phe·no·lic

phe·nol·phtha·lein

phe·nol·sul·fon·phtha·lein

phe·nol·tet·ra·io·do·phtha·lein

phe·nom·e·no·log·i·cal

phe.nom.e.nol.o.gy
pl phe.nom.e.nol.o.gies

phe.no.thi.azine

phe.no.type

phe.no.typ.ic
also phe.no.typ.i.cal

phen.ox.ide

phe.noxy

phe.noxy.ace.tic

phe.noxy.ben.za.mine

phe.noxy.meth.yl

phen.sux.i.mide

phen.ter.mine

phen.tet.io.tha.lein

phen.tol.amine

phe.nyl

phe.nyl.acet.amide

phe.nyl.ace.tic

phe.nyl.al.a.nine

phen.yl.bu.ta.zone

phen.yl.ene

phen.yl.eph.rine

phe.nyl.eth.yl

phe.nyl.eth.yl.amine

phe.nyl.eth.y.lene

phe.nyl.hy.dra.zine

phe.nyl.ic

phe.nyl.ke.ton.uria

phe.nyl.ke.ton.uric

phen.yl.mer.cu.ric

phen.yl.pro.pa.nol.amine

phe.nyl.py.ru.vate

phe.nyl.py.ru.vic

phen.yl.thio.car.ba.mide

phen.yl.thio.urea

phe.nyt.o.in

pheo.chrome

pheo.chro.mo.blast

pheo.chro.mo.cyte

pheo.chro.mo.cy.to.ma
pl pheo.chro.mo.cy.to.mas
or pheo.chro.mo.cy.to.ma.ta

pheo.phor.bide

pheo.phy.tin

phe.ren.ta.sin

phe.re.sis
pl phe.re.ses

pher.o.mon.al

pher.o.mone

phi.al

Phi.a.loph.o.ra

phil.ter

phil.trum
pl phil.tra

phi.mo.sis
pl phi.mo.ses

phi phe.nom.e.non

phleb.ec.ta.sia

phle.bit.ic

phle.bi.tis
pl phle.bit.i.des

phle.bo.cly.sis
pl phle.bo.cly.ses

phle.bo.gram

phle.bo.graph

phle.bo.graph.ic

phle.bog.ra.phy
pl phle.bog.ra.phies

phle.bo.lith

phle.bol.o.gy
pl phle.bol.o.gies

phle.bor.rha.phy
pl phle.bor.rha.phies

phle.bo.scle.ro.sis
pl phle.bo.scle.ro.ses

phle.bo.scle.rot.ic

phle.bo.throm.bo.sis
pl phle.bo.throm.bo.ses

phle.bot.o.mist

phle.bot.o.mize
phle.bot.o.mized
phle.bot.o.miz.ing

phle.bot.o.mus
pl phle.bot.o.mi
also phle.bot.o.mus.es

phle.bot.o.my
pl phle.bot.o.mies

phlegm

phleg.ma.sia al.ba do.lens

phleg.ma.sia ce.ru.lea do.lens

phleg·mat·ic
phleg·mat·i·cal·ly
phleg·mon
phleg·mon·ous
phlo·gis·tic
phlog·o·gen·ic
  also phlo·gog·e·nous

phlor·e·tin
phlo·ri·zin
  or phlo·rhi·zin
  or phlo·rid·zin
phlo·ri·zin·ized
  also phlo·rhi·zin·ized
  or phlo·rid·zin·ized

phlor·o·glu·cin·ol
phlox·ine
phlyc·ten·u·lar
phlyc·te·nule
pho·bia
pho·bic
pho·bo·pho·bia
pho·co·me·lia
pho·co·me·lic
pho·com·e·lus
  pl pho·com·e·li

phon
pho·nate
  pho·nat·ed
  pho·nat·ing
pho·na·tion
pho·na·to·ry
pho·neme
pho·ne·mic
pho·ne·mi·cal·ly
pho·nen·do·scope
pho·net·ic
pho·net·i·cal·ly

pho·net·ics
pho·ni·at·rics
pho·ni·a·try
  pl pho·ni·a·tries

pho·nic
pho·ni·cal·ly
pho·nics
pho·no·car·dio·
  gram
pho·no·car·dio·
  graph
pho·no·car·dio·
  graph·ic
pho·no·car·di·og·
  ra·phy
  pl pho·no·car·di·og·
  ra·phies

pho·no·log·i·cal
  also pho·no·log·ic

pho·nol·o·gy
  pl pho·nol·o·gies

phor·bol
pho·ria
Phor·mia
pho·rom·e·ter
phos·gene
phos·pha·gen
phos·pha·tase
phos·phate
phos·pha·tide
phos·pha·tid·ic
phos·pha·ti·dyl·
  cho·line
phos·pha·ti·dyl·
  eth·a·nol·amine
phos·pha·ti·dyl·ser·
  ine

phos·pha·tu·ria
phos·phene
phos·phide
phos·phine
phos·phite
phos·pho·ar·gi·
  nine
phos·pho·cre·atine
phos·pho·di·es·ter·
  ase
phos·pho·enol·py·
  ru·vate
phos·pho·enol·py·
  ru·vic
phos·pho·fruc·to·
  ki·nase
phos·pho·glu·co·
  mu·tase
phos·pho·glu·co·
  nate
phos·pho·glyc·er·
  al·de·hyde
phos·pho·glyc·er·
  ate
phos·pho·gly·cer·ic
phos·pho·hexo·
  isom·er·ase
phos·pho·ino·si·
  tide
phos·pho·ki·nase
phos·pho·li·pase
phos·pho·lip·id
  also phos·pho·lip·ide

phos·pho·mono·es·
  ter·ase

phos·pho·ne·cro·
sis
pl phos·pho·ne·cro·
ses

phos·pho·ni·um
phos·pho·pro·tein
phos·pho·py·ru·
vate
phos·phor
also phos·phore

phos·pho·res·cence
phos·pho·res·cent
phos·pho·ri·bo·syl·
py·ro·phos·phate
phos·pho·ri·bo·syl·
trans·fer·ase
phos·pho·ric
phos·pho·rized
phos·pho·rol·y·sis
pl phos·pho·rol·y·ses

phos·pho·ro·lyt·ic
phos·pho·rous
adjective (see phospho-
rus)

phos·pho·rus
noun (see phospho-
rous)

phos·pho·ryl
phos·phor·y·lase
phos·phor·y·late
phos·phor·y·lat·
ed
phos·phor·y·lat·
ing
phos·phor·y·la·tion
phos·phor·y·la·tive

phos·pho·ryl·cho·
line
phos·pho·trans·fer·
ase
phos·pho·tung·
state
phos·pho·tung·stic
phos·sy jaw
phos·vi·tin
pho·tic
pho·ti·cal·ly
pho·tism
pho·to·al·ler·gic
pho·to·al·ler·gy
pl pho·to·al·ler·gies

pho·to·bi·o·log·i·
cal
also pho·to·bi·o·log·ic

pho·to·bi·ol·o·gist
pho·to·bi·ol·o·gy
pl pho·to·bi·ol·o·gies

pho·to·ca·tal·y·sis
pl pho·to·ca·tal·y·ses

pho·to·cat·a·lyst
pho·to·cat·a·lyze
pho·to·cat·a·
lyzed
pho·to·cat·a·lyz·
ing
pho·to·chem·i·cal
pho·to·chem·is·try
pl pho·to·chem·is·
tries

pho·to·che·mo·
ther·a·py
pl pho·to·che·mo·
ther·a·pies

pho·to·chro·mic
pho·to·chro·mism
pho·to·chro·mo·
gen
pho·to·chro·mo·
gen·ic
pho·to·chro·mo·ge·
nic·i·ty
pl pho·to·chro·mo·ge·
nic·i·ties

pho·to·co·ag·u·la·
tion
pho·to·co·ag·u·la·
tor
pho·to·con·vul·sive
pho·to·de·com·po·
si·tion
pho·to·der·ma·ti·tis
pl pho·to·der·ma·ti·
tis·es
or pho·to·der·ma·tit·i·
des

pho·to·der·ma·to·
sis
pl pho·to·der·ma·to·
ses

pho·to·dy·nam·ic
pho·to·dy·nam·i·
cal·ly
pho·to·elec·tric
pho·to·elec·tri·cal·
ly
pho·to·elec·tric·i·ty
pl pho·to·elec·tric·i·
ties

pho·to·flu·o·ro·
gram

pho·to·fluo·o·ro·
 graph·ic
pho·to·fluo·o·rog·ra·
 phy
 pl pho·to·flu·o·rog·ra·
 phies
pho·to·gen·ic
pho·to·in·ac·ti·va·
 tion
pho·to·ki·ne·sis
 pl pho·to·ki·ne·ses
pho·to·ki·net·ic
pho·to·ky·mo·
 graph
pho·to·ky·mo·
 graph·ic
pho·to·lu·mi·nes·
 cence
pho·to·lu·mi·nes·
 cent
pho·tol·y·sis
 pl pho·tol·y·ses
pho·to·lyt·ic
pho·to·lyt·i·cal·ly
pho·to·lyz·able
pho·to·lyze
 pho·to·lyzed
 pho·to·lyz·ing
pho·to·mac·ro·
 graph
pho·to·mac·ro·
 graph·ic
pho·to·mac·rog·ra·
 phy
 pl pho·to·mac·rog·ra·
 phies
pho·tom·e·ter

pho·to·met·ric
pho·to·met·ri·cal·ly
pho·tom·e·try
 pl pho·tom·e·tries
pho·to·mi·cro·
 graph
pho·to·mi·crog·ra·
 pher
pho·to·mi·cro·
 graph·ic
pho·to·mi·cro·
 graph·i·cal·ly
pho·to·mi·crog·ra·
 phy
 pl pho·to·mi·crog·ra·
 phies
pho·to·mi·cro·
 scope
pho·to·mul·ti·pli·er
pho·ton
pho·ton·ic
pho·to·ox·i·da·tion
pho·to·ox·i·da·tive
pho·to·ox·i·dize
 pho·to·ox·i·dized
 pho·to·ox·i·diz·
 ing
pho·to·patch test
pho·to·pe·ri·od
pho·to·pe·ri·od·ic
pho·to·pe·ri·od·i·
 cal·ly
pho·to·pe·ri·od·ic·i·
 ty
 pl pho·to·pe·ri·od·ic·
 i·ties
pho·to·pe·ri·od·ism

pho·to·phil·ic
 or pho·toph·i·lous
 also pho·to·phile

pho·to·pho·bia
pho·to·pho·bic
pho·to·phos·phor·
 y·la·tion
phot·oph·thal·mia
phot·opic
pho·to·pig·ment
pho·to·pro·duc·
 tion
pho·top·sia
pho·to·re·ac·tion
pho·to·re·ac·ti·vat·
 ing
pho·to·re·ac·ti·va·
 tion
pho·to·re·cep·tion
pho·to·re·cep·tive
pho·to·re·cep·tor
pho·to·roent·gen
 or pho·to·roent·gen·o·
 graph·ic

pho·to·roent·gen·o·
 gram
pho·to·scan
 pho·to·scanned
 pho·to·scan·ning
pho·to·scan·ner
pho·to·scope
pho·to·sen·si·tive
pho·to·sen·si·tiv·i·
 ty
 pl pho·to·sen·si·tiv·i·
 ties

pho·to·sen·si·ti·za·
tion
pho·to·sen·si·tize
 pho·to·sen·si·
 tized
 pho·to·sen·si·tiz·
 ing
pho·to·sen·si·tiz·er
pho·to·sta·bil·i·ty
 pl pho·to·sta·bil·i·ties
pho·to·sta·ble
pho·to·syn·the·sis
 pl pho·to·syn·the·ses
pho·to·syn·the·size
 pho·to·syn·the·
 sized
 pho·to·syn·the·
 siz·ing
pho·to·syn·thet·ic
pho·to·syn·thet·i·
 cal·ly
pho·to·tac·tic
pho·to·tac·ti·cal·ly
pho·to·tax·is
 pl pho·to·tax·es
pho·to·ther·a·py
 pl pho·to·ther·a·pies
pho·to·tim·er
pho·to·tox·ic
pho·to·tox·ic·i·ty
 pl pho·to·tox·ic·i·ties
pho·to·troph·ic
pho·to·tro·pic
pho·tot·ro·pism
phrag·mo·plast
phren·em·phrax·is
 pl phren·em·phrax·es

phren·ic
phren·i·cec·to·my
 pl phren·i·cec·to·mies
phren·i·co·ex·er·e·
 sis
 pl phren·i·co·ex·er·e·
 ses
phren·i·co·li·en·al
phren·i·cot·o·my
 pl phren·i·cot·o·mies
phre·nol·o·gy
 pl phre·nol·o·gies
phren·o·sin
phry·no·der·ma
phthal·ate
phtha·lein
phthal·ic
phthal·yl·sul·fa·thi·
 a·zole
phthi·o·col
phthi·o·ic
phthi·ri·a·sis
 pl phthi·ri·a·ses
Phthir·i·us
Phthi·rus
phthi·sic
 or phthi·si·cal
phthis·io·gen·e·sis
 pl phthis·io·gen·e·ses
phthis·io·gen·ic
phthis·i·ol·o·gist
phthis·i·ol·o·gy
 pl phthis·i·ol·o·gies
phthis·io·pho·bia
phthis·io·ther·a·py
 pl phthis·io·ther·a·
 pies

phthi·sis
 pl phthi·ses
phthi·sis bul·bi
phy·co·cy·a·nin
phy·co·er·y·thrin
phy·co·log·i·cal
phy·col·o·gist
phy·col·o·gy
 pl phy·col·o·gies
phy·co·my·cete
Phy·co·my·ce·tes
phy·co·my·ce·tous
phy·co·my·co·sis
 pl phy·co·my·co·ses
phy·lac·tic
phy·let·ic
phy·let·i·cal·ly
phyl·lode
phyl·lo·er·y·thrin
phyl·lo·qui·none
phy·lo·gen·e·sis
 pl phy·lo·gen·e·ses
phy·lo·ge·net·ic
phy·lo·ge·net·i·cal·
 ly
phy·log·e·ny
 pl phy·log·e·nies
phy·lum
 pl phy·la
phy·sa·lia
phy·sa·lif·e·rous
Phy·sa·lop·tera
phy·ses
 pl of phy·sis
phys·iat·rics
phys·iat·rist
phys·ic

phys·i·cal
phy·si·cian
phys·i·cist
phys·i·co·chem·i·cal
phys·ics
phys·i·o·chem·i·cal
phys·i·o·log·i·cal
or phys·i·o·log·ic
phys·i·ol·o·gist
phys·i·ol·o·gy
pl phys·i·ol·o·gies
phys·io·path·o·log·ic
or phys·io·path·o·log·i·cal
phys·io·pa·thol·o·gy
pl phys·io·pa·thol·o·gies
phys·io·ther·a·pist
phys·io·ther·a·py
pl phys·io·ther·a·pies
phy·sique
phy·sis
pl phy·ses
phy·so·stig·mine
phy·tan·ic
phy·tase
phy·tate
phy·tic
phy·to·be·zoar
phy·to·hem·ag·glu·ti·nin
phy·to·hor·mone
phy·tol
phy·to·na·di·one

phy·ton·cid·al
phy·ton·cide
phy·to·patho·gen
phy·to·patho·gen·ic
phy·to·pa·thol·o·gist
phy·to·phar·ma·col·o·gy
pl phy·to·phar·ma·col·o·gies
phy·to·pho·to·der·ma·ti·tis
pl phy·to·pho·to·der·ma·ti·ti·ses
or phy·to·pho·to·der·ma·tit·i·des
phy·tos·ter·ol
phy·to·ther·a·py
pl phy·to·ther·a·pies
phy·to·tox·ic
phy·to·tox·ic·i·ty
pl phy·to·tox·ic·i·ties
phy·to·tox·in
phy·tyl
pia
pia-arach·noid
also pia-arach·noid·al
or pi·arach·noid
pi·al
pia ma·ter
pi·an
pi·a·nist's cramp
pi·blok·to
pi·ca
pi·chi
Pick's dis·ease
Pick·wick·ian syn·drome

pi·clo·ram
pi·co·far·ad
pi·co·gram
pic·o·line
pic·o·lin·ic
pi·co·mo·lar
pi·co·mole
pi·cor·na·vi·rus
pi·co·sec·ond
pic·ram·ic
pic·rate
pic·ric
pic·ro·car·mine
pic·ro·lon·ic
pic·ro·podo·phyl·lin
pic·ro·tox·in
pic·ro·tox·in·in
pic·ryl
pie·dra
Pierre Ro·bin syn·drome
pi·ezo·chem·is·try
pl pi·ezo·chem·is·tries
pi·ezo·elec·tric
pi·ezo·elec·tric·i·ty
pl pi·ezo·elec·tric·i·ties
pi·ezom·e·ter
pi·ezo·met·ric
pi·ezom·e·try
pl pi·ezom·e·tries
pi·geon breast
pi·geon-breast·ed
pi·geon-toed
pig·ment

pig·men·tary
pig·men·ta·tion
pig·ment·ed
pig·men·to·phage
pig·men·tum ni·
grum
pig·my
var of pygmy
Pi·gnet in·dex
pig·weed
pi·la·ry
pi·las·ter
pi·li
pl of pi·lus
pil·lar
pil·let
pi·lo·car·pi·dine
pi·lo·car·pine
pi·lo·car·pus
pl pi·lo·car·pus·es
pi·lo·erec·tion
pi·lo·mo·tor
pi·lo·ni·dal
pi·lose
pi·lo·se·ba·ceous
pi·los·i·ty
pl pi·los·i·ties
pil·u·lar
or pil·lu·lar
pil·ule
or pil·lule
pi·lus
pl pi·li
pi·mar·i·cin
pi·mel·ic
pim·o·zide
pim·ple

pim·pled
pim·ply
pi·ne·al
pi·ne·a·lec·to·mize
pi·ne·a·lec·to·
mized
pi·ne·a·lec·to·
miz·ing
pi·ne·al·ec·to·my
pl pi·ne·al·ec·to·mies
pin·e·a·lo·cyte
pin·e·a·lo·ma
pl pin·e·a·lo·mas
or pin·e·a·lo·ma·ta
pi·nene
pin·guec·u·la
also pin·guic·u·la
pl pin·guec·u·lae
also pin·guic·u·lae
pink·eye
pink·root
pin·na
pl pin·nae
or pin·nas
pin·nal
pi·no·cy·to·sis
pl pi·no·cy·to·ses
pi·no·cy·tot·ic
or pi·no·cyt·ic
pi·no·cy·tot·i·cal·ly
pin·ta
pin·tid
pin·to
pin·worm
Pi·oph·i·la
Pi·per
pi·per·a·zine

pip·er·ine
pi·per·o·caine
pi·per·o·nyl bu·tox·
ide
pip·er·ox·an
pi·pette
or pi·pet
pi·pet·ted
pi·pet·ting
pip·sis·se·wa
pir·i·form
or pyr·i·form
pir·i·for·mis
or pyr·i·for·mis
piro·plasm
or piro·plas·ma
pl piro·plasms
or piro·plas·ma·ta
Piro·plas·ma
piro·plas·mic
piro·plas·mo·sis
pl piro·plas·mo·ses
Pir·quet test
pi·si·form
pitch·blende
pitch·er's el·bow
pith·e·coid
pith·i·a·tism
pith·i·at·ric
pi·tot tube
pit·ting
pi·tu·i·cyte
pi·tu·itary
pl pi·tu·itar·ies
pi·tu·itary ba·soph·
i·lism

pit·y·ri·a·sis
  pl pit·y·ri·a·ses

pit·y·ri·a·sis ro·sea

pit·y·ri·a·sis ru·bra
  pi·lar·is

pit·y·ri·a·sis ver·si·
  col·or

piv·ot

pla·ce·bo
  pl pla·ce·bos

pla·cen·ta
  pl pla·cen·tas
  or pla·cen·tae

pla·cen·tal

plac·en·ta·lia

pla·cen·ta pre·via
  pl pla·cen·tae previ·ae

pla·cen·ta·tion

plac·en·ti·tis
  pl plac·en·tit·i·des

plac·en·tog·ra·phy
  pl plac·en·tog·ra·
  phies

plac·en·to·ma
  pl plac·en·to·mas
  or plac·en·to·ma·ta

plac·ode

placque
  var of plaque

pla·gi·o·ceph·a·ly
  pl pla·gi·o·ceph·a·lies

Pla·gi·or·chis

plague

pla·nar·ia

pla·nar·i·an

Plan·a·ri·idae

plan·chet

pla·ni·gram

pla·nig·ra·phy
  pl pla·nig·ra·phies

pla·nim·e·ter

pla·no

pla·no·cel·lu·lar

pla·no·con·cave

pla·no·con·vex

pla·nor·bid

Pla·nor·bi·dae

Pla·nor·bis

plan·ta·go

plan·tain

plan·tar

plan·tar·is
  pl plan·tar·es

plan·ti·grade

plaque
  also placque

plasm

plas·ma

plas·ma·blast

plas·ma·cyte

plas·ma·cy·toid

plas·ma·cy·to·ma
  also plas·mo·cy·to·ma
  pl plas·ma·cy·to·mas
  or plas·ma·cy·to·ma·
  ta
  also plas·mo·cy·to·
  mas
  or plas·mo·cy·to·ma·
  ta

plas·ma·cy·to·sis
  pl plas·ma·cy·to·ses

plas·ma·gel

plas·ma·gene

plas·ma·lem·ma

plas·mal·o·gen

plas·ma·pher·e·sis
  pl plas·ma·pher·e·ses

plas·ma·sol

plas·mat·ic

plas·mic

plas·mid

plas·min

plas·min·o·gen

plas·mo·cy·to·ma
  var of plasmacytoma

plas·mo·di·al
  also plas·mod·ic

plas·mo·di·cid·al

plas·mo·di·cide

Plas·mo·di·idae

plas·mo·di·tro·pho·
  blast

plas·mo·di·um
  pl plas·mo·dia

Plas·mod·ro·ma

plas·mog·a·my
  pl plas·mog·a·mies

plas·mol·y·sis

plas·mo·lyt·ic

plas·mo·lyz·abil·i·
  ty
  pl plas·mo·lyz·abil·i·
  ties

plas·mo·lyz·able

plas·mo·lyze
  plas·mo·lyzed
  plas·mo·lyz·ing

plas·mon
  also plas·mone

plas·mop·ty·sis
  pl plas·mop·ty·ses

plas·mo·some
  also plas·ma·some

plas·mot·o·my
  pl plas·mot·o·mies

plas·tein

plas·ter of par·is

plas·tic

plas·tic·i·ty
  pl plas·tic·i·ties

plas·ti·ci·za·tion

plas·ti·cize
  plas·ti·cized
  plas·ti·ciz·ing

plas·ti·ciz·er

plas·tid

plas·tid·i·al

plas·tog·a·my
  pl plas·tog·a·mies

plas·to·qui·none

plas·ty
  pl plas·ties

plate·let

plat·i·num

plat·ode

platy·ba·sia

platy·ce·phal·ic

platy·ceph·a·ly
  pl platy·ceph·a·lies

platy·cne·mia

platy·cne·mic

platy·cne·my
  pl platy·cne·mies

platy·hel·minth
  pl platy·hel·minths

Platy·hel·min·thes

platy·hel·min·thic

platy·hi·er·ic

platy·mer·ic

platy·pel·lic

platy·pel·loid

platy·pel·ly
  pl platy·pel·lies

plat·yr·rhine

pla·tys·ma
  pl pla·tys·ma·ta
  also pla·tys·mas

pla·tys·mal

pled·get

ple·gia

pleio·tro·pic

plei·ot·ro·py
  pl plei·ot·ro·pies

pleo·chro·ic

ple·och·ro·ism

pleo·cy·to·sis
  pl pleo·cy·to·ses

pleo·mor·phic
  also pleio·mor·phic

pleo·mor·phism

ple·op·tics

ple·ro·cer·coid

pleth·o·ra

ple·tho·ric

ple·thys·mo·gram

ple·thys·mo·graph

ple·thys·mo·graph·
  ic

ple·thys·mo·graph·
  i·cal·ly

pleth·ys·mog·ra·
  phy
  pl pleth·ys·mog·ra·
    phies

pleu·ra
  pl pleu·rae
  or pleu·ras

pleu·ral

pleu·rec·to·my
  pl pleu·rec·to·mies

pleu·ri·sy
  pl pleu·ri·sies

pleu·rit·ic

pleu·ri·tis
  pl pleu·rit·i·des

pleu·ro·dyn·ia

pleu·ro·peri·car·di·
  tis
  pl pleu·ro·peri·car·
    dit·i·des

pleu·ro·peri·to·ne·
  al

pleu·ro·pneu·mo·
  nia

pleu·ro·pneu·mo·
  nia-like or·gan·
  ism

pleu·ro·pul·mo·
  nary

pleu·ro·thot·o·nos

plex·ec·to·my
  pl plex·ec·to·mies

plexi·form

plex·im·e·ter

plex·op·a·thy
  pl plex·op·a·thies

plex·or

plex·us
pli·ca
  pl pli·cae
pli·ca cir·cu·la·ris
  pl pli·cae cir·cu·la·res
pli·ca fim·bri·a·ta
  pl pli·cae fim·bri·a·tae
pli·cal
pli·ca semi·lu·na·ris
  pl pli·cae semi·lu·na·res
pli·ca sub·lin·gua·lis
  pl pli·cae sub·lin·gua·les
pli·cate
  pli·cat·ed
  pli·cat·ing
pli·ca·tion
ploi·dy
  pl ploi·dies
plom·bage
plug·ger
plum·ba·gin
plum·bic
plum·bism
Plum·mer-Vin·son syn·drome
plump·er
plu·ri·glan·du·lar
plu·rip·o·tent
plu·ri·po·ten·tial
plu·ri·po·ten·ti·al·i·ty
  pl plu·ri·po·ten·ti·al·i·ties

plu·to·ni·um
ply·lo·ric
pneu·mat·ic
pneu·mat·i·cal·ly
pneu·ma·ti·za·tion
pneu·ma·tized
pneu·ma·to·cele
pneu·ma·to·graph
pneu·ma·to·sis
  pl pneu·ma·to·ses
pneu·ma·tu·ria
pneu·mo·ba·cil·lus
  pl pneu·mo·ba·cil·li
pneu·mo·coc·cal
pneu·mo·coc·ce·mia
pneu·mo·coc·cic
pneu·mo·coc·cus
  pl pneu·mo·coc·ci
pneu·mo·co·ni·o·sis
  pl pneu·mo·co·ni·o·ses
pneu·mo·cys·tic
Pneu·mo·cys·tis
Pneu·mo·cys·tis ca·ri·nii pneu·mo·nia
pneu·mo·cyte
pneu·mo·en·ceph·a·li·tis
  pl pneu·mo·en·ceph·a·lit·i·des
pneu·mo·en·ceph·a·lo·gram
pneu·mo·en·ceph·a·lo·graph·ic

pneu·mo·en·ceph·a·log·ra·phy
  pl pneu·mo·en·ceph·a·log·ra·phies

pneu·mo·gas·tric
pneu·mo·gram
pneu·mo·graph
pneu·mo·graph·ic
pneu·mog·ra·phy
  pl pneu·mog·ra·phies

pneu·mo·hy·dro·tho·rax
  pl pneu·mo·hy·dro·tho·rax·es
  or pneu·mo·hy·dro·tho·ra·ces

pneu·mol·y·sis
  pl pneu·mol·y·ses

pneu·mo·me·di·as·ti·num
  pl pneu·mo·me·di·as·ti·na

pneu·mo·my·co·sis
  pl pneu·mo·my·co·ses

pneu·mo·nec·to·my
  pl pneu·mo·nec·to·mies

pneu·mo·nia
pneu·mon·ic
pneu·mo·ni·tis
  pl pneu·mo·nit·i·des

pneu·mo·no·cen·te·sis
  pl pneu·mo·no·cen·te·ses

pneu·mo·no·co·ni·
o·sis
pl pneu·mo·no·co·ni·
o·ses

pneu·mo·nol·y·sis
pl pneu·mo·nol·y·ses

pneu·mop·a·thy
pl pneu·mop·a·thies

pneu·mo·peri·car·
di·um
pl pneu·mo·peri·car·
dia

pneu·mo·peri·to·
ne·um
pl pneu·mo·peri·to·
ne·ums
or pneu·mo·peri·to·
nea

pneu·mo·roent·
gen·og·ra·phy
pl pneu·mo·roent·
gen·og·ra·phies

pneu·mo·scle·ro·
sis
pl pneu·mo·scle·ro·
ses

pneu·mo·tacho·
gram

pneu·mo·tacho·
graph

pneu·mo·tax·ic

pneu·mo·tho·rax
pl pneu·mo·tho·rax·es
or pneu·mo·tho·ra·
ces

pneu·mo·tro·pic

pneu·mot·ro·pism

pock·mark

pock·marked

po·dag·ra

po·dal·ic

po·di·at·ric

po·di·a·trist

po·di·a·try
pl po·di·a·tries

podo·derm

podo·der·ma·ti·tis
pl podo·der·ma·ti·tis·
es
or podo·der·ma·tit·i·
des

podo·phyl·lin

podo·phyl·lo·tox·in

podo·phyl·lum
pl podo·phyl·li
or podo·phyl·lums

po·go·ni·on

poi·kilo·cyte

poi·kilo·cy·to·sis
pl poi·kilo·cy·to·ses

poi·kilo·der·ma
pl poi·kilo·der·mas
or poi·kilo·der·ma·ta

poi·kil·os·mot·ic

poi·ki·lo·therm

poi·ki·lo·ther·mic

poise

Poi·seuille's law

poi·son

poi·soned

poi·son·ing

poi·son·ous

poke·weed

po·lar

po·lar·im·e·ter

po·lari·met·ric

po·lar·im·e·try
pl po·lar·im·e·tries

po·lari·scope

po·lari·scop·ic

po·lari·scop·i·cal·ly

po·lar·i·ty
pl po·lar·i·ties

po·lar·iz·abil·i·ty
pl po·lar·iz·abil·i·ties

po·lar·iz·able

po·lar·iza·tion

po·lar·ize

po·lar·ized

po·lar·iz·ing

po·lar·iz·er

po·lar·o·gram

po·laro·graph·ic

po·laro·graph·i·cal·
ly

po·lar·og·ra·phy
pl po·lar·og·ra·phies

Po·len·ske val·ue

po·lice·man
pl po·lice·men

pol·i·clin·ic
outpatient dispensary
(*see* polyclinic)

po·lio

po·lio·dys·tro·phy
pl po·lio·dys·tro·phies

po·lio·en·ceph·a·li·
tis
pl po·lio·en·ceph·a·
lit·i·des

po·lio·en·ceph·alo·
  my·eli·tis
  pl po·lio·en·ceph·alo·
  my·elit·i·des
po·lio·my·elit·ic
po·lio·my·eli·tis
  pl po·lio·my·elit·i·des
po·li·o·sis
  pl po·li·o·ses
po·lio·vi·rus
po·litz·er bag
pol·len
pol·li·ci·za·tion
pol·li·no·sis
  or pol·le·no·sis
  pl pol·li·no·ses
  or pol·le·no·ses
pol·lut·ant
pol·lute
  pol·lut·ed
  pol·lut·ing
pol·lut·er
pol·lu·tion
pol·lu·tive
po·lo·ni·um
pol·toph·a·gy
  pl pol·toph·a·gies
poly
  pl pol·ys
poly(A)
poly·ac·id
poly·acryl·amide
poly·ad·e·nyl·ate
poly·ad·e·nyl·at·ed
poly·ad·e·nyl·a·
  tion
poly·ad·e·nyl·ic

poly·am·ide
poly·amine
poly·ar·ter·i·tis
poly·ar·thri·tis
  pl poly·ar·thrit·i·des
poly·ar·tic·u·lar
poly·ba·sic
poly·ba·sic·i·ty
  pl poly·ba·sic·i·ties
poly·blast
poly·blas·tic
poly·bro·mi·nat·ed
poly(C)
poly·cen·tric
poly·chlo·ri·nat·ed
poly·chro·ma·sia
poly·chro·mat·ic
poly·chro·mato·
  phil·ic
poly·cis·tron·ic
poly·clin·ic
  hospital (see policlinic)
poly·clo·nal
poly·cy·clic
poly·cys·tic
poly·cy·the·mia
poly·cy·the·mia ve·
  ra
poly·cy·the·mic
poly·cyt·i·dyl·ic
poly·dac·tyl
poly·dac·tyl·ia
poly·dac·tyl·ism
poly·dac·ty·lous
poly·dac·ty·ly
  pl poly·dac·ty·lies
poly·dip·sia

poly·dip·sic
poly·dis·perse
poly·dis·per·si·ty
  pl poly·dis·per·si·ties
poly·drug
poly·elec·tro·lyte
poly·em·bry·on·ic
poly·em·bry·o·ny
  pl poly·em·bry·o·nies
poly·en·do·crine
poly·ene
poly·enic
poly·es·trous
poly·ga·lac·tia
poly·ga·lac·tu·ro·
  nase
poly·gene
poly·ge·nic
poly·gen·i·cal·ly
poly·glan·du·lar
poly·graph
poly·graph·ic
poly·graph·i·cal·ly
poly·hy·dram·ni·os
poly·hy·droxy
poly I:C
poly·ino·sin·ic
poly I·poly C
poly·ly·sine
poly·men·or·rhea
poly·mer
poly·mer·ase
poly·mer·ic
poly·mer·i·cal·ly
po·ly·mer·ism
po·ly·mer·iza·tion

po·ly·mer·ize
  po·ly·mer·ized
  po·ly·mer·iz·ing
poly·meth·yl
poly·mi·cro·bi·al
poly·morph
poly·mor·phic
poly·mor·phi·cal·ly
poly·mor·phism
poly·mor·pho·nu·
  cle·ar
poly·mor·phous
poly·my·al·gia
  rheu·mat·i·ca
poly·myo·si·tis
poly·myx·in
poly·neu·rit·ic
poly·neu·ri·tis
  pl poly·neu·rit·i·des
  or poly·neu·ri·tis·es
poly·neu·ro·pa·thy
  pl poly·neu·ro·pa·
    thies
poly·nu·cle·ar
poly·nu·cle·o·tide
poly·ol
poly·oma
poly·os·tot·ic
pol·yp
pol·yp·ec·to·my
  pl pol·yp·ec·to·mies
poly·pep·tide
poly·pep·tid·ic
poly·pha·gia
poly·phar·ma·cy
  pl poly·phar·ma·cies
poly·pha·sic

poly·phy·let·ic
poly·phy·let·i·cal·ly
poly·ploid
poly·ploi·dy
  pl poly·ploi·dies
po·lyp·nea
po·lyp·ne·ic
pol·yp·oid
pol·yp·o·sis
  pl pol·yp·o·ses
pol·yp·ous
poly·pus
  pl poly·pi
  or poly·pus·es
poly·ri·bo·nu·cle·o·
  tide
poly·ri·bo·som·al
poly·ri·bo·some
poly·sac·cha·ride
poly·se·ro·si·tis
poly·some
poly·so·my
  pl poly·so·mies
poly·sor·bate
poly·sper·mic
poly·sper·my
  pl poly·sper·mies
poly·sty·rene
poly·syn·ap·tic
poly·syn·ap·ti·cal·
  ly
poly·tene
poly·te·ny
  pl poly·te·nies
poly·tet·ra·flu·o·ro·
  eth·yl·ene
poly·the·lia

poly·thi·a·zide
po·lyt·o·cous
poly·to·mo·gram
poly·to·mog·ra·phy
  pl poly·to·mog·ra·
    phies
poly·typ·ic
poly(U)
poly·un·sat·u·rate
poly·un·sat·u·rat·
  ed
poly·uria
poly·uri·dyl·ic
poly·va·lence
poly·va·lent
poly·vi·nyl
poly·vi·nyl·pyr·rol·
  i·done
poly·zo·ot·ic
po·made
po·man·der
pom·pho·lyx
pon·der·al
pons
  pl pon·tes
pons Va·ro·lii
  pl pon·tes Va·ro·lii
pon·tic
pon·tile
pon·tine
pon·to·cer·e·bel·lar
pop·li·te·al
pop·li·te·us
  pl pop·li·tei
pop·py
  pl pop·pies
pop·u·la·tion

por·ce·lain
por·cine
por·en·ceph·a·ly
  pl por·en·ceph·a·lies
po·ri·on
  pl po·ria
  or po·ri·ons
po·ro·ceph·a·li·a·sis
  pl po·ro·ceph·a·li·a·ses
Po·ro·ce·phal·i·dae
Po·ro·ceph·a·lus
po·ro·sis
  pl po·ro·ses
  or po·ro·sis·es
po·ros·i·ty
  pl po·ros·i·ties
po·rot·ic
po·rous
por·phin
  also por·phine
por·pho·bi·lin·o·gen
por·phyr·ia
por·phy·rin
por·phy·rin·uria
por·phy·rop·sin
por·ta
  pl por·tae
por·ta·ca·val
por·ta hep·a·tis
por·tal
por·tio
  pl por·ti·o·nes
por·tog·ra·phy
  pl por·tog·ra·phies

Por·tu·guese man-of-war
  pl Por·tu·guese men-of-war
port-wine stain
po·si·tion
po·si·tion·al
pos·i·tive
pos·i·tron
po·sol·o·gy
  pl po·sol·o·gies
post·abor·tal
post·abor·tion
post·ab·sorp·tion
post·ad·e·noid·ec·to·my
post·ad·o·les·cent
post·anal
post·an·es·thet·ic
post·an·ox·ic
post·ax·i·al
post·bran·chi·al
post·ca·nine
post·cap·il·lary
post·car·di·nal
post·ca·va
post·ca·val
post·cen·tral
post·cho·le·cys·tec·to·my
post·ci·bal
post·co·ital
post·em·bry·on·ic
post·en·ceph·a·li·tic
pos·te·ri·or
pos·tero·an·te·ri·or

pos·tero·in·ter·nal
pos·tero·lat·er·al
pos·tero·me·di·al
post·fix
post·fix·a·tion
post·gan·gli·on·ic
post·glen·oid
post·hem·or·rhag·ic
pos·thi·tis
  pl pos·thit·i·des
post·hu·mous
post·hu·mous·ly
post·hyp·not·ic
post·ic·tal
post·in·farc·tion
post·isch·emic
post·junc·tion·al
post·ma·ture
post·mei·ot·ic
post·meno·paus·al
post·mi·tot·ic
post·mor·tal
post·mor·tem
post·na·sal
post·na·tal
post·nor·mal
post·nor·mal·i·ty
  pl post·nor·mal·i·ties
post·op·er·a·tive
post·oral
post·or·bit·al
post·par·tum
post·phle·bit·ic
post·pi·tu·itary
post·pran·di·al
post·pu·ber·tal

post·ra·di·a·tion
post·sur·gi·cal
post·syn·ap·tic
post·syn·ap·ti·cal·ly
post·tran·scrip·tion·al
post·trans·fu·sion
post·trans·la·tion·al
post·trau·mat·ic
post·treat·ment
pos·tur·al
pos·ture
post·vac·ci·nal
po·ta·ble
pot·ash
po·tas·si·um
po·ten·cy
  pl po·ten·cies
po·tent
po·ten·tial
po·ten·ti·ate
  po·ten·ti·at·ed
  po·ten·ti·at·ing
po·ten·ti·a·tion
po·ten·ti·a·tor
po·ten·ti·om·e·ter
po·ten·tio·met·ric
po·tion
Pott's dis·ease
Pott's frac·ture
pouch of Doug·las
poul·tice
  poul·ticed
  poul·tic·ing

Pou·part's lig·a·ment
po·vi·done
pow·der
pow·er
pox
  pl pox
  or pox·es
pox·vi·rus
PP fac·tor
prac·ti·cal nurse
prac·tice
  prac·ticed
  prac·tic·ing
prac·ti·tio·ner
prac·to·lol
Pra·der-Wil·li syn·drome
pral·i·dox·ime
pra·seo·dym·i·um
Praus·nitz-Küst·ner re·ac·tion
pra·ze·pam
pra·zo·sin
pre·ad·mis·sion
pre·ad·o·les·cence
pre·ad·o·les·cent
pre·adult
pre·an·es·thet·ic
pre·aor·tic
pre·au·ric·u·lar
pre·ax·i·al
pre·can·cer·o·sis
  pl pre·can·cer·o·ses
pre·can·cer·ous
pre·cap·il·lary
  pl pre·cap·il·lar·ies

pre·car·ti·lage
pre·cen·tral
pre·cep·tee
pre·cep·tor
pre·chord·al
pre·cip·i·ta·bil·i·ty
  pl pre·cip·i·ta·bil·i·ties
pre·cip·i·ta·ble
pre·cip·i·tant
pre·cip·i·tate
  pre·cip·i·tat·ed
  pre·cip·i·tat·ing
pre·cip·i·ta·tion
pre·cip·i·tin
pre·cip·i·tin·o·gen
pre·cip·i·tin·o·gen·ic
pre·clin·i·cal
pre·co·cious
pre·coc·i·ty
  pl pre·coc·i·ties
pre·co·ital
pre·con·scious
pre·cor·dial
pre·cor·di·um
  pl pre·cor·dia
pre·cur·sor
pre·den·tal
pre·den·tin
  or pre·den·tine
pre·di·a·be·tes
pre·di·a·bet·ic
pre·di·gest
pre·di·ges·tion

pre·dis·pose
  pre·dis·posed
  pre·dis·pos·ing
pre·dis·po·si·tion
pre·dis·po·si·tion·al
pred·nis·o·lone
pred·ni·sone
pre·drug
pre·eclamp·sia
pre·eclamp·tic
pree·mie
  or pre·mie
pre·erup·tive
pre·eryth·ro·cyt·ic
pre·for·ma·tion
pre·fron·tal
pre·gan·gli·on·ic
pre·gen·i·tal
preg·nan·cy
  pl preg·nan·cies
preg·nane
preg·nane·di·ol
preg·nant
preg·nene
preg·nen·in·o·lone
preg·nen·o·lone
pre·hen·sile
pre·hen·sil·i·ty
  pl pre·hen·sil·i·ties
pre·hen·sion
pre·hos·pi·tal
pre·im·plan·ta·tion
pre·in·cu·bate
  pre·in·cu·bat·ed
  pre·in·cu·bat·ing
pre·in·cu·ba·tion

pre·in·fec·tion
pre·in·jec·tion
pre·in·va·sive
pre·leu·ke·mia
pre·leu·ke·mic
pre·ma·lig·nant
pre·mar·i·tal
pre·ma·ture
pre·ma·tu·ri·ty
  pl pre·ma·tu·ri·ties
pre·max·il·la
  pl pre·max·il·lae
pre·max·il·lary
pre·med
pre·med·i·cal
pre·med·i·cate
  pre·med·i·cat·ed
  pre·med·i·cat·ing
pre·med·i·ca·tion
pre·mei·ot·ic
pre·men·ar·che
pre·men·ar·che·al
pre·meno·paus·al
pre·men·stru·al
pre·men·stru·um
  pl pre·men·stru·ums
  or pre·men·strua
pre·mie
  var of preemie
pre·mo·lar
pre·mon·i·to·ry
pre·mor·bid
pre·mor·tal
pre·mor·tem
pre·mo·tor
pre·mu·ni·tion

pre·my·elo·cyte
pre·na·tal
pre·neo·plas·tic
pre·nor·mal
pre·nor·mal·i·ty
  pl pre·nor·mal·i·ties
pre·oe·di·pal
pre·op·er·a·tive
pre·op·tic
pre·ovu·la·to·ry
pre·ox·y·gen·ation
prep
  prepped
  prep·ping
prep·a·ra·tion
pre·pare
  pre·pared
  pre·par·ing
pre·par·tum
pre·pa·tel·lar
pre·pa·tent
pre·phe·nic
pre·po·ten·cy
  pl pre·po·ten·cies
pre·po·tent
pre·po·ten·tial
pre·psy·chot·ic
pre·pu·ber·al
pre·pu·ber·tal
pre·pu·ber·ty
  pl pre·pu·ber·ties
pre·pu·bes·cence
pre·pu·bes·cent
pre·puce
pre·pu·tial
pre·py·lo·ric
pre·re·nal

pre·rep·li·cat·ive
pre·re·pro·duc·tive
pre·ret·i·nal
pre·sa·cral
pres·by·cu·sis
  pl pres·by·cu·ses
pres·by·ope
pres·byo·phre·nia
pres·byo·phren·ic
pres·by·opia
pres·by·opic
pre·schizo·phren·ic
pre·scribe
  pre·scribed
  pre·scrib·ing
pre·scrip·tion
pre·se·nile
pre·se·nil·i·ty
  pl pre·se·nil·i·ties
pre·sen·ta·tion
pre·sent·ing
pre·ser·va·tive
pre·serve
  pre·served
  pre·serv·ing
pre·so·mite
pre·sphe·noid
  also pre·sphe·noi·dal
pres·sor
pres·so·re·cep·tor
pres·sure
pre·su·bic·u·lum
  pl pre·su·bic·u·la
pre·sump·tive
pre·sur·gi·cal
pre·syn·ap·tic

pre·syn·ap·ti·cal·ly
pre·sys·to·le
pre·sys·tol·ic
pre·tec·tal
pre·term
pre·ter·mi·nal
pre·tib·i·al
pre·treat
pre·treat·ment
prev·a·lence
pre·ven·ta·tive
pre·ven·tive
pre·ven·to·ri·um
  pl pre·ven·to·ria
  also pre·ven·to·ri·ums

pre·ver·te·bral
pre·vi·able
pri·a·pism
Price-Jones curve
prick·le cell
prick·ly heat
pri·mal scene
pri·ma·quine
pri·ma·ry
  pl pri·ma·ries

pri·mate
Pri·ma·tes
pri·ma·to·log·i·cal
pri·ma·tol·o·gy
  pl pri·ma·tol·o·gies

prim·er
pri·mi·done
pri·mi·grav·id
pri·mi·grav·i·da
  pl pri·mi·grav·i·das
  or pri·mi·grav·i·dae

pri·mip·a·ra
  pl pri·mip·a·ras
  or pri·mip·a·rae

pri·mip·a·rous
prim·i·tive
pri·mor·di·al
pri·mor·di·um
  pl pri·mor·dia

prin·ci·ple
P-R in·ter·val
prism
pris·mat·ic
pri·vate
pro·abor·tion
pro·abor·tion·ist
pro·ac·cel·er·in
pro·ac·tive
pro·am·ni·on
  pl pro·am·ni·ons
  or pro·am·nia

pro·am·ni·ot·ic
pro·bac·te·rio·phage
pro·band
pro·bang
pro·bar·bi·tol
probe
  probed
  prob·ing
pro·ben·e·cid
pro·bos·cis
  pl pro·bos·cis·es
  also pro·bos·ci·des

pro·cain·amide
pro·caine
pro·car·ba·zine

pro·cary·ote
var of prokaryote

pro·cary·ot·ic
var of prokaryotic

pro·ce·dure

pro·cer·coid

pro·ce·rus
pl pro·ce·ri
or pro·ce·rus·es

pro·ces·sus
pl pro·ces·sus

pro·ces·sus vag·i·na·lis

pro·chlor·per·azine

pro·chro·mo·some

pro·ci·den·tia

proc·li·na·tion

pro·co·ag·u·lant

pro·col·la·gen

pro·con·ver·tin

pro·cre·ate
pro·cre·at·ed
pro·cre·at·ing

pro·cre·ation

pro·cre·ative

proc·tec·to·my
pl proc·tec·to·mies

proc·ti·tis

proc·toc·ly·sis
pl proc·toc·ly·ses

proc·to·co·li·tis

proc·to·de·al
or proc·to·dae·al

proc·to·de·um
or proc·to·dae·um
pl proc·to·dea
or proc·to·de·ums
or proc·to·daea
or proc·to·dae·ums

proc·to·log·ic
or proc·to·log·i·cal

proc·tol·o·gist

proc·tol·o·gy
pl proc·tol·o·gies

proc·to·pexy
pl proc·to·pex·ies

proc·to·plas·ty
pl proc·to·plas·ties

proc·to·scope
proc·to·scoped
proc·to·scop·ing
proc·to·scop·ic
proc·to·scop·i·cal·ly

proc·tos·co·py
pl proc·tos·co·pies

proc·to·sig·moid·ec·to·my
pl proc·to·sig·moid·ec·to·mies

proc·to·sig·moid·itis

proc·to·sig·moid·o·scope

proc·to·sig·moid·o·scop·ic

proc·to·sig·moid·os·co·py
pl proc·to·sig·moid·os·co·pies

proc·tot·o·my
pl proc·tot·o·mies

pro·cum·bent

pro·dig·i·o·sin

prod·ro·ma
pl prod·ro·mas
or pro·dro·ma·ta

pro·dro·mal
also pro·dro·mic

pro·drome

pro·duc·tive

pro·en·zyme

pro·eryth·ro·blast

pro·eryth·ro·blas·tic

pro·eryth·ro·cyte

pro·es·tro·gen

pro·es·trous

pro·es·trus
or pro·es·trum

pro·fer·ment

pro·fes·sion

pro·fes·sion·al

pro·fi·bri·no·ly·sin

pro·file
pro·filed
pro·fil·ing

pro·fla·vine
also pro·fla·vin

pro·flu·o·ri·da·tion·ist

pro·found·ly

pro·fun·da

pro·fun·da fem·o·ris

pro·gen·i·tor

prog·e·ny
  pl prog·e·nies

pro·ge·ria

pro·ges·ta·tion·al

pro·ges·ter·one

pro·ges·tin

pro·ges·to·gen
  also pro·ges·ta·gen

pro·ges·to·gen·ic
  also pro·ges·ta·gen·ic

pro·glot·tid

pro·glot·tis
  pl pro·glot·ti·des

prog·na·thic

prog·na·thism

prog·na·thous

prog·no·sis
  pl prog·no·ses

prog·nos·tic

prog·nos·ti·cate
  prog·nos·ti·cat·ed
  prog·nos·ti·cat·ing

prog·nos·ti·ca·tion

pro·gran·u·lo·cyte

pro·grav·id

pro·gres·sive

pro·guan·il

pro·hor·mone

pro·in·su·lin

pro·ject

pro·jec·tion

pro·jec·tive

pro·kary·ote
  also pro·cary·ote

pro·kary·ot·ic
  also pro·cary·ot·ic

pro·la·bi·um
  pl pro·la·bia

pro·lac·tin

pro·la·min
  or pro·la·mine

pro·lan

pro·lapse
  pro·lapsed
  pro·laps·ing

pro·lap·sus

pro·lif·er·ate
  pro·lif·er·at·ed
  pro·lif·er·at·ing

pro·lif·er·a·tion

pro·lif·er·a·tive

pro·line

pro·lym·pho·cyte

pro·mas·ti·gote

pro·ma·zine

pro·mega·kary·o·cyte

pro·meg·a·lo·blast

pro·meta·phase

pro·meth·a·zine

pro·me·thi·um

prom·i·nence

pro·mono·cyte

prom·on·to·ry
  pl prom·on·to·ries

pro·mote
  pro·mot·ed
  pro·mot·ing

pro·mot·er

pro·my·elo·cyte

pro·my·elo·cyt·ic

pro·nase

pro·nate

pro·nat·ed
  pro·nat·ing

pro·na·tion

pro·na·tor

pro·na·tor qua·dra·tus

pro·na·tor te·res

pro·neph·ric

pro·neph·ros

pro·neth·a·lol

pro·no·grade

pro·nor·mo·blast

pron·to·sil

pron·to·sil al·bum

pron·to·sil ru·brum

pro·nu·cle·us
  pl pro·nu·clei
  also pro·nu·cle·us·es

prop·a·gate
  prop·a·gat·ed
  prop·a·gat·ing

prop·a·ga·tion

pro·pam·i·dine

pro·pane

pro·pa·no·ic

pro·pa·nol

pro·pan·o·lol

pro·pan·the·line

pro·par·a·caine

pro·pene

pro·per·din

pro·peri·to·ne·al

pro·phage

pro·phase

pro·pha·sic

pro·phy·lac·tic

pro·phy·lac·ti·cal·ly

pro·phy·lax·is
pl pro·phy·lax·es

pro·pio·lac·tone
or β-pro·pio·lac·tone

pro·pi·o·ma·zine

pro·pi·o·nate

pro·pi·oni·bac·te·ri·um
pl pro·pi·oni·bac·te·ria

pro·pi·on·ic

pro·pio·phe·none

pro·pos·i·ta
pl pro·pos·i·tae

pro·pos·i·tus
pl pro·pos·i·ti

pro·poxy·phene

pro·pran·o·lol

pro·pri·etary
pl pro·pri·etar·ies

pro·prio·cep·tion

pro·prio·cep·tive

pro·prio·cep·tor

pro·prio·spi·nal

pro·pto·sis
pl pro·pto·ses

pro·pyl

pro·pyl·ene

pro·pyl·hex·e·drine

pro·pyl·par·a·ben

pro·pyl·thio·ura·cil

pro·sec·tor

pro·sec·to·ri·al

pros·en·ce·phal·ic

pros·en·ceph·a·lon

pros·op·ag·no·sia

pros·ta·cy·clin

pros·ta·glan·din

pros·tate

pros·ta·tec·to·my
pl pros·ta·tec·to·mies

pros·tat·ic

pros·ta·tism

pros·ta·ti·tis

pros·ta·to·li·thot·o·my
pl pros·ta·to·li·thot·o·mies

pros·ta·tor·rhea

pros·ta·tot·o·my
pl pros·ta·tot·o·mies

pros·the·sis
pl pros·the·ses

pros·thet·ic

pros·thet·i·cal·ly

pros·thet·ics

pros·the·tist

pros·thi·on

prosth·odon·tics

prosth·odon·tist

pros·trate
　pros·trat·ed
　pros·trat·ing

pros·tra·tion

prot·ac·tin·i·um
also pro·to·ac·tin·i·um

prot·amine

prot·anom·a·lous

prot·anom·a·ly
pl prot·anom·a·lies

prot·a·nope

prot·an·opia

pro·te·an

pro·te·ase

pro·tec·tive

pro·tei
pl of proteus

pro·te·ic

pro·teid

pro·tein

pro·tein·aceous

pro·tein·ase

pro·tein·ate

pro·tein·oid

pro·tein·o·sis
pl pro·tein·o·ses
or pro·tein·o·sis·es

pro·tein·uria

pro·tein·uric

pro·teo·gly·can

pro·teo·lip·id
also pro·teo·lip·ide

pro·te·ol·y·sis
pl pro·te·ol·y·ses

pro·teo·lyt·ic

pro·teo·lyt·i·cal·ly

pro·teo·lyzed

pro·teo·lyose

pro·te·us
pl pro·tei

proth·e·sis
pl proth·e·ses

pro·thet·ic

pro·throm·bic

pro·throm·bin

pro·throm·bino·pe·
   nia
pro·tide
pro·ti·re·lin
pro·tist
Pro·tis·ta
pro·tis·tan
pro·ti·um
pro·to·ac·tin·i·um
   var of protactinium
pro·to·col
pro·to·cone
pro·to·co·nid
pro·to·di·as·to·le
pro·to·di·a·stol·ic
pro·to·fil·a·ment
pro·to·gen
pro·to·heme
pro·to·he·min
pro·to·mo·nad
Pro·to·mon·a·di·na
pro·ton
pro·ton·ic
pro·to·on·co·gene
pro·to·path·ic
pro·to·pec·tin
pro·to·pine
pro·to·plasm
pro·to·plas·mat·ic
pro·to·plas·mic
pro·to·plast
pro·to·por·phyr·ia
pro·to·por·phy·rin
Pro·to·stron·gy·lus
pro·to·tax·ic

Pro·to·the·ca
pro·to·the·co·sis
   pl pro·to·the·co·ses
pro·to·troph
pro·to·tro·phic
pro·tot·ro·phy
   pl pro·tot·ro·phies
pro·to·tro·pic
pro·tot·ro·py
   pl pro·tot·ro·pies
pro·to·ver·a·trine
pro·to·zoa
   pl of protozoon
Pro·to·zoa
   animal phylum or
   subkingdom
pro·to·zo·a·ci·dal
pro·to·zo·a·cide
pro·to·zo·al
pro·to·zo·an
pro·to·zo·i·a·sis
   pl pro·to·zo·i·a·ses
pro·to·zoo·log·i·
   cal
pro·to·zo·ol·o·gist
pro·to·zo·ol·o·gy
   pl pro·to·zo·ol·o·gies
pro·to·zo·on
   pl pro·to·zoa
pro·tract
pro·trac·tion
pro·trip·ty·line
pro·trude
   pro·trud·ed
   pro·trud·ing
pro·tru·sion
pro·tru·sive

pro·tu·ber·ance
pro·tu·ber·ant
pro·ven·tric·u·
   lus
   pl pro·ven·tric·u·li
pro·vi·ral
pro·vi·rus
pro·vi·ta·min
prov·o·ca·tion
pro·voc·a·tive
pro·voke
   pro·voked
   pro·vok·ing
prox·e·mics
prox·i·mad
prox·i·mal
prox·i·mate
pro·zone
pru·na·sin
Pru·nus
pru·rig·i·nous
pru·ri·go
pru·rit·ic
pru·ri·tus
pru·ri·tus ani
pru·ri·tus vul·
   vae
Prus·sian blue
prus·si·ate
prus·sic
psal·te·ri·um
   pl psal·te·ria
psam·mo·ma
   pl psam·mo·mas
   or psam·mo·ma·ta
psam·mo·ma·
   tous

pseud·ar·thro·sis
also pseu·do·ar·thro·
sis
pl pseud·ar·thro·ses
also pseu·do·ar·thro·
ses

pseu·do·ag·glu·ti·
na·tion
pseu·do·al·lele
pseu·do·al·le·lic
pseu·do·al·lel·ism
pseu·do·an·eu·
rysm
pseu·do·bul·bar
pseu·do·cho·lin·es·
ter·ase
pseu·do·cow·pox
pseu·do·cy·e·sis
pl pseu·do·cy·e·ses

pseu·do·cyst
pseu·do·ephed·
rine
pseu·do·glob·u·lin
pseu·do·gout
pseu·do·hal·lu·ci·
na·tion
pseu·do·he·mo·
phil·ia
pseu·do·her·maph·
ro·dism
pseu·do·her·maph·
ro·dite
pseu·do·her·maph·
ro·dit·ic
pseu·do·her·maph·
ro·dit·ism

pseu·do·hy·per·tro·
phic
pseu·do·hy·per·tro·
phy
pl pseu·do·hy·per·tro·
phies

pseu·do·hy·po·
para·thy·roid·
ism
pseu·do·iso·chro·
mat·ic
pseu·do·ker·a·tin
pseu·do·leu·ke·mia
pseu·do·leu·ke·mic
pseu·do·mem·
brane
pseu·do·mem·bra·
nous
pseu·do·mo·nad
pseu·do·mo·nas
pl pseu·do·mo·na·des

pseu·do·neu·rot·ic
pseu·do·pa·ral·y·sis
pl pseu·do·pa·ral·y·
ses

pseu·do·par·a·site
pseu·do·par·a·sit·ic
Pseu·do·phyl·lid·ea
pseu·do·phyl·lid·e·
an
pseu·do·plague
pseu·do·pod
pseu·dop·o·dal
or pseu·do·po·di·al

pseu·do·po·di·um
pl pseu·do·po·dia

pseu·do·preg·nan·
cy
pl pseu·do·preg·nan·
cies

pseu·do·preg·nant
pseu·do·ra·bies
pseu·do·re·ac·tion
pseu·do·sci·ence
pseu·do·sci·en·tif·
ic
pseu·do·scle·ro·sis
pl pseu·do·scle·ro·ses

pseu·do·strat·i·fi·
ca·tion
pseu·do·strat·i·fied
pseu·do·tu·ber·cu·
lo·sis
pl pseu·do·tu·ber·cu·
lo·ses

pseu·do·tu·mor
pseu·do·tu·mor·al
pseu·do·tu·mor
cer·e·bri
pseu·do·uri·dine
pseu·do·xan·tho·
ma elas·ti·cum
psi·lo·cin
psi·lo·cy·bin
psi·lo·sis
pl psi·lo·ses

psit·ta·co·sis
pl psit·ta·co·ses

psit·ta·co·tic
pso·as
pl pso·ai
or pso·ae

pso·ra·len

psychopathic

pso·ri·a·si·form
pso·ri·a·sis
  pl pso·ri·a·ses

pso·ri·a·sis ar·thro·
  path·i·ca
pso·ri·at·ic
Pso·rop·tes
pso·rop·tic
psych·as·the·nia
psych·as·then·ic
psy·che
psy·che·del·ic
psy·che·del·i·cal·ly
psy·chi·at·ric
psy·chi·at·ri·cal·ly
psy·chi·a·trist
psy·chi·a·try
  pl psy·chi·a·tries

psy·chic
  also psy·chi·cal

psy·chi·cal·ly
psy·cho·acous·tics
psy·cho·ac·tive
psy·cho·anal·y·sis
  also psych·anal·y·sis
  pl psy·cho·anal·y·ses
  also psych·anal·y·ses

psy·cho·an·a·lyst
psy·cho·an·a·lyt·ic
  also psy·cho·an·a·lyt·
  i·cal

psy·cho·an·a·lyze
  psy·cho·an·a·
  lyzed
  psy·cho·an·a·lyz·
  ing

psy·cho·bi·o·log·i·
  cal
  also psy·cho·bio·log·ic
psy·cho·bi·ol·o·gist
psy·cho·bi·ol·o·gy
  pl psy·cho·bi·ol·o·gies
psy·cho·chem·i·cal
psy·cho·chem·is·
  try
  pl psy·cho·chem·is·
  tries

psy·cho·di·ag·nos·
  tics
psy·cho·dra·ma
psy·cho·dra·mat·ic
psy·cho·dy·nam·ic
psy·cho·dy·nam·i·
  cal·ly
psy·cho·dy·nam·ics
psy·cho·ed·u·ca·
  tion·al
psy·cho·gal·van·ic
psy·cho·gal·va·
  nom·e·ter
psy·cho·gal·va·no·
  met·ric
psy·cho·gen·e·sis
  pl psy·cho·gen·e·ses
psy·cho·ge·net·ic
psy·cho·ge·net·i·
  cal·ly
psy·cho·gen·ic
psy·cho·gen·i·cal·ly
psy·cho·ge·ri·at·
  rics
psy·cho·ki·ne·sis
  pl psy·cho·ki·ne·ses

psy·cho·ki·net·ic
psy·cho·lep·sy
  pl psy·cho·lep·sies
psy·cho·lep·tic
psy·cho·lin·guis·
  tics
psy·cho·log·i·cal
  also psy·cho·log·ic
psy·cho·log·i·cal·ly
psy·chol·o·gist
psy·chol·o·gize
  psy·chol·o·gized
  psy·chol·o·giz·
  ing
psy·chol·o·gy
  pl psy·chol·o·gies
psy·cho·met·ric
psy·cho·met·ri·cal·
  ly
psy·cho·me·tri·
  cian
psy·chom·e·trist
psy·chom·e·try
  pl psy·chom·e·tries
psy·cho·mi·met·ic
psy·cho·mo·til·i·ty
  pl psy·cho·mo·til·i·
  ties

psy·cho·mo·tion
psy·cho·mo·tor
psy·cho·neu·ral
psy·cho·neu·ro·sis
  pl psy·cho·neu·ro·ses

psy·cho·neu·rot·ic
psy·cho·path
psy·cho·path·ia
psy·cho·path·ic

psy·cho·path·i·cal·ly

psy·cho·patho·log·i·cal
  or psy·cho·patho·log·ic

psy·cho·pa·thol·o·gist

psy·cho·pa·thol·o·gy

psy·chop·a·thy
  pl psy·chop·a·thies

psy·cho·phar·ma·ceu·ti·cal

psy·cho·phar·ma·co·log·ic
  or psy·cho·phar·ma·co·log·i·cal

psy·cho·phar·ma·col·o·gist

psy·cho·phar·ma·col·o·gy
  pl psy·cho·phar·ma·col·o·gies

psy·cho·phon·as·the·nia

psy·cho·phys·i·cal

psy·cho·phys·i·cist

psy·cho·phys·ics

psy·cho·phys·i·o·log·i·cal
  also psy·cho·phys·i·o·log·ic

psy·cho·phys·i·ol·o·gist

psy·cho·phys·i·ol·o·gy
  pl psy·cho·phys·i·ol·o·gies

psy·cho·sen·so·ry

psy·cho·sex·u·al

psy·cho·sex·u·al·i·ty
  pl psy·cho·sex·u·al·i·ties

psy·cho·sis
  pl psy·cho·ses
  mental illness (see sycosis)

psy·cho·so·cial

psy·cho·so·mat·ic

psy·cho·so·mat·i·cal·ly

psy·cho·so·mat·i·cist

psy·cho·so·mat·ics

psy·cho·sur·geon

psy·cho·sur·gery
  pl psy·cho·sur·ger·ies

psy·cho·sur·gi·cal

psy·cho·syn·the·sis
  pl psy·cho·syn·the·ses

psy·cho·tech·ni·cal
  also psy·cho·tech·nic

psy·cho·tech·nics

psy·cho·tech·no·log·i·cal

psy·cho·tech·nol·o·gist

psy·cho·tech·nol·o·gy
  pl psy·cho·tech·nol·o·gies

psy·cho·ther·a·peu·tic

psy·cho·ther·a·peu·ti·cal·ly

psy·cho·ther·a·peu·tics

psy·cho·ther·a·pist

psy·cho·ther·a·py
  pl psy·cho·ther·a·pies

psy·chot·ic

psy·chot·i·cal·ly

psy·chot·o·gen

psy·choto·gen·ic

psy·choto·mi·met·ic

psy·choto·mi·met·i·cal·ly

psy·cho·tox·ic

psy·cho·tro·pic

psy·chrom·e·ter

psy·chro·met·ric

psy·chrom·e·try
  pl psy·chrom·e·tries

psy·chro·phile

psy·chro·phil·ic

psyl·li·um

pter·i·dine

pter·in

pter·i·on

pte·ro·ic

pter·o·yl·glu·tam·ic

pte·ryg·i·um
  pl pte·ryg·i·ums
  or pte·ryg·ia

pter·y·goid

pter·y·goi·de·us
  pl pter·y·goi·dei

pter·y·go·man·dib·
  u·lar
pter·y·go·max·il·
  lary
pter·y·go·pal·a·tine
pter·y·go·spi·nous
pto·maine
ptosed
pto·sis
  pl pto·ses
ptot·ic
pty·a·lin
pty·a·lism
pu·ber·al
pu·ber·tal
pu·ber·tas prae·cox
pu·ber·ty
  pl pu·ber·ties
pu·ber·u·lic
pu·ber·u·lon·ic
pu·bes
  pl pu·bes
pu·bes
  pl of pubis
pu·bes·cence
pu·bes·cent
pu·bic
pu·bi·ot·o·my
  pl pu·bi·ot·o·mies
pu·bis
  pl pu·bes
pu·bo·cap·su·lar
pu·bo·coc·cy·geal
pu·bo·coc·cy·ge·us
  pl pu·bo·coc·cy·gei
pu·den·dal

pu·den·dum
  pl pu·den·da
pu·dic
pu·er·per·al
puff·er
Pu·lex
Pu·lic·i·dae
pul·lo·rum dis·
  ease
pul·mo·nary
pul·mon·ic
pul·mo·tor
pulp·al
pulp·ec·to·my
  pl pulp·ec·to·mies
pulp·i·tis
  pl pulp·it·i·des
pulp·ot·o·my
  pl pulp·ot·o·mies
pulpy
  pulp·i·er
  pulp·i·est
pul·sate
  pul·sat·ed
  pul·sat·ing
pul·sa·tile
pul·sa·til·la
pul·sa·tion
pulse
  pulsed
  puls·ing
pul·sion
pul·sus al·ter·nans
pul·sus par·a·dox·
  us
pul·ta·ceous
pul·ver·i·za·tion

pul·ver·ize
  pul·ver·ized
  pul·ver·iz·ing
pul·ver·u·lent
pul·vi·nar
pum·ice
punch-drunk
punc·tate
punc·ta·tion
punc·ti·form
punc·tum
  pl punc·ta
punc·ture
  punc·tured
  punc·tur·ing
pun·gen·cy
  pl pun·gen·cies
pun·gent
pu·pa
  pl pu·pae
  or pu·pas
pu·pal
  relating to a pupa
pu·pil
  *opening in the iris of
  the eye*
pu·pil·lary
  also pu·pi·lary
pu·pil·lo·di·la·tor
pu·pil·log·ra·phy
  pl pu·pil·log·ra·phies
pu·pil·lom·e·ter
pu·pil·lom·e·try
  pl pu·pil·lom·e·tries
pu·pil·lo·mo·tor
pure·bred
pur·ga·tion

pur.ga.tive

purge
 purged
 purg.ing

pu.rine

pu.ri.ty

Pur.kin.je af.ter.
 image

Pur.kin.je cell

Pur.kin.je fi.ber

Pur.kin.je phe.
 nom.e.non

Pur.kin.je's net.
 work

Pur.kin.je's sys.
 tem

Pur.kin.je's tis.sue

pu.ro.my.cin

pur.ple
 pur.pler
 pur.plest

pur.pu.ra

pur.pu.ra hem.or.
 rhag.i.ca

pur.pu.ra rheu.
 mat.i.ca

pur.pu.rate

pur.pu.ric

pur.pu.rin

purse-string su.
 ture

pu.ru.lence

pu.ru.lent

pus.sy
 pus.si.er
 pus.si.est

pus.tu.lant

pus.tu.lar

pus.tu.lat.ed

pus.tule

pu.ta.men
 pl pu.tam.i.na

pu.tam.i.nous

pu.tre.fac.tion

pu.tre.fac.tive

pu.tre.fy
 pu.tre.fied
 pu.tre.fy.ing

pu.tres.cent

pu.tres.ci.bil.i.ty
 pl pu.tres.ci.bil.i.ties

pu.tres.ci.ble

pu.tres.cine

pu.trid

pu.trid.i.ty
 pl pu.trid.i.ties

P wave

py.ar.thro.sis
 pl py.ar.thro.ses

pyc.nic
 var of pyknic

pyc.no.dys.os.to.sis
 var of pyknodysostosis

pyc.nom.e.ter
 or pyk.nom.e.ter

pyc.no.met.ric
 or pyk.no.met.ric

pyc.nom.e.try
 or pyk.nom.e.try
 pl pyc.nom.e.tries
 or pyk.nom.e.tries

pyc.no.sis
 var of pyknosis

pyc.not.ic
 var of pyknotic

py.el.ec.ta.sis
 pl py.el.ec.ta.ses

py.eli.tis

py.elo.gram

py.elo.graph.ic

py.elog.ra.phy
 pl py.elog.ra.phies

py.elo.li.thot.o.my
 pl py.elo.li.thot.o.
 mies

py.elo.ne.phrit.ic

py.elo.ne.phri.tis
 pl py.elo.ne.phrit.i.
 des

py.elo.plas.ty
 pl py.elo.plas.ties

py.e.los.to.my
 pl py.e.los.to.mies

py.e.lot.o.my
 pl py.e.lot.o.mies

py.elo.ure.ter.o.
 gram

py.elo.ure.ter.og.
 ra.phy
 pl py.elo.ure.ter.og.
 ra.phies

py.elo.ve.nous

py.emia

py.emic

Py.emo.tes

pyg.ma.lion.ism

pyg.my
 also pig.my
 pl pyg.mies
 also pig.mies

py·gop·a·gus
  pl py·gop·a·gi

pyk·nic
  also pyc·nic

pyk·no·dys·os·to·
sis
  or pyc·no·dys·os·to·
  sis
  pl pyk·no·dys·os·to·
  ses
  or pyc·no·dys·os·to·
  ses

pyk·no·ep·i·lep·sy
  pl pyk·no·ep·i·lep·
  sies

pyk·no·lep·sy
  pl pyk·no·lep·sies

pyk·nom·e·ter
  var of pycnometer

pyk·no·met·ric
  var of pycnometric

pyk·nom·e·try
  var of pycnometry

pyk·no·sis
  also pyc·no·sis

pyk·not·ic
  also pyc·not·ic

py·le·phle·bi·tis
  pl py·le·phle·bit·i·des

py·lon

py·lo·rec·to·my
  pl py·lo·rec·to·mies

py·lo·ric

py·lo·ro·du·o·de·
nal

py·lo·ro·my·ot·o·
my
  pl py·lo·ro·my·ot·o·
  mies

py·lo·ro·plas·ty
  pl py·lo·ro·plas·ties

py·lo·ro·spasm

py·lo·rus
  pl py·lo·ri

pyo·cele

pyo·coc·cus
  pl pyo·coc·ci

pyo·col·pos

pyo·cy·a·nase

pyo·cy·a·ne·us
  also pyo·cy·a·ne·ous
  or pyo·cy·an·ic

pyo·cy·a·nin
  or pyo·cy·a·nine

pyo·der·ma
  also pyo·der·mia

pyo·der·ma·to·sis
  pl pyo·der·ma·to·ses

pyo·der·mic

py·o·gen

pyo·gen·ic

pyo·me·tra

pyo·myo·si·tis

pyo·ne·phro·sis
  pl pyo·ne·phro·ses

pyo·ne·phrot·ic

pyo·pneu·mo·tho·
rax
  pl pyo·pneu·mo·tho·
  rax·es
  or pyo·pneu·mo·tho·
  ra·ces

py·or·rhea

py·or·rhea al·ve·o·
lar·is

py·or·rhe·ic

pyo·sal·pinx
  pl pyo·sal·pin·ges

pyo·sep·ti·ce·mia

pyo·sep·ti·ce·mic

pyo·tho·rax
  pl pyo·tho·rax·es
  or pyo·tho·ra·ces

pyr·a·mid

py·ram·i·dal

py·ram·i·da·lis
  pl py·ram·i·da·les
  or py·ram·i·da·lis·es

py·ram·i·dot·o·my
  pl py·ram·i·dot·o·
  mies

pyr·a·mis
  pl pyr·a·mi·des

py·ran

py·ra·nose

py·ran·tel

pyr·a·zin·amide

pyr·azole

py·raz·o·line

py·raz·o·lone

py·re·thrum

pyr·e·to·ther·a·py
  pl pyr·e·to·ther·a·pies

py·rex·ia

py·rex·i·al

py·rex·ic

pyr·i·dine

pyr·i·do·stig·mine

pyr·i·dox·al

pyr·i·dox·amine

pyr·i·dox·ic ac·id
or 4-pyr·i·dox·ic ac·id

pyr·i·dox·ine

pyr·i·form
var of piriform

pyr·i·for·mis
var of piriformis

py·ril·amine

py·ri·meth·amine

py·rim·i·dine

py·ro·cat·e·chol

py·ro·gal·lic

py·ro·gal·lol

py·ro·gen

py·ro·gen·ic

py·ro·ge·nic·i·ty
pl py·ro·ge·nic·i·ties

py·rol·y·sis
pl py·rol·y·ses

py·ro·lyt·ic

py·ro·ma·nia

py·ro·ma·ni·ac

py·ro·ma·ni·a·cal

py·ro·nine

py·ro·ni·no·phil·ic

py·ro·pho·bia

py·ro·pho·bic

py·ro·phos·pha·tase

py·ro·phos·phate

py·ro·phos·pho·ric

py·ro·sis

py·rox·y·lin

pyr·role

pyr·ro·lic

py·ruv·al·de·hyde

py·ru·vate

py·ru·vic

py·uria

Q

qat
var of khat

Q fe·ver

QRS com·plex

Q-T in·ter·val

quack·ery
pl quack·er·ies

quad·rant

quad·rate

qua·dra·tus
pl qua·dra·ti

qua·dra·tus fem·o·ris

qua·dra·tus la·bii su·pe·ri·or·is

qua·dra·tus lum·bor·um

qua·dra·tus plan·tae

quad·ri·ceps

quad·ri·ceps fem·o·ris

quad·ri·gem·i·nal

qua·drip·a·ra

quad·ri·ple·gia

quad·ri·ple·gic

quad·ri·va·lent

qua·dru·plet

quan·tal

quan·ti·ta·tive

quan·tum
pl quan·ta

quar·an·tin·able

quar·an·tine
quar·an·tined
quar·an·tin·ing

quart

quar·tan

quartz

quas·sia

quas·sin

quat
var of khat

qua·ter·na·ry

qua·ter·ni·za·tion

qua·ter·nize
qua·ter·nized
qua·ter·niz·ing

que·brach·a·mine

que·brach·ine

que·brach·i·tol

que·bra·cho

Queck·en·stedt test

quel·lung

quer·ce·tin

quer·ci·mer·i·trin

quer·ci·trin

Quer·cus

quer·u·lent
also quer·u·lant

quick·en
quick·ened
quick·en·ing

quick·lime

quick·sil·ver

qui·es·cent

quil·la·ic

quil·la·ja

qui·na

quin·a·crine
quin·al·bar·bi·tone
quin·al·dine
quin·a·mine
Quin·cke's dis·
 ease
Quin·cke's ede·ma
quin·eth·a·zone
qui·ne·tum
quin·hy·drone
quin·ic
quin·i·cine
quin·i·dine
qui·nine
qui·nin·ic
quin·oid
 var of quinonoid
quin·o·line
quin·o·lin·ol
qui·none
qui·no·noid
 or quin·oid
quino·tox·ine
qui·no·vin
qui·no·vose
quin·que·va·lent
quin·sy
 pl quin·sies
quint
quin·tu·plet
qui·nu·cli·dine
qui·nu·cli·di·nyl
 ben·zi·late
quit·tor
quo·tid·i·an
quo·tient
Q wave

R

ra·bid
ra·bies
 pl ra·bies
rac·e·mase
ra·ce·mic
ra·ce·mi·za·tion
ra·ce·mize
 ra·ce·mized
 ra·ce·miz·ing
ra·ce·mose
ra·chis·chi·sis
 pl ra·chis·chi·ses
ra·chit·ic
ra·chi·tis
 also rha·chi·tis
 pl ra·chit·i·des
 or rha·chit·i·des
rach·i·to·gen·ic
rad
ra·di·a·bil·i·ty
 pl ra·di·a·bil·i·ties
ra·di·al
ra·di·ant
ra·di·ate
 ra·di·at·ed
 ra·di·at·ing
ra·di·a·tion
rad·i·cal
ra·di·ces
 pl of radix
rad·i·cle
ra·dic·u·lar
ra·dic·u·li·tis
ra·dic·u·lop·a·thy
 pl ra·dic·u·lop·a·thies

ra·dii
 pl of radius
ra·dio·ac·tive
ra·dio·ac·tiv·i·ty
 pl ra·dio·ac·tiv·i·ties
ra·dio·al·ler·go·sor·
 bent
ra·dio·as·say
ra·dio·au·to·graph
ra·dio·au·to·graph·
 ic
ra·dio·au·tog·ra·
 phy
 pl ra·dio·au·tog·ra·
 phies
ra·dio·bi·o·log·i·cal
 also ra·dio·bi·o·log·ic
ra·dio·bi·o·log·i·
 cal·ly
ra·dio·bi·ol·o·gist
ra·dio·bi·ol·o·gy
 pl ra·dio·bi·ol·o·gies
ra·dio·car·bon
ra·dio·chem·i·cal
ra·dio·chem·ist
ra·dio·chem·is·try
 pl ra·dio·chem·is·tries
ra·dio·chro·mato·
 gram
ra·dio·chro·ma·to·
 graph·ic
ra·dio·chro·ma·tog·
 ra·phy
 pl ra·dio·chro·ma·tog·
 ra·phies
ra·dio·chro·mi·um
ra·dio·co·balt

ra·dio·col·loid
ra·dio·col·loi·dal
ra·dio·den·si·ty
  pl ra·dio·den·si·ties
ra·dio·der·ma·ti·tis
  pl ra·dio·der·ma·ti·
  tis·es
  or ra·dio·der·ma·tit·i·
  des
ra·dio·di·ag·no·sis
  pl ra·dio·di·ag·no·ses
ra·dio·el·e·ment
ra·dio·en·zy·mat·ic
ra·dio·en·zy·mat·i·
  cal·ly
ra·dio·fre·quen·cy
  pl ra·dio·fre·quen·
  cies
ra·dio·gen·ic
ra·dio·gold
ra·dio·gram
ra·dio·graph
ra·di·og·ra·pher
ra·dio·graph·ic
ra·dio·graph·i·cal·
  ly
ra·di·og·ra·phy
  pl ra·di·og·ra·phies
ra·dio·im·mu·no·
  as·say
ra·dio·im·mu·no·
  as·say·able
ra·dio·im·mu·no·
  elec·tro·pho·re·
  sis
  pl ra·dio·im·mu·no·
  elec·tro·pho·re·ses

ra·dio·im·mu·no·
  elec·tro·pho·ret·
  ic
ra·dio·im·mu·no·
  log·i·cal
  also ra·dio·im·mu·no·
  log·ic
ra·dio·io·din·at·ed
ra·dio·io·din·ation
ra·dio·io·dine
ra·dio·iron
ra·dio·iso·tope
ra·dio·iso·to·pic
ra·dio·iso·to·pi·cal·
  ly
ra·dio·la·bel
ra·dio·la·beled
  or ra·dio·la·belled
ra·dio·la·bel·ing
  or ra·dio·la·bel·
  ling
ra·dio·lead
ra·di·o·log·i·cal
  or ra·di·o·log·ic
ra·dio·log·i·cal·ly
ra·di·ol·o·gist
ra·di·ol·o·gy
  pl ra·di·ol·o·gies
ra·dio·lu·cen·cy
  pl ra·dio·lu·cen·cies
ra·dio·lu·cent
ra·di·ol·y·sis
  pl ra·di·ol·y·ses
ra·di·om·e·ter
ra·dio·met·ric
ra·dio·met·ri·cal·ly

ra·di·om·e·try
  pl ra·di·om·e·tries
ra·dio·mi·met·ic
ra·dio·ne·cro·sis
  pl ra·dio·ne·cro·ses
ra·dio·ne·crot·ic
ra·dio·nu·clide
ra·dio·opac·i·ty
  pl ra·dio·opac·i·ties
ra·di·opaque
ra·dio·par·ent
ra·dio·phar·ma·
  ceu·ti·cal
ra·dio·phos·pho·
  rus
ra·dio·pro·tec·tion
ra·dio·pro·tec·tive
ra·dio·pro·tec·tor
  also ra·dio·pro·tec·tor·
  ant
ra·dio·re·sis·tance
ra·dio·re·sis·tant
ra·dio·re·spi·ro·
  met·ric
ra·dio·sen·si·tive
ra·dio·sen·si·tiv·i·
  ty
  pl ra·dio·sen·si·tiv·i·
  ties
ra·dio·sen·si·ti·za·
  tion
ra·dio·sen·si·tiz·er
ra·dio·sen·si·tiz·ing
ra·dio·so·di·um
ra·dio·ster·il·iza·
  tion
ra·dio·ster·il·ized

ra·dio·stron·tium
ra·dio·sur·gery
  pl ra·dio·sur·ger·ies
ra·dio·tele·met·ric
ra·dio·te·lem·e·try
  pl ra·dio·te·lem·e·tries
ra·dio·ther·a·peut·ic
ra·dio·ther·a·peut·i·cal·ly
ra·dio·ther·a·pist
ra·dio·ther·a·py
  pl ra·dio·ther·a·pies
ra·dio·tho·ri·um
ra·dio·tox·emia
ra·dio·tox·ic·i·ty
  pl ra·dio·tox·ic·i·ties
ra·dio·trac·er
ra·dio·trans·par·ent
ra·dio·ul·nar
ra·di·um
ra·di·us
  pl ra·dii
  also ra·di·us·es
ra·dix
  pl ra·di·ces
  or ra·dix·es
ra·don
rad·u·la
  pl rad·u·lae
  also rad·u·las
rad·u·lar
raf·fi·nose
rag·sort·er's dis·ease

rag·weed
Rail·lie·ti·na
rale
Ra·man ef·fect
ram·i·fi·ca·tion
ram·i·fy
  ram·i·fied
  ram·i·fy·ing
ra·mose
Rams·den eye·piece
ram·u·lus
  pl ram·u·li
ra·mus
  pl ra·mi
ra·mus com·mu·ni·cans
  pl ra·mi com·mu·ni·can·tes
Ra·na
ran·cid
ran·cid·i·fy
  ran·cid·i·fied
  ran·cid·i·fy·ing
ran·cid·i·ty
  pl ran·cid·i·ties
ra·nine
ran·u·la
Ra·oult's law
rape
  raped
  rap·ing
rape·seed
ra·phe
  also rha·phe
rap·ist
rap·port

rap·tus
rar·efac·tion
rar·efac·tion·al
rar·efy
  also rar·i·fy
  rar·efied
    also rar·i·fied
  rar·efy·ing
    also rar·i·fy·ing
rash
ras·pa·to·ry
  pl ras·pa·to·ries
rat-bite fe·ver
Rath·ke's pouch
rat·i·cid·al
rat·i·cide
ra·tio
  pl ra·tios
ra·tion
  ra·tioned
  ra·tion·ing
ra·tio·nal
ra·tio·nal·i·ty
  pl ra·tio·nal·i·ties
ra·tio·nal·iza·tion
ra·tio·nal·ize
  ra·tio·nal·ized
  ra·tio·nal·iz·ing
ra·tio·nal·iz·er
rat·tle
rat·tle·snake
Rat·tus
rau·wol·fia
Ray·naud's dis·ease
re·ab·sorb
re·ab·sorp·tion

re·act
re·ac·tance
re·ac·tant
re·ac·tion
re·ac·ti·vate
  re·ac·ti·vat·ed
  re·ac·ti·vat·ing
re·ac·ti·va·tion
re·ac·tive
re·ac·tiv·i·ty
  pl re·ac·tiv·i·ties
re·ac·tor
re·ad·just
re·agent
re·ag·gre·gate
  re·ag·gre·gat·ed
  re·ag·gre·gat·ing
re·ag·gre·ga·tion
re·agin
re·agin·ic
re·al·i·ty
  pl re·al·i·ties
ream·er
re·am·pu·ta·tion
Re·au·mur
re·base
  re·based
  re·bas·ing
re·bound
re·cal·ci·fi·ca·tion
re·cal·ci·fied
re·cal·ci·trant
re·call
re·can·a·li·za·tion
re·can·a·lize
  re·can·a·lized
  re·can·a·liz·ing

re·ca·pit·u·la·tion
re·cep·tac·u·lum
  chy·li
re·cep·tive
re·cep·tiv·i·ty
  pl re·cep·tiv·i·ties
re·cep·tor
re·cess
re·ces·sion
re·ces·sive
re·ces·sus
re·cid·i·vate
  re·cid·i·vat·ed
  re·cid·i·vat·ing
re·cid·i·va·tion
re·cid·i·vism
re·cid·i·vist
re·cid·i·vis·tic
rec·i·pe
re·cip·i·ent
Reck·ling·hau·
  sen's dis·ease
re·com·bi·nant
re·com·bi·na·tion
re·com·bine
  re·com·bined
  re·com·bin·ing
Rec·om·mend·ed
  Dai·ly Al·low·
  ance
re·com·pres·sion
re·con
re·con·sti·tute
  re·con·sti·tut·ed
  re·con·sti·tut·ing
re·con·sti·tu·tion
re·con·struct

re·con·struc·tion
re·con·struc·tive
re·cov·er
  re·cov·ered
  re·cov·er·ing
re·cov·er·able
re·cov·ery
  pl re·cov·er·ies
re·cru·desce
  re·cru·desced
  re·cru·desc·ing
re·cru·des·cence
re·cru·des·cent
re·cruit·ment
re·crys·tal·li·za·
  tion
re·crys·tal·lize
  re·crys·tal·lized
  re·crys·tal·liz·ing
rec·ta
  pl of rectum
rec·tal
rec·ti
  pl of rectus
rec·ti·fi·ca·tion
rec·ti·fy
  rec·ti·fied
  rec·ti·fy·ing
rec·to·cele
rec·to·co·li·tis
rec·to·scope
rec·to·sig·moid
rec·to·ure·thral
rec·to·uter·ine
rec·to·vag·i·nal
rec·to·ves·i·cal

rec·tum
  pl rec·tums
  or rec·ta
rec·tus
  pl rec·ti
rec·tus ab·do·mi·nis
rec·tus ca·pi·tis pos·te·ri·or ma·jor
rec·tus ca·pi·tis pos·te·ri·or mi·nor
rec·tus fe·mo·ris
rec·tus in·fe·ri·or
rec·tus lat·e·ra·lis
rec·tus me·di·a·lis
rec·tus oc·u·li
rec·tus su·pe·ri·or
re·cum·bent
re·cu·per·ate
  re·cu·per·at·ed
  re·cu·per·at·ing
re·cu·per·a·tion
re·cu·per·a·tive
re·cur
  re·curred
  re·cur·ring
re·cur·rence
re·cur·rent
red·bird cac·tus
red-blind
red-green blind·ness
re·dia
  pl re·di·ae
  also re·di·as

re·di·al
red·in·te·gra·tion
red·in·te·gra·tive
re·dis·solve
  re·dis·solved
  re·dis·solv·ing
red·out
re·dox
re·duce
  re·duced
  re·duc·ing
re·duc·i·bil·i·ty
  pl re·duc·i·bil·i·ties
re·duc·ible
re·duc·tant
re·duc·tase
re·duc·tion
re·duc·tive
re·dun·dant
re·du·pli·cate
  re·du·pli·cat·ed
  re·du·pli·cat·ing
re·du·pli·ca·tion
re·du·vi·id
Red·u·vi·idae
Re·du·vi·us
Reed-Stern·berg cell
re·ed·u·cate
  re·ed·u·cat·ed
  re·ed·u·cat·ing
re·ed·u·ca·tion
re·en·try
  pl re·en·tries
re·ex·plo·ra·tion
re·fec·tion

re·fer
  re·ferred
  re·fer·ring
re·fer·able
  also re·fer·rable
ref·er·ence
re·fer·ral
re·fill
re·fill·able
re·fine
  re·fined
  re·fin·ing
re·flect
re·flec·tance
re·flec·tion
re·flec·tor
re·flex
re·flex·ive
re·flexo·gen·ic
  or re·flex·og·e·nous
re·flex·ol·o·gist
re·flex·ol·o·gy
  pl re·flex·ol·o·gies
re·flux
re·fract
re·frac·tile
re·frac·tion
re·frac·tion·ist
re·frac·tive
re·frac·tiv·i·ty
  pl re·frac·tiv·i·ties
re·frac·tom·e·ter
re·frac·to·met·ric
re·frac·tom·e·try
  pl re·frac·tom·e·tries
re·frac·to·ri·ness
re·frac·to·ry

re·frac·ture
  re·frac·tured
  re·frac·tur·ing
re·fran·gi·bil·i·ty
  pl re·fran·gi·bil·i·ties
re·frig·er·ant
re·frig·er·a·tion
re·frin·gent
Ref·sum's dis·ease
re·gen·er·a·ble
re·gen·er·ate
  re·gen·er·at·ed
  re·gen·er·at·ing
re·gen·er·a·tion
re·gen·er·a·tive
re·gime
reg·i·men
re·gion
re·gion·al
reg·is·tered
reg·is·trar
reg·is·try
  pl reg·is·tries
re·gress
re·gres·sion
re·gres·sive
reg·u·lar
reg·u·lar·i·ty
  pl reg·u·lar·i·ties
reg·u·late
  reg·u·lat·ed
  reg·u·lat·ing
reg·u·la·tion
reg·u·la·tive
reg·u·la·tor
reg·u·la·tory
re·gur·gi·tant

re·gur·gi·tate
  re·gur·gi·tat·ed
  re·gur·gi·tat·ing
re·gur·gi·ta·tion
re·hab
re·ha·bil·i·tant
re·ha·bil·i·tate
  re·ha·bil·i·tat·ed
  re·ha·bil·i·tat·ing
re·ha·bil·i·ta·tion
re·ha·bil·i·ta·tive
re·ha·bil·i·tee
Reh·fuss tube
re·hy·drate
  re·hy·drat·ed
  re·hy·drat·ing
re·hy·dra·tion
Rei·chert-Meissl
  num·ber
Rei·chert val·ue
re·im·plant
re·im·plan·ta·tion
rei·nec·kate
Rei·nec·ke salt
re·in·fec·tion
re·in·force
  re·in·forced
  re·in·forc·ing
re·in·force·able
re·in·force·ment
re·in·forc·er
re·in·ner·vate
  re·in·ner·vat·ed
  re·in·ner·vat·ing
re·in·ner·va·tion

re·in·oc·u·late
  re·in·oc·u·lat·ed
  re·in·oc·u·lat·ing
re·in·oc·u·la·tion
re·in·te·grate
  re·in·te·grat·ed
  re·in·te·grat·ing
re·in·te·gra·tion
re·in·te·gra·tive
Reiss·ner's mem·
  brane
Rei·ter's syn·
  drome
re·ject
re·jec·tion
re·lapse
  re·lapsed
  re·laps·ing
re·late
  re·lat·ed
  re·lat·ing
re·la·tion
re·la·tion·al
re·la·tion·ship
re·lax
re·lax·ant
re·lax·ation
re·lax·in
re·leas·er
re·li·a·bil·i·ty
  pl re·li·a·bil·i·ties
re·li·a·ble
re·lief
re·lieve
  re·lieved
  re·liev·ing
re·liev·er

Re·mak's fi·ber
re·me·di·a·ble
re·me·di·al
re·me·di·a·tion
rem·e·dy
　pl rem·e·dies
rem·e·dy
　rem·e·died
　rem·e·dy·ing
re·min·er·al·iza·
　tion
re·mis·sion
re·mit
　re·mit·ted
　re·mit·ting
re·mit·tent
REM sleep
re·nal
re·na·tur·a·tion
re·na·ture
　re·na·tured
　re·na·tur·ing
Ren·du-Os·ler-We·
　ber dis·ease
re·nin
　enzyme of the kidney
　(see rennin)

ren·net
ren·nin
　milk-coagulating
　enzyme (see renin)

re·no·gram
re·no·graph·ic
re·nog·ra·phy
　pl re·nog·ra·phies
re·no·pri·val
re·no·re·nal

re·no·tro·pic
　or re·no·tro·phic
re·no·vas·cu·lar
Ren·shaw cell
reo·vi·rus
re·pair
re·pand
re·par·a·tive
re·peat
re·pel·lent
　also re·pel·lant
rep·e·ti·tion
re·plant
re·plan·ta·tion
re·ple·tion
rep·li·ca·ble
rep·li·case
rep·li·cate
　rep·li·cat·ed
　rep·li·cat·ing
rep·li·ca·tion
rep·li·ca·tive
rep·li·con
re·po·lar·iza·tion
re·po·lar·ize
　re·po·lar·ized
　re·po·lar·iz·ing
re·port·able
re·po·si·tion
re·pos·i·to·ry
re·press
re·press·ibil·i·ty
　pl re·press·ibil·i·ties
re·press·ible
re·pres·sion
re·pres·sive
re·pres·sor

re·pro·duce
　re·pro·duced
　re·pro·duc·ing
re·pro·duc·tion
re·pro·duc·tive
re·pul·sion
res·azur·in
res·cin·na·mine
re·sect
re·sect·abil·i·ty
　pl re·sect·abil·i·ties
re·sect·able
re·sec·tion
re·sec·to·scope
re·ser·pine
re·ser·pin·iza·tion
re·ser·pin·ized
re·serve
res·er·voir
res·i·den·cy
　pl res·i·den·cies
res·i·dent
re·sid·u·al
res·i·due
re·sid·u·um
　pl re·sid·ua
　also re·sid·u·ums
re·sil·ience
re·sil·ien·cy
　pl re·sil·ien·cies
re·sil·ient
res·in
res·in·ous
re·sist·ance
re·sis·tant
　also re·sist·ent

re·sis·tiv·i·ty
  pl re·sis·tiv·i·ties
re·so·cial·iza·tion
res·o·lu·tion
re·solv·able
re·solve
  re·solved
  re·solv·ing
re·sol·vent
res·o·nance
res·o·nant
re·sorb
res·or·cin
res·or·cin·ol
re·sorp·tion
re·sorp·tive
re·spi·ra·ble
res·pi·ra·tion
res·pi·ra·tor
res·pi·ra·to·ry
re·spire
  re·spired
  re·spir·ing
res·pi·rom·e·ter
res·pi·ro·met·ric
res·pi·rom·e·try
  pl res·pi·rom·e·tries
re·spond
re·spon·dent
re·spond·er
re·sponse
res·ti·form
res·to·ra·tion
re·stor·ative
re·store
  re·stored
  re·stor·ing

re·straint
re·stric·tion
re·sus·ci·tate
  re·sus·ci·tat·ed
  re·sus·ci·tat·ing
re·sus·ci·ta·tion
re·sus·ci·ta·tive
re·sus·ci·ta·tor
re·syn·the·sis
  pl re·syn·the·ses
re·syn·the·size
  re·syn·the·sized
  re·syn·the·siz·ing
re·tain
re·tain·er
re·tar·date
re·tar·da·tion
re·tard·ed
re·te
  pl re·tia
re·ten·tion
re·te tes·tis
  pl re·tia tes·ti·um
re·tia
  pl of rete
re·tic·u·la
  pl of reticulum
re·tic·u·lar
re·tic·u·lin
re·tic·u·lo·cyte
re·tic·u·lo·cyt·ic
re·tic·u·lo·cy·to·pe·nia
re·tic·u·lo·cy·to·sis
  pl re·tic·u·lo·cy·to·ses
re·tic·u·lo·en·do·the·li·al

re·tic·u·lo·en·do·the·li·o·sis
  pl re·tic·u·lo·en·do·the·li·o·ses
re·tic·u·lo·en·do·the·li·um
  pl re·tic·u·lo·en·do·the·lia
re·tic·u·lo·sar·co·ma
  pl re·tic·u·lo·sar·co·mas
  or re·tic·u·lo·sar·co·ma·ta
re·tic·u·lo·sis
  pl re·tic·u·lo·ses
re·tic·u·lo·spi·nal
re·tic·u·lum
  pl re·tic·u·la
ret·i·na
  pl ret·i·nas
  or ret·i·nae
ret·i·nac·u·lum
  pl ret·i·nac·u·la
ret·i·nal
ret·i·nene
ret·i·ni·tis
  pl re·ti·ni·ti·des
ret·i·ni·tis pig·men·to·sa
ret·i·ni·tis pro·lif·er·ans
ret·i·no·blas·to·ma
  pl ret·i·no·blas·to·mas
  or ret·i·no·blas·to·ma·ta
ret·i·no·cho·roid·i·tis

ret·i·no·ic
ret·i·noid
ret·i·nol
ret·i·nop·a·thy
  pl ret·i·nop·a·thies
ret·i·nos·chi·sis
  pl ret·i·nos·chi·ses
ret·i·no·scope
ret·i·no·scop·ic
ret·i·nos·co·py
  pl ret·i·nos·co·pies
ret·i·no·tec·tal
re·tort
re·tract
re·trac·tile
re·trac·tion
re·trac·tor
ret·ro·ac·tive
ret·ro·bul·bar
ret·ro·ca·val
ret·ro·cli·na·tion
ret·ro·fec·tion
ret·ro·flex·ion
ret·ro·gnath·ic
ret·ro·gnath·ism
ret·ro·grade
ret·ro·gres·sion
ret·ro·gres·sive
ret·ro·len·tal
ret·ro·len·tic·u·lar
ret·ro·lin·gual
ret·ro·man·dib·u·
  lar
ret·ro·mo·lar
ret·ro-or·bit·al
ret·ro·per·i·to·ne·al

ret·ro·per·i·to·ne·
  um
  pl ret·ro·per·i·to·ne·
    ums
  or ret·ro·per·i·to·nea
ret·ro·pha·ryn·geal
ret·ro·pu·bic
ret·ro·pul·sion
ret·ro·spec·tive
ret·ro·stal·sis
  pl ret·ro·stal·ses
ret·ro·stal·tic
ret·ro·ster·nal
ret·ro·ver·sion
ret·ro·vi·ral
ret·ro·vi·rus
re·trude
  re·trud·ed
  re·trud·ing
re·tru·sion
re·tru·sive
re·up·take
re·vac·ci·na·tion
re·vas·cu·lar·iza·
  tion
re·verse tran·scrip·
  tase
re·vers·ibil·i·ty
  pl re·vers·ibil·i·ties
re·vers·ible
re·vers·ibly
re·ver·sion
re·ver·tant
re·viv·able
re·vive
  re·vived
  re·viv·ing

re·viv·i·fi·ca·tion
re·ward
Reye's syn·drome
  also Reye syn·drome
R fac·tor
rhab·dit·i·form
Rhab·di·tis
rhab·di·toid
rhab·do·my·ol·y·sis
  pl rhab·do·my·ol·y·
    ses
rhab·do·my·o·ma
  pl rhab·do·my·o·mas
  or rhab·do·my·o·ma·
    ta
rhab·do·myo·sar·
  co·ma
  pl rhab·do·myo·sar·
    co·mas
  or rhab·do·myo·sar·
    co·ma·ta
rhab·do·vi·rus
rha·chi·tis
  var of rachitis
rhag·a·des
rham·nose
rham·no·side
Rham·nus
rha·phe
  var of raphe
rhat·a·ny
  pl rhat·a·nies
rhe·ni·um
rheo·base
rheo·ba·sic
rhe·ol·o·gy
  pl rhe·ol·o·gies
rheo·stat

rheo·stat·ic

rheo·tax·is
  pl rheo·tax·es

rhe·ot·ro·pism

rhe·sus mon·key

rheum

Rhe·um

rheu·mat·ic

rheu·ma·tism

rheu·ma·toid

rheu·ma·tol·o·gist

rheu·ma·tol·o·gy
  pl rheu·ma·tol·o·gies

rheumy

rhex·is
  pl rhex·es

Rh fac·tor

rhi·nal

rhin·en·ce·pha·lic

rhin·en·ceph·a·lon
  pl rhin·en·ceph·a·la

rhi·ni·tis
  pl rhi·nit·i·des

rhi·no·gen·ic

rhi·no·la·lia

rhi·no·lith

rhi·nol·o·gist

rhi·nol·o·gy
  pl rhi·nol·o·gies

rhi·no·pha·ryn·
  geal

rhi·no·phar·yn·gi·
  tis
  pl rhi·no·phar·yn·git·
  i·des

rhi·no·phy·ma
  pl rhi·no·phy·mas
  or rhi·no·phy·ma·ta

rhi·no·plas·tic

rhi·no·plas·ty
  pl rhi·no·plas·ties

rhi·nor·rhea

rhi·no·scle·ro·ma
  pl rhi·no·scle·ro·ma·
  ta

rhi·no·scop·ic

rhi·nos·co·py
  pl rhi·nos·co·pies

rhi·no·spo·rid·i·o·
  sis
  pl rhi·no·spo·rid·i·o·
  ses

rhi·no·spo·rid·i·um
  pl rhi·no·spo·rid·ia

rhi·not·o·my
  pl rhi·not·o·mies

rhi·no·tra·che·itis

rhi·no·vi·rus

Rhipi·ceph·a·lus

rhi·zoid

rhi·zoi·dal

rhi·zo·ma·tous

rhi·zome

rhi·zo·plast

rhi·zo·pod

Rhi·zop·o·da

rhi·zo·pus

rhi·zot·o·my
  pl rhi·zot·o·mies

Rh-neg·a·tive

rho·da·mine

rho·da·nese

rho·di·um

Rhod·ni·us

rho·dop·sin

Rho·do·tor·u·la

rhomb·en·ceph·a·
  lon

rhom·boi·de·us
  pl rhom·boi·dei

rhon·chus
  pl rhon·chi

rho·ta·cism

Rh-pos·i·tive

rhu·barb

rhus
  pl rhus·es
  or rhus

rhythm

rhyth·mic
  or rhyth·mi·cal

rhyth·mic·i·ty
  pl rhyth·mic·i·ties

rhyt·i·dec·to·my
  pl rhyt·i·dec·to·mies

ri·ba·vi·rin

ri·bi·tol

ri·bo·fla·vin
  also ri·bo·fla·vine

ri·bo·nu·cle·ase

ri·bo·nu·cle·ic

ri·bo·nu·cleo·pro·
  tein

ri·bo·nu·cle·o·side

ri·bo·nu·cle·o·tide

ri·bose

ri·bo·side

ri·bo·som·al

ri·bo·some

ri·cin
ri·cin·ole·ic
ric·i·nus
rick·ets
rick·etts·emia
rick·ett·sia
  pl rick·ett·sias
  or rick·ett·si·ae
  also rick·ett·sia
Rick·ett·si·a·ce·ae
Rick·ett·si·al
Rick·ett·si·a·les
rick·ett·si·al·pox
rick·ett·si·ol·o·gy
  pl rick·ett·si·ol·o·gies
rick·ett·si·o·sis
  pl rick·ett·si·o·ses
rick·ett·sio·stat·ic
rick·ety
Ri·de·al-Walk·er
  test
ridge·ling
  or ridg·ling
Rie·del's dis·ease
ri·fam·pin
  or ri·fam·pi·cin
rif·a·my·cin
Rift Val·ley fe·ver
Riggs' dis·ease
right-eyed
right-hand·ed
ri·gid·i·ty
  pl ri·gid·i·ties
rig·or
rig·or mor·tis
ri·ma
  pl ri·mae

ri·ma glot·ti·dis
rin·der·pest
ring·bone
Ring·er's so·lu·tion
  also Ring·er so·lu·tion
ring·hals
ring·worm
Rin·ne's test
  or Rin·ne test
ri·so·ri·us
  pl ri·so·rii
ris·to·ce·tin
ri·sus sar·do·ni·cus
rit·o·drine
RNase
  or RNA·ase
Rob·ert·so·ni·an
Rob·i·son es·ter
Ro·chelle salt
Rocky Moun·tain
  spot·ted fe·ver
ro·dent
Ro·den·tia
ro·den·ti·ci·dal
ro·den·ti·cide
rod of Cor·ti
roent·gen
  also rönt·gen
roent·gen·ky·mo·
  graph·ic
roent·gen·ky·mog·
  ra·phy
  pl roent·gen·ky·mog·
  ra·phies
roent·gen·o·gram
roent·gen·o·graph

roent·gen·o·graph·
  ic
roent·gen·o·graph·
  i·cal·ly
roent·gen·og·ra·
  phy
  pl roent·gen·og·ra·
  phies
roent·gen·o·log·ic
  or roent·gen·o·log·i·
  cal
roent·gen·ol·o·gist
roent·gen·ol·o·gy
  pl roent·gen·ol·o·gies
roent·gen·o·scope
roent·gen·o·scop·ic
roent·gen·os·co·py
  pl roent·gen·os·co·
  pies
roent·gen·ther·a·py
  pl roent·gen·ther·a·
  pies
Rog·er·ian
Ro·lan·dic
rolf
rolf·er
rolf·ing
ro·li·tet·ra·cy·cline
Ro·ma·now·sky
  stain
  or Ro·ma·now·sky's
  stain
  also Ro·ma·nov·sky
  stain
  or Ro·ma·nov·sky's
  stain
Rom·berg's sign
  or Rom·berg sign

Rom·berg's test
 or Rom·berg test

ron·geur
ron·nel
rönt·gen
 var of roentgen
room·ing-in
root·ed
root·let
rop·i·ness
ropy
 also rop·ey
 rop·i·er
 rop·i·est

Ror·schach
ro·sa·cea
ros·an·i·line
ro·sa·ry pea
rose ben·gal
ro·se·o·la
ro·se·o·la in·fan·
 tum
ro·se·o·lar
ro·sette
ros·in
ro·sol·ic
ros·tel·lum
ros·trad
ros·tral
ros·trum
 pl ros·trums
 or ros·tra

ro·ta·me·ter
ro·ta·tion
ro·ta·tion·al

ro·ta·tor
 pl ro·ta·tors
 or ro·ta·to·res
ro·ta·vi·rus
ro·te·none
Rou·get cell
rough·age
rou·leau
 pl rou·leaux
 or rou·leaus

round-shoul·dered
round·worm
Rous sar·co·ma
ru·be·an·ic
ru·be·fa·cient
ru·bel·la
ru·be·o·la
ru·be·o·lar
ru·bid·i·um
Ru·bin test
ru·bor
ru·bri·blast
ru·bri·cyte
ru·bro·spi·nal
ru·di·ment
ru·di·men·ta·ry
Ruf·fi·ni's cor·pus·
 cle
 or Ruf·fi·ni cor·pus·
 cle

ru·ga
 pl ru·gae
ru·gos·i·ty
 pl ru·gos·i·ties

ru·men
 pl ru·mi·na
 or ru·mens

ru·men·ot·o·my
 pl ru·men·ot·o·mies
ru·mi·nal
ru·mi·nant
ru·mi·nate
 ru·mi·nat·ed
 ru·mi·nat·ing
ru·mi·na·tion
ru·mi·na·tive
Rum·pel-Leede
 test
ru·pia
ru·pi·al
rup·ture
 rup·tured
 rup·tur·ing
ru·the·ni·um
ruth·er·ford
ru·tin
ru·tin·ose
R wave

S

sab·a·dil·la
Sa·bin vac·cine
sab·u·lous
sac
sac·cade
sac·cad·ic
sac·cate
sac·cha·rase
sac·cha·rate
sac·cha·rat·ed
sac·char·ic
sac·cha·ride
sac·cha·rif·er·ous

sac·char·i·fi·ca·tion
sac·char·i·fy
  sac·char·i·fied
  sac·char·i·fy·ing
sac·char·im·e·ter
sac·char·i·met·ric
sac·cha·rim·e·try
  pl sac·cha·rim·e·tries
sac·cha·rin
sac·cha·rine
sac·cha·ro·gen·ic
sac·cha·ro·lyt·ic
sac·cha·rom·e·ter
Sac·cha·ro·my·ces
Sac·cha·ro·my·ce·
  ta·ce·ae
sac·cha·rose
sac·ci·form
sac·cu·lar
sac·cu·lat·ed
  also sac·cu·late
sac·cu·la·tion
sac·cule
sac·cu·lus
  pl sac·cu·li
sac·cus
  pl sac·ci
sa·cra
  pl of sacrum
sa·cral
sa·cral·iza·tion
sa·cro·coc·cy·geal
sa·cro·coc·cy·ge·us
  dor·sa·lis
sa·cro·coc·cy·ge·us
  ven·tra·lis
sa·cro·il·i·ac

sa·cro·il·i·i·tis
sa·cro·spi·na·lis
sa·cro·spi·nous
sa·cro·tu·ber·ous
sa·cro·uter·ine
sa·crum
  pl sa·cra
sad·dle·nose
sa·dism
sa·dist
sa·dis·tic
sa·dis·ti·cal·ly
sa·do·mas·och·ism
sa·do·mas·och·ist
sa·do·mas·och·ist·
  ic
safe·ty
  pl safe·ties
saf·flow·er
saf·fron
saf·ra·nine
  or saf·ra·nin
saf·role
  also saf·rol
sag·it·tal
sa·go
  pl sa·gos
Saint An·tho·ny's
  fire
Saint-Ig·na·tius's-
  bean
Saint Lou·is en·
  ceph·a·li·tis
Saint Vi·tus' dance
  also Saint Vi·tus's
  dance
sal·abra·sion

sal am·mo·ni·ac
sal·bu·ta·mol
sa·lep
sal·i·cin
sal·i·cyl·al·de·hyde
sal·i·cyl·amide
sal·i·cyl·an·il·ide
sa·lic·y·late
sa·lic·y·lat·ed
sal·i·cyl·azo·sul·fa·
  pyr·i·dine
sal·i·cyl·ic
sal·i·cyl·ism
sal·i·cyl·uric
sa·lim·e·ter
sa·line
sa·lin·i·ty
  pl sa·lin·i·ties
sa·li·va
sal·i·vary
sal·i·vate
  sal·i·vat·ed
  sal·i·vat·ing
sal·i·va·tion
sal·i·va·to·ry
Salk vac·cine
sal·mine
sal·mo·nel·la
  pl sal·mo·nel·lae
  or sal·mo·nel·las
  or sal·mo·nel·la
sal·mo·nel·lal
sal·mo·nel·lo·sis
  pl sal·mo·nel·lo·ses
sal·ol
sa·lom·e·ter

sal·pin·gec·to·my
  pl sal·pin·gec·to·mies

sal·pin·gi·tis
  pl sal·pin·gi·tis·es

sal·pin·gog·ra·phy
  pl sal·pin·gog·ra·phies

sal·pin·gol·y·sis
  pl sal·pin·gol·y·ses

sal·pin·go-oo·pho·rec·to·my
  pl sal·pin·go-oo·pho·rec·to·mies

sal·pin·go-oo·pho·ri·tis

sal·pin·go·pha·ryn·ge·us

sal·pin·gos·to·my
  pl sal·pin·gos·to·mies

sal·ta·to·ry

salt·pe·ter

sa·lu·bri·ous

sa·lu·bri·ty
  pl sa·lu·bri·ties

sal·uret·ic

sal·uret·i·cal·ly

sal·u·tary

sal·via

sal vo·la·ti·le

sa·mar·i·um

sam·ple

san·a·to·ri·um
  pl san·a·to·ri·ums
  or san·a·to·ria

sand·fly fe·ver

Sand·hoff-Jatz·ke·witz dis·ease

Sand·hoff's dis·ease
  or Sand·hoff dis·ease

san·gui·nar·ia

san·guin·a·rine

san·guine

san·guin·e·ous

san·guin·o·lent

san·gui·no·pu·ru·lent

san·i·tar·i·an

san·i·tari·ly

san·i·tar·i·um
  pl san·i·tar·i·ums
  or san·i·tar·ia

san·i·tary

san·i·tate
  san·i·tat·ed
  san·i·tat·ing

san·i·ta·tion

san·i·ti·za·tion

san·i·tize
  san·i·tized
  san·i·tiz·ing

san·i·to·ri·um
  pl san·i·to·ri·ums
  or san·i·to·ria

san·i·ty
  pl san·i·ties

San Joa·quin fe·ver

San Joa·quin val·ley fe·ver

S-A node

san·ta·lol

san·ton·i·ca

san·to·nin

San·to·ri·ni's duct

sa·phe·na

sa·phe·no·fem·o·ral

sa·phe·nous

sap·id

sa·po
  pl sa·pos

sa·po·ge·nin

sap·o·na·ceous

sap·o·nat·ed

sa·pon·i·fi·able

sa·pon·i·fi·ca·tion

sa·pon·i·fy
  sa·pon·i·fied
  sa·pon·i·fy·ing

sa·po·nin

sap·o·tox·in

sap·phic

sap·phism

sap·phist

sa·pre·mia

sa·proph·i·lous

sap·ro·phyte

sap·ro·phyt·ic

sap·ro·phyt·i·cal·ly

sap·ro·zo·ic

sar·al·a·sin

sar·ci·na
  pl sar·ci·nas
  or sar·ci·nae

sar·co·blast

sar·co·cyst

sar·co·cys·tis
  pl sar·co·cys·tis
  or sar·co·cys·tis·es

Sar·co·di·na

scalpel

sar·co·din·i·an
sar·coid
sar·coid·o·sis
  pl sar·coid·o··ses

sar·co·lac·tic
sar·co·lem·ma
sar·co·lem·mal
sar·co·ly·sin
  or sar·co·ly·sine

sar·co·ma
  pl sar·co·mas
  or sar·co·ma·ta

sar·co·ma·gen·ic
sar·co·ma·to·sis
  pl sar·co·ma·to·ses

sar·co·ma·tous
sar·co·mere
sar·co·mer·ic
Sar·coph·a·ga
sar·coph·a·gid
sar·co·plasm
sar·co·plas·mic
  also sar·co·plas·mat·ic

Sar·cop·tes
sar·cop·tic
sar·cop·ti·cide
Sar·cop·ti·dae
Sar·cop·toi·dea
sar·co·sine
sar·co·som·al
sar·co·some
Sar·co·spo·rid·ia
sar·co·spo·rid·ian
sar·co·spo·rid·i·o·
  sis
  pl sar·co·spo·rid·i·o·
    ses

sar·co·tu·bu·lar
sar·don·ic laugh
sa·rin
sar·men·to·cy·ma·
  rin
sar·men·to·gen·in
sar·men·tose
sar·sa·pa·ril·la
sar·sa·sap·o·gen·in
sar·sa·sap·o·nin
  also sar·sap·o·nin

sar·to·ri·us
  pl sar·to·rii

sat·el·lite
sat·el·lit·ed
sat·el·lit·ism
sat·el·lit·o·sis
  pl sat·el·lit·o·ses

sa·ti·ety
  pl sa·ti·eties

sat·u·ra·ble
sat·u·rate
  sat·u·rat·ed
  sat·u·rat·ing
sat·u·ra·tion
sat·ur·nine
sat·urn·ism
sa·ty·ri·a·sis
  pl sa·ty·ri·a·ses

sau·cer·iza·tion
sau·cer·ize
  sau·cer·ized
  sau·cer·iz·ing
sav·in
saxi·tox·in

scab·by
scab·bi·er
scab·bi·est
sca·bi·ci·dal
sca·bi·cide
sca·bies
  pl sca·bies

sca·bi·et·ic
  also sca·bet·ic

sca·la
  pl sca·lae

sca·la me·dia
  pl sca·lae me·di·ae

sca·la tym·pa·ni
  pl sca·lae tym·pa·no·
    rum

sca·la ves·tib·u·li
  pl sca·lae ves·tib·u·lo·
    rum

scald·ed-skin syn·
  drome
scale
  scaled
  scal·ing
sca·lene
sca·le·not·o·my
  also sca·le·ni·ot·o·my
  pl sca·le·not·o·mies
  also sca·le·ni·ot·o·
    mies

sca·le·nus
  pl sca·le·ni

sca·le·nus an·ti·cus
sca·le·nus me·di·us
scal·er
scal·i·ness
scal·pel

scaly
  scal·i·er
  scal·i·est
scam·mo·ny
  pl scam·mo·nies
scan·di·um
scan·ner
Scan·zo·ni ma·neu·ver
  also Scan·zo·ni's ma·neu·ver
sca·pha
scaph·o·ceph·a·ly
  pl scaph·o·ceph·a·lies
scaph·oid
scap·u·la
  pl scap·u·lae
  or scap·u·las
scap·u·lar
scarf·skin
scar·i·fi·ca·tion
scar·i·fy
  scar·i·fied
  scar·i·fy·ing
scar·la·ti·na
scar·la·ti·nal
scar·la·ti·ni·form
scar·la·ti·no·gen·ic
scar·let fe·ver
Scar·pa's fas·cia
Scar·pa's fo·ra·men
Scar·pa's tri·an·gle
scat·o·log·i·cal
  also scat·o·log·ic
sca·tol·o·gy
  pl sca·tol·o·gies

sca·toph·a·gy
  pl sca·toph·a·gies
scat·ter
scat·ter·ing
Scha·fer meth·od
  or Schae·fer meth·od
  also Scha·fer's meth·od
Scham·berg's dis·ease
Schar·ding·er dex·trin
Schar·ding·er en·zyme
Schatz·ki ring
Schee·le's green
Scheie syn·drome
sche·ma
  pl sche·ma·ta
  also sche·mas
sche·mat·ic
sche·mat·i·cal·ly
Scheuer·mann's dis·ease
Schick test
Schiff re·ac·tion
Schiff's re·agent
  or Schiff re·agent
Schil·der's dis·ease
Schil·der's en·ceph·a·li·tis
Schil·ler's test
Schil·ling in·dex
Schil·ling test
Schim·mel·busch's dis·ease

schin·dy·le·sis
  pl schin·dy·le·ses
schis·to·cyte
schis·to·so·ma
schis·to·so·mal
Schis·to·so·mat·i·dae
Schis·to·so·ma·toi·dea
schis·to·some
schis·to·so·mi·a·sis
  pl schis·to·so·mi·a·ses
schis·to·so·mi·a·sis hae·ma·to·bi·um
schis·to·so·mi·a·sis ja·pon·i·ca
schis·to·so·mi·a·sis man·soni
Schis·to·so·moph·o·ra
schis·to·som·u·lum
  pl schis·to·som·u·la
schizo
  pl schiz·os
schizo·af·fec·tive
schi·zog·o·nous
  or schizo·gon·ic
schi·zog·o·ny
  pl schi·zog·o·nies
schiz·oid
schiz·oid·ism
Schizo·my·ce·tes
schiz·ont
schi·zon·ti·ci·dal
schi·zon·ti·cide
schizo·pha·sia
schizo·phrene

schizo·phre·nia
schizo·phren·ic
schiz·o·phren·i·
form
schiz·o·phreno·
gen·ic
schizo·thy·mic
Schizo·tryp·a·num
Schlemm's ca·nal
Schön·lein-Hen·
och
Schön·lein's dis·
ease
schra·dan
Schuff·ner's dots
Schül·ler-Chris·
tian dis·ease
Schwann cell
schwan·no·ma
 pl schwan·no·mas
 or schwan·no·ma·ta
sci·at·ic
sci·at·i·ca
sci·ence
sci·en·tif·ic
sci·en·tif·i·cal·ly
sci·en·tist
scil·li·ro·side
scin·ti·gram
scin·ti·graph·ic
scin·tig·ra·phy
 pl scin·tig·ra·phies
scin·til·late
 scin·til·lat·ed
 scin·til·lat·ing
scin·til·la·tion
scin·til·la·tor

scin·til·lom·e·ter
scin·ti·scan
scin·ti·scan·ner
scin·ti·scan·ning
scir·rhoid
scir·rhous
scir·rhus
 pl scir·rhi
scis·sile
scis·sion
scis·sors
sclera
scler·al
scle·rec·to·my
 pl scle·rec·to·mies
scle·re·ma neo·na·
to·rum
scle·ri·tis
sclero·cor·ne·al
sclero·dac·tyl·ia
sclero·dac·ty·ly
 pl sclero·dac·ty·lies
sclero·der·ma
 pl sclero·der·mas
 or sclero·der·ma·ta
sclero·der·ma·tous
sclero·ker·a·ti·tis
 pl sclero·ker·a·tit·i·
 des
scle·ro·ma
 pl scle·ro·mas
 or scle·ro·ma·ta
sclero·pro·tein
scle·rose
 scle·rosed
 scle·ros·ing

scle·ro·sis
 pl scle·ro·ses
scle·ro·stome
sclero·ther·a·py
 pl sclero·ther·a·pies
scle·rot·ic
scle·ro·tium
 pl scle·ro·tia
sclero·tome
sclero·tom·ic
scle·rot·o·my
 pl scle·rot·o·mies
sco·lex
 pl sco·li·ces
 also scol·e·ces
 or sco·lex·es
sco·li·o·sis
 pl sco·li·o·ses
sco·li·ot·ic
scom·broid
sco·po·la
sco·pol·amine
sco·po·le·tin
sco·po·phil·ia
 or scop·to·phil·ia
sco·po·phil·i·ac
 or scop·to·phil·i·ac
sco·po·phil·ic
 or scop·to·phil·ic
scor·bu·tic
scor·bu·tus
scor·pi·on
sco·to·ma
 pl sco·to·mas
 or sco·to·ma·ta
sco·to·pic
scra·pie

screw·worm
scrof·u·la
scrof·u·lo·der·ma
scrof·u·lous
scro·tal
scro·to·cele
scro·to·plas·ty
 pl scro·to·plas·ties
scro·tum
 pl scro·ta
 or scro·tums

scrub
 scrubbed
 scrub·bing
scru·ple
scurf
scurfy
scur·vy
 pl scur·vies
scu·tu·lum
 pl scu·tu·la
scyb·a·lous
scyb·a·lum
 pl scyb·a·la

Scyph·o·zoa
scyph·o·zo·an
seal·ant
sea on·ion
sea·sick·ness
seat·worm
se·ba·ceous
seb·or·rhea
seb·or·rhe·al
seb·or·rhe·ic
se·bum
seco·bar·bi·tal
sec·ond·ary

sec·ond-de·gree
 burn
se·cre·ta·gogue
 also se·cre·to·gogue

se·crete
 se·cret·ed
 se·cret·ing
se·cre·tin
se·cre·tion
se·cre·to·gogue
 var of secretagogue

se·cre·tor
se·cre·to·ry
sec·tion
 sec·tioned
 sec·tion·ing
se·cun·di·grav·i·da
 pl se·cun·di·grav·i·
 das
 or se·cun·di·grav·i·
 dae

sec·un·dines
sec·un·dip·a·ra
 pl sec·un·dip·a·ras
 or sec·un·dip·a·rae
se·date
 se·dat·ed
 se·dat·ing
se·da·tion
sed·a·tive
sed·i·ment
sed·i·ment·able
sed·i·men·ta·tion
se·do·hep·tose
se·do·hep·tu·lose
seg·ment
seg·men·tal

seg·men·ta·tion
seg·men·tec·to·my
 pl seg·men·tec·to·
 mies

seg·ment·ed
seg·ment·er
Seg·men·ti·na
seg·re·gant
seg·re·gate
 seg·re·gat·ed
 seg·re·gat·ing
seg·re·ga·tion
seg·re·gat·or
Seid·litz pow·ders
Sei·gnette salt
 or Sei·gnette's salt

sei·zure
sel·a·chyl
se·lec·tion
se·lec·tion·ist
se·lec·tive
se·lec·tiv·i·ty
 pl se·lec·tiv·i·ties

sel·e·nif·er·ous
se·le·ni·ous
se·le·ni·um
se·len·odont
sel·e·no·sis
self-abuse
self-anal·y·sis
 pl self-anal·y·ses

self-an·a·lyt·i·cal
 or self-an·a·lyt·ic
self-as·sem·bly
 pl self-as·sem·blies

self-aware·ness
self-con·cept

self-dif·fer·en·ti·a·
tion
self-ex·am·i·na·
tion
self-hyp·no·sis
pl self-hyp·no·ses

self-in·duced
self-lim·it·ed
self-lim·it·ing
self-med·i·ca·tion
self-rec·og·ni·tion
self-rep·li·cat·ing
self-rep·li·ca·tion
self-stim·u·la·tion
self-stim·u·la·to·ry
self-tol·er·ance
self-treat·ment
sel·la
pl sel·las
or sel·lae

sel·lar
sel·la tur·ci·ca
pl sel·lae tur·ci·cae

se·men
semi·car·ba·zide
semi·cir·cu·lar
semi·co·ma
semi·co·ma·tose
semi·con·scious
semi·con·ser·va·
tive
semi·dom·i·nant
semi·le·thal
semi·lu·nar

semi·mem·bra·no·
sus
pl semi·mem·bra·no·
si

sem·i·nal
semi·nif·er·ous
sem·i·no·ma
pl sem·i·no·mas
or sem·i·no·ma·ta

semi·per·me·abil·i·
ty
pl semi·per·me·abil·i·
ties

semi·per·me·able
semi·pri·vate
semi·sol·id
semi·spi·na·lis
pl semi·spi·na·les

semi·spi·na·lis cap·
i·tis
semi·spi·na·lis cer·
vi·cis
semi·spi·na·lis tho·
ra·cis
semi·syn·thet·ic
sem·i·ten·di·no·sus
pl sem·i·ten·di·no·si

Sem·li·ki For·est
vi·rus
Sen·dai vi·rus
se·ne·cio
pl se·ne·cios

se·ne·ci·o·sis
pl se·ne·ci·o·ses

sen·e·ga
se·nes·cence
se·nes·cent

se·nile
se·nil·i·ty
pl se·nil·i·ties

se·ni·um
sen·na
sen·no·side
sen·sa·tion
sense
sensed
sens·ing
sen·si·bil·i·ty
pl sen·si·bil·i·ties

sen·si·ble
sen·si·tive
sen·si·tiv·i·ty
pl sen·si·tiv·i·ties

sen·si·ti·za·tion
sen·si·tize
sen·si·tized
sen·si·tiz·ing
sen·si·tiz·er
sen·sor
sen·so·ri·al
sen·so·ri·mo·tor
sen·so·ri·neu·ral
sen·so·ri·um
pl sen·so·ri·ums
or sen·so·ria

sen·so·ry
sen·su·al·ism
sen·su·al·ist
sen·su·al·i·ty
pl sen·su·al·i·ties

sen·tient
sen·ti·ment
sen·ti·nel

sep·a·rate
  sep·a·rat·ed
  sep·a·rat·ing
sep·a·ra·tion
sep·a·ra·tor
sep·sis
  pl sep·ses
sep·tal
sep·tate
sep·ta·tion
sep·tec·to·my
  pl sep·tec·to·mies
sep·tic
sep·ti·ce·mia
sep·ti·ce·mic
sep·ti·co·py·emia
sep·ti·co·py·emic
sep·to·mar·gin·al
sep·tos·to·my
  pl sep·tos·to·mies
sep·tum
  pl sep·ta
sep·tum pel·lu·ci·
  dum
  pl sep·ta pel·lu·ci·da
sep·tum trans·ver·
  sum
  pl sep·ta trans·ver·sa
sep·tup·let
se·quela
  pl se·quel·ae
se·quence
  se·quenced
  se·quenc·ing
se·quenc·er
se·quen·tial
se·ques·ter

se·ques·trant
se·ques·tra·tion
se·ques·trec·to·my
  pl se·ques·trec·to·
  mies
se·ques·trum
  pl se·ques·trums
  also se·ques·tra
se·ra
  pl of serum
ser·e·noa
se·ri·al·o·graph
  or se·rio·graph
se·ri·al·og·ra·phy
  pl se·ri·al·og·ra·phies
se·ries
ser·ine
se·ro·con·ver·sion
se·ro·di·ag·no·sis
  pl se·ro·di·ag·no·ses
se·ro·di·ag·nos·tic
se·ro·ep·i·de·mi·o·
  log·ic
  or se·ro·ep·i·de·mi·o·
  log·i·cal
se·ro·ep·i·de·mi·ol·
  o·gy
  pl se·ro·ep·i·de·mi·ol·
  o·gies
se·ro·fi·brin·ous
se·ro·group
se·ro·log·i·cal
  or se·ro·log·ic
se·rol·o·gist
se·rol·o·gy
  pl se·rol·o·gies
se·ro·mu·coid

se·ro·neg·a·tive
se·ro·neg·a·tiv·i·ty
  pl se·ro·neg·a·tiv·i·
  ties
se·ro·pos·i·tive
se·ro·pos·i·tiv·i·ty
  pl se·ro·pos·i·tiv·i·ties
se·ro·pu·ru·lent
se·ro·re·ac·tion
se·ro·re·sis·tance
se·ro·re·sis·tant
se·ro·sa
  pl se·ro·sas
  also se·ro·sae
se·ro·sal
se·ro·san·guin·e·
  ous
  or se·ro·san·guin·ous
se·ro·si·tis
se·ro·ther·a·py
  pl se·ro·ther·a·pies
se·ro·to·ner·gic
  or se·ro·to·nin·er·gic
se·ro·to·nin
se·ro·type
  se·ro·typed
  se·ro·typ·ing
se·rous
ser·o·var
ser·pen·tar·ia
ser·pig·i·nous
ser·rat·ed
Ser·ra·tia
ser·ra·tus
  pl ser·ra·ti
ser·ra·tus mag·nus
serre·fine

sideroblast

Ser·to·li cell
  also Ser·to·li's cell

se·rum
  pl se·rums
  or se·ra

se·rum·al

ses·a·me

ses·a·moid

ses·a·moid·itis

ses·qui·ter·pene

ses·sile

Se·tar·ia

set·fast

se·ton

sex-lim·it·ed

sex-link·age

sex-linked

sex·o·log·i·cal

sex·ol·o·gist

sex·ol·o·gy
  pl sex·ol·o·gies

sex·ti·grav·i·da
  pl sex·ti·grav·i·das
  or sex·ti·grav·i·dae

sex·tu·plet

sex·u·al

sex·u·al·i·ty
  pl sex·u·al·i·ties

Se·za·ry cell

Se·za·ry syn·drome
  or Se·za·ry's syn·drome

shad·ow-cast·ing

shaft
  pl shafts

Shar·pey's fi·ber

sheath
  pl sheaths

sheathed

sheath of Hert·wig

sheath of Schwann

Shee·han's syn·drome

shell-shocked

shi·at·su
  also shi·at·zu

Shi·ga ba·cil·lus

shi·gel·la
  pl shi·gel·lae
  also shi·gel·las

shig·el·lo·sis
  pl shig·el·lo·ses

shi·kim·ic

shin·bone

shin·er

shin·gles

shin·splints

ship·ping fe·ver

shiv·er

shiv·er·ing

Shope pap·il·lo·ma
  also Shope's pap·il·lo·ma

short·sight·ed

short·wave

shoul·der

shoul·der-hand syn·drome

shut-in

si·al·ad·e·ni·tis
  also si·al·o·ad·e·ni·tis

si·al·a·gogue

si·al·ic

si·a·lo·ad·e·nec·to·my
  pl si·a·lo·ad·e·nec·to·mies

si·a·lo·do·cho·plas·ty
  pl si·a·lo·do·cho·plas·ties

si·a·lo·gly·co·pro·tein

si·a·lo·gram

si·a·log·ra·phy
  pl si·a·log·ra·phies

si·a·lo·lith

si·a·lo·li·thi·a·sis
  pl si·a·lo·li·thi·a·ses

si·a·lo·li·thot·o·my
  pl si·a·lo·li·thot·o·mies

si·al·or·rhea

Si·a·mese twin

sib·i·lant

sib·ling

sib·ship

sic·ca syn·drome

sick·bed

sick·en

sick·le
  sick·led
  sick·ling

sick·le-cell ane·mia

sick·le-cell trait

sick·le·mia

sick·le·mic

sick·ler

side·bone

sid·er·o·blast

sid·ero·blas·tic
sid·ero·cyte
sid·ero·pe·nia
sid·ero·pe·nic
sid·er·oph·i·lin
sid·er·o·sis
sid·er·ot·ic
sight·ed
sig·ma fac·tor
sig·ma·tism
sig·moid
sig·moid·ec·to·my
  pl sig·moid·ec·to·mies
sig·moid·itis
sig·moid·o·pexy
  pl sig·moid·o·pex·ies
sig·moid·o·scope
sig·moid·o·scop·ic
sig·moid·os·co·py
  pl sig·moid·os·co·pies
sig·moid·os·to·my
  pl sig·moid·os·to·mies
sig·na
sig·na·ture
sig·net ring
si·lent
si·lex
sil·i·ca
sil·i·cate
si·li·ceous
  also si·li·cious
si·lic·ic
sil·i·co·flu·o·ride
sil·i·con
sil·i·cone

sil·i·con·ize
sil·i·con·ized
sil·i·con·iz·ing
sil·i·co·sis
  pl sil·i·co·ses
sil·i·cot·ic
sil·i·co·tu·ber·cu·
  lo·sis
  pl sil·i·co·tu·ber·cu·
  lo·ses
sil·ver
si·meth·i·cone
Sim·monds' dis·
  ease
sim·u·late
sim·u·lat·ed
sim·u·lat·ing
sim·u·la·tion
sim·u·la·tor
Sim·u·li·i·dae
Si·mu·li·um
si·nal
sin·ci·put
  pl sin·ci·puts
  or sin·cip·i·ta
Sind·bis vi·rus
sin·gle-blind
sin·gul·tus
si·nis·tral
sin·is·tral·i·ty
  pl sin·is·tral·i·ties
si·no·atri·al
  also si·nu·atri·al
si·nus
si·nus·itis
si·nus of Mor·ga·
  gni

si·nus of Val·sal·va
si·nu·soid
si·nu·soi·dal
si·nus·ot·o·my
  pl si·nus·ot·o·mies
si·nus rhom·boi·
  da·lis
si·nus ter·mi·na·lis
si·nus ve·no·sus
si·nus ve·no·sus
  scle·rae
Si·phon·ap·tera
Sip·py di·et
sir·up
  var of syrup
sir·upy
  var of syrupy
Sis·tru·rus
sit·fast
si·tos·ter·ol
sit·u·a·tion
sit·u·a·tion·al
si·tus in·ver·sus
sitz bath
six-o-six
  or 606
six-year mo·lar
Sjö·gren's syn·
  drome
  also Sjö·gren syn·
  drome
ska·tole
  also ska·tol
skel·e·tal
skel·e·ton
skene·i·tis
  also sken·i·tis

Skene's gland
skia·gram
skia·graph
skia·scope
Skin·ner box
Skin·ner·ian
skull·cap
sleep·ing pill
sleep·walk
sleep·walk·er
slit lamp
slough
slow-wave sleep
sludge
slur·ry
   pl slur·ries
small·pox
smec·tic
smeg·ma
smell·ing salts
Smith frac·ture
  or Smith's frac·ture
Smith-Pe·ter·sen
  nail
smok·er
snake·bite
snake·root
sneeze
  sneezed
  sneez·ing
Snel·len chart
snif·fles
snore
  snored
  snor·ing
snow-blind
snow blind·ness

snuf·fles
so·cial
so·cial·iza·tion
so·cial·ize
  so·cial·ized
  so·cial·iz·ing
so·cio·bio·log·i·cal
so·cio·bi·ol·o·gist
so·cio·bi·ol·o·gy
  pl so·cio·bi·ol·o·gies
so·cio·drama
so·cio·dra·mat·ic
so·cio·log·i·cal
  also so·cio·log·ic
so·ci·ol·o·gist
so·ci·ol·o·gy
  pl so·ci·ol·o·gies
so·cio·med·i·cal
so·cio·path
so·cio·path·ic
so·ci·op·a·thy
  pl so·ci·op·a·thies
so·cio·psy·cho·log·
  i·cal
so·cio·sex·u·al
sock·et
so·da
so·di·um
so·do·ku
sod·om·ite
sod·omit·ic
  or sod·omit·i·cal
sod·omy
  pl sod·om·ies
sol
So·la·na·ce·ae
so·la·na·ceous

so·la·nine
  or so·la·nin
so·lar·i·um
  pl so·lar·ia
  also so·lar·i·ums
so·lar plex·us
So·le·nog·ly·pha
So·le·nop·sis
sole·print
so·le·us
  pl so·lei
  also so·le·us·es
sol·i·da·go
  pl sol·i·da·gos
sol·u·bil·i·ty
  pl sol·u·bil·i·ties
sol·u·bi·li·za·tion
sol·u·bi·lize
  sol·u·bi·lized
  sol·u·bi·liz·ing
sol·u·bi·liz·er
sol·u·ble
sol·ute
so·lu·tion
sol·vate
  sol·vat·ed
  sol·vat·ing
sol·va·tion
sol·vent
sol·vol·y·sis
  pl sol·vol·y·ses
sol·vo·lyt·ic
so·ma
  pl so·ma·ta
  or so·mas
so·mat·ic
so·mat·i·cal·ly

so·ma·ti·za·tion
so·ma·tize
  so·ma·tized
  so·ma·tiz·ing
so·ma·to·gen·ic
so·ma·to·log·i·cal
so·ma·tol·o·gy
  pl so·ma·tol·o·gies
so·ma·to·me·din
so·ma·to·met·ric
so·ma·tom·e·try
  pl so·ma·tom·e·tries
so·ma·to·plasm
so·ma·to·pleure
so·ma·to·pleu·ric
so·ma·to·psy·chic
so·ma·to·sen·so·ry
so·ma·to·stat·in
so·ma·to·ther·a·peu·tic
so·ma·to·ther·a·py
  pl so·ma·to·ther·a·pies
so·ma·to·to·nia
so·ma·to·ton·ic
so·ma·to·top·ic
so·ma·to·top·i·cal·ly
so·ma·to·trop·ic
  or so·ma·to·tro·phic
so·ma·to·tro·pin
  also so·ma·to·tro·phin
so·ma·to·type
  so·ma·to·typed
  so·ma·to·typ·ing
so·ma·to·typ·ic

so·ma·to·typ·i·cal·ly
som·es·the·sis
  pl som·es·the·sis·es
som·es·thet·ic
so·mite
so·mit·ic
som·nam·bu·lance
som·nam·bu·lant
som·nam·bu·lism
som·nam·bu·list
som·nam·bu·lis·tic
som·ni·fa·cient
som·nif·er·ous
som·no·lence
som·no·lent
sone
son·ic
son·i·cal·ly
son·i·cate
  son·i·cat·ed
  son·i·cat·ing
son·i·ca·tion
sono·gram
so·nog·ra·pher
sono·graph·ic
so·nog·ra·phy
  pl so·nog·ra·phies
soph·o·rine
so·por
so·po·rif·ic
sor·bate
sor·bic
sor·bi·tan
sor·bi·tol
sor·bose

sor·des
  pl sor·des
sore
  sor·er
  sor·est
sore·head
so·ta·lol
souf·fle
space of Fon·tana
space of Ret·zi·us
spac·er
Span·ish fly
spar·ga·no·sis
  pl spar·ga·no·ses
spar·ga·num
  pl spar·ga·na
  also spar·ga·nums
spar·te·ine
spasm
spas·mod·ic
spas·mod·i·cal·ly
spas·mo·gen·ic
spas·mo·lyt·ic
spas·mo·lyt·i·cal·ly
spas·mo·phile
  or spas·mo·phil·ic
spas·mo·phil·ia
spas·tic
spas·ti·cal·ly
spas·tic·i·ty
  pl spas·tic·i·ties
spa·tial
spa·tia zon·u·lar·ia
spat·u·la
spat·u·late
  spat·u·lat·ed
  spat·u·lat·ing

sphenoethmoidal

spat·u·la·tion
spav·in
spav·ined
spay
  spayed
  spay·ing
spear·mint
spe·cial·ist
spe·cial·iza·tion
spe·cial·ize
  spe·cial·ized
  spe·cial·iz·ing
spe·cial·ty
  pl spe·cial·ties

spe·cies
  pl spe·cies

spe·cies-spe·cif·ic
spe·cif·ic
spec·i·fic·i·ty
  pl spec·i·fic·i·ties

spec·i·men
spec·ta·cles
spec·ti·no·my·cin
spec·tra
  pl of spectrum

spec·tral
spec·tro·chem·i·cal
spec·tro·chem·is·try
  pl spec·tro·chem·is·tries

spec·tro·flu·o·rom·e·ter
  also spec·tro·flu·o·rim·e·ter

spec·tro·flu·o·ro·met·ric

spec·tro·flu·o·rom·e·try
  pl spec·tro·flu·o·rom·e·tries

spec·tro·gram
spec·tro·graph
spec·tro·graph·ic
spec·tro·graph·i·cal·ly
spec·trog·ra·phy
  pl spec·trog·ra·phies

spec·trom·e·ter
spec·tro·met·ric
spec·trom·e·try
  pl spec·trom·e·tries

spec·tro·pho·tom·e·ter
spec·tro·pho·to·met·ric
spec·tro·pho·to·met·ri·cal·ly
spec·tro·pho·tom·e·try
  pl spec·tro·pho·tom·e·tries

spec·tro·po·lar·im·e·ter
spec·tro·scope
spec·tro·scop·ic
spec·tro·scop·i·cal·ly
spec·tros·co·pist
spec·tros·co·py
  pl spec·tros·co·pies

spec·trum
  pl spec·tra
  or spec·trums

spec·u·lum
  pl spec·u·la
  also spec·u·lums

sperm
  pl sperm
  or sperms

sper·ma·ce·ti
sper·mat·ic
sper·ma·tid
sper·mato·cele
sper·mato·cid·al
sper·mato·cide
sper·mato·cyte
sper·mato·gen·e·sis
  pl sper·mato·gen·e·ses

sper·mato·gen·ic
sper·mato·go·ni·al
sper·mato·go·ni·um
  pl sper·mato·go·nia

sper·ma·tor·rhea
sper·ma·to·zo·al
sper·ma·to·zo·an
sper·ma·to·zo·on
  pl sper·ma·to·zoa

sper·mi·cid·al
sper·mi·cide
sper·mi·dine
sperm·ine
sper·mio·gen·e·sis
  pl sper·mio·gen·e·ses

Sphae·roph·o·rus
sphag·num
sphe·no·eth·moid
  or sphe·no·eth·moi·dal

sphe·noid
   or sphe·noi·dal

sphe·noid·itis

sphe·no·man·dib·
   u·lar

sphe·no·max·il·
   lary

sphe·no·oc·cip·i·tal

sphe·no·pal·a·tine

sphe·no·pa·ri·etal

spher·i·cal

sphe·ro·cyte

sphe·ro·cyt·ic

sphe·ro·cy·to·sis

sphe·roi·dal
   also spher·oid

sphe·rom·e·ter

sphe·ro·plast

sphinc·ter

sphinc·ter·al

sphinc·ter ani ex·
   ter·nus

sphinc·ter ani in·
   ter·nus

sphinc·ter·ic

sphinc·ter of Od·di

sphinc·tero·plas·ty
   pl sphinc·tero·plas·
      ties

sphinc·ter·ot·o·my
   pl sphinc·ter·ot·o·
      mies

sphinc·ter pu·pil·
   lae

sphinc·ter ure·
   thrae

sphinc·ter va·gi·
   nae

sphin·go·lip·id

sphin·go·lip·i·do·
   sis
   pl sphin·go·lip·i·do·
      ses

sphin·go·my·elin

sphin·go·my·elin·
   ase

sphin·go·sine

sphyg·mic

sphyg·mo·gram

sphyg·mo·graph

sphyg·mo·ma·
   nom·e·ter

sphyg·mo·ma·
   nom·e·try
   pl sphyg·mo·ma·nom·
      e·tries

spi·ca
   pl spi·cae
   or spi·cas

spic·ule

Spiel·mey·er-Vogt
   dis·ease

spi·ge·lia

spi·ge·lian

spi·na
   pl spi·nae

spi·na bi·fi·da

spi·na bi·fi·da oc·
   cul·ta

spi·nal

spi·nal·is
   pl spi·na·les

spi·na·lis ca·pi·tis

spi·na·lis cer·vi·cis

spi·na·lis tho·ra·cis

spin·dle

spinn·bar·keit

spi·no·cer·e·bel·lar

spi·no·ol·i·vary

spi·nose

spi·no·tec·tal

spi·no·tha·lam·ic

spi·nous

spiny-head·ed
   worm

spi·ral

spi·reme

Spi·ril·la·ce·ae

spi·ril·li·ci·dal

spi·ril·lo·sis
   pl spi·ril·lo·ses
   or spi·ril·lo·sis·es

spi·ril·lum
   pl spi·ril·la

spir·it of harts·
   horn
   or spir·its of harts·
      horn

spir·its of wine
   or spir·it of wine

Spi·ro·cer·ca

Spi·ro·chae·ta

Spi·ro·chae·ta·ce·
   ae

Spi·ro·chae·ta·les

spi·ro·chet·al

spi·ro·chete

spi·ro·chet·emia

spi·ro·che·ti·ci·dal

spi·ro·che·ti·cide

spi·ro·chet·ol·y·sis
 pl spi·ro·chet·ol·y·ses

spi·ro·chet·osis
 pl spi·ro·chet·oses

spi·ro·gram

spi·ro·graph

spi·ro·graph·ic

spi·rog·ra·phy
 pl spi·rog·ra·phies

spi·rom·e·ter

spi·ro·met·ric

spi·rom·e·try
 pl spi·rom·e··tries

spi·ro·no·lac·tone

Spi·ru·ri·da

spit·ting co·bra

spit·tle

splanch·nic

splanch·ni·cec·to·
 my
 pl splanch·ni·cec·to·
 mies

splanch·ni·cot·o·
 my
 pl splanch·ni·cot·o·
 mies

splanch·nol·o·gy
 pl splanch·nol·o·gies

splanch·no·meg·a·
 ly
 pl splanch·no·meg·a·
 lies

splanch·no·mi·cria

splanch·no·pleure

splanch·no·pleu·
 ric

splay·foot

spleen

sple·nec·to·mize
 sple·nec·to·
 mized
 sple·nec·to·miz·
 ing

sple·nec·to·my
 pl sple·nec·to·mies

splen·ic

sple·ni·tis

sple·ni·um
 pl sple·nia

sple·ni·us
 pl sple·nii

sple·ni·us cap·i·tis

sple·ni·us cer·vi·
 cis

sple·ni·za·tion

sple·no·cyte

spleno·meg·a·ly
 pl spleno·meg·a·lies

sple·nop·a·thy
 pl sple·nop·a·thies

spleno·por·to·gram

spleno·por·tog·ra·
 phy
 pl spleno·por·tog·ra·
 phies

spleno·re·nal

sple·no·sis
 pl sple·no·ses
 or sple·no·sis·es

splint·age

splin·ter
 splin·tered
 splin·ter·ing

split-brain

spon·dy·lit·ic

spon·dy·li·tis

spon·dy·lo·lis·the·
 sis

spon·dy·lol·y·sis
 pl spon·dy·lol·y·ses

spon·dy·lop·a·thy
 pl spon·dy·lop·a·thies

spon·dy·lo·sis
 pl spon·dy·lo·ses
 or spon·dy·lo·sis·es

spon·gi·form

spon·gin

spong·i·ness

spon·gi·o·blast

spon·gi·o·blas·to·
 ma
 pl spon·gi·o·blas·to·
 mas
 or spon·gi·o·blas·to·
 ma·ta

spon·gi·o·cyte

spon·gi·o·sa

spon·gi·o·sis

spongy
 spong·i·er
 spong·i·est

spon·ta·ne·ous

spo·rad·ic

spo·rad·i·cal·ly

spo·ran·gial

spo·ran·gio·phore

spo·ran·gio·spore

spo·ran·gi·um
 pl spo·ran·gia

spore
  spored
  spor·ing
spo·ri·cide
spo·rid·i·al
spo·rid·i·um
  pl spo·rid·ia
spo·ro·blast
spo·ro·cyst
spo·ro·gen·e·sis
  pl spo·ro·gen·e·ses
spo·rog·e·nous
spo·ro·gon·ic
  also spo·rog·o·nous
spo·rog·o·ny
  pl spo·rog·o·nies
spo·ront
spo·ro·phore
spo·ro·phyte
spo·ro·phyt·ic
spo·ro·tri·cho·sis
  pl spo·ro·tri·cho·ses
spo·ro·tri·chot·ic
spo·rot·ri·chum
  pl spo·rot·ri·cha
spo·ro·zoa
spo·ro·zo·an
spo·ro·zo·ite
spor·u·late
  spor·u·lat·ed
  spor·u·lat·ing
spor·u·la·tion
spot·ted fe·ver
sprain
sprue
spur
  spurred

spu·tum
  pl spu·ta
squa·lene
squa·ma
  pl squa·mae
squame
squa·mo·co·lum·nar
squa·mo·sal
squa·mous
squill
squint
sta·bi·late
sta·bile
sta·bil·i·ty
  pl sta·bil·i·ties
sta·bi·li·za·tion
sta·bi·lize
  sta·bi·lized
  sta·bi·liz·ing
sta·bi·liz·er
sta·ble
  sta·bler
  sta·blest
stachy·bot·ryo·tox·i·co·sis
  pl stachy·bot·ryo·tox·i·co·ses
stach·y·drine
stach·y·ose
Sta·der splint
staff of Aes·cu·la·pi·us
stag·gers
stag·horn cal·cu·lus

stain·abil·i·ty
  pl stain·abil·i·ties
stain·able
stal·ag·mom·e·ter
sta·lag·mo·met·ric
stam·i·na
stam·mer
  stam·mered
  stam·mer·ing
stam·mer·er
stanch
  also staunch
stand·still
Stan·ford-Bi·net test
stan·nic
stan·nous
stan·o·lone
stan·o·zo·lol
sta·pe·dec·to·my
  pl sta·pe·dec·to·mies
sta·pe·di·al
sta·pe·di·us
  pl sta·pe·dii
sta·pes
  pl sta·pes
  or sta·pe·des
staph
staph·i·sa·gria
staph·y·lec·to·my
  pl staph·y·lec·to·mies
staph·y·lo·co·ag·u·lase
staph·y·lo·coc·cal
  also staph·y·lo·coc·cic
staph·y·lo·coc·ce·mia

staph·y·lo·coc·ce·
mic
staph·y·lo·coc·co·
sis
staph·y·lo·coc·cus
pl staph·y·lo·coc·ci
staph·y·lo·ki·nase
staph·y·lol·y·sin
staph·y·lo·ma
staph·y·lo·tox·in
starchy
starch·i·er
starch·i·est
Star·ling's hy·poth·
e·sis
Star·ling's law
star·va·tion
starve
starved
starv·ing
sta·sis
pl sta·ses

stat
stat·am·pere
stat·cou·lomb
stat·im
stato·co·nia
stato·ki·net·ic
stato·lith
stat·ure
sta·tus
pl sta·tus·es
sta·tus asth·mat·i·
cus
sta·tus ep·i·lep·ti·
cus

sta·tus lym·phat·i·
cus
sta·tus thy·mi·co·
lym·phat·i·cus
staunch
var of stanch
staves·acre
ste·ap·sin
stea·rate
stea·ric
stea·rin
also stea·rine
stea·rop·tene
stea·ryl
ste·a·ti·tis
ste·ato·py·gia
ste·ato·py·gic
also ste·ato·py·gous
ste·at·or·rhea
ste·a·to·sis
pl ste·a·to·ses
stego·my·ia
Stein·mann pin
stel·late
stel·lec·to·my
pl stel·lec·to·mies
Sten·der dish
steno·car·dia
ste·nosed
ste·nos·ing
ste·no·sis
pl ste·no·ses
ste·not·ic
Sten·sen's duct
also Sten·son's duct
stent
also stint

Steph·a·no·fi·lar·ia
steph·a·no·fil·a·ri·
a·sis
pl steph·a·no·fil·a·ri·
a·ses

Steph·a·nu·rus
step·page
ster·co·bi·lin
ster·co·bi·lin·o·gen
ster·co·ra·ceous
ster·co·ral
ster·cu·lia
ste·reo·cam·pim·e·
ter
ste·reo·chem·i·cal
ste·reo·chem·is·try
pl ste·reo·chem·is·
tries
ste·reo·cil·i·um
pl ste·reo·cil·ia
ste·re·og·no·sis
ste·re·og·nos·tic
ste·reo·gram
ste·reo·graph
ste·reo·iso·mer
ste·reo·iso·mer·ic
ste·reo·isom·er·ism
ste·reo·log·i·cal
also ste·reo·log·ic
ste·re·ol·o·gy
pl ste·re·ol·o·gies
ste·reo·pho·to·mi·
cro·graph
ste·re·op·sis
ste·reo·ra·dio·
graph

ste·reo·ra·dio·
  graph·ic
ste·reo·ra·di·og·ra·
  phy
  pl ste·reo·ra·di·og·ra·
    phies
ste·reo·roent·gen·
  og·ra·phy
  pl ste·reo·roent·gen·
    og·ra·phies
ste·reo·scope
ste·reo·scop·ic
ste·reo·scop·i·cal·ly
ste·re·os·co·py
  pl ste·re·os·co·pies
ste·reo·se·lec·tive
ste·reo·se·lec·tiv·i·
  ty
  pl ste·reo·se·lec·tiv·i·
    ties
ste·reo·spe·cif·ic
ste·reo·spe·cif·i·
  cal·ly
ste·reo·spec·i·fic·i·
  ty
  pl ste·reo·spec·i·fic·i·
    ties
ste·reo·tac·tic
ste·reo·tac·ti·cal·ly
ste·reo·tax·ic
ste·reo·tax·i·cal·ly
ste·reo·tax·is
  pl ste·reo·tax·es
ste·reo·type
  ste·reo·typed
  ste·reo·typ·ing
ste·reo·typ·i·cal
  also ste·reo·typ·ic

ste·reo·ty·py
  pl ste·reo·ty·pies
ste·ric
ste·ri·cal·ly
ste·rig·ma
  pl ste·rig·ma·ta
  also ste·rig·mas
ste·rig·ma·to·cys·
  tin
ster·il·ant
ster·ile
ste·ril·i·ty
  pl ste·ril·i·ties
ster·il·iza·tion
ster·il·ize
  ster·il·ized
  ster·il·iz·ing
ster·il·iz·er
ster·na
  pl of sternum
ster·nal
ster·na·lis
  pl ster·na·les
Stern·berg cell
Stern·berg-Reed
  cell
ster·ne·bra
  pl ster·ne·brae
ster·no·cla·vic·u·
  lar
ster·no·clei·do·
  mas·toid
ster·no·clei·do·
  mas·toi·de·us
  pl ster·no·clei·do·
    mas·toi·dei
ster·no·cos·tal

ster·no·hy·oid
ster·no·hy·oi·de·us
  pl ster·no·hy·oi·dei
ster·no·mas·toid
ster·no·thy·roid
ster·no·thy·roi·de·
  us
  pl ster·no·thy·roi·dei
ster·not·o·my
  pl ster·not·o·mies
ster·num
  pl ster·nums
  or ster·na
ster·nu·ta·tion
ster·nu·ta·tor
ste·roid
ste·roi·dal
ste·roido·gen·e·sis
  pl ste·roido·gen·e·ses
ste·roido·gen·ic
ste·rol
ster·tor
ster·to·rous
stetho·scope
stetho·scop·ic
stetho·scop·i·cal·ly
Ste·vens-John·son
  syn·drome
sthen·ic
stib·amine
stib·o·phen
stiff-man syn·
  drome
sti·fle
stig·ma
  pl stig·ma·ta
  or stig·mas

stig·mas·ter·ol
stig·mat·ic
stig·mat·i·cal·ly
stilb·am·i·dine
stil·bene
stil·bes·trol
Stiles-Craw·ford
    ef·fect
sti·let
    or sti·lette

sti·let·ted
still·birth
still·born
Still's dis·ease
stim·u·lant
stim·u·late
    stim·u·lat·ed
    stim·u·lat·ing
stim·u·la·tion
stim·u·la·tive
stim·u·la·tor
stim·u·la·to·ry
stim·u·lus
    pl stim·u·li

sting·er
stint
    var of stent

stip·pled
stip·pling
stir·rup
sto·chas·tic
sto·chas·ti·cal·ly
stock·i·nette
    or stock·i·net

stoi·chi·o·met·ric
stoi·chi·om·e·try
    pl stoi·chi·om·e·tries

Stokes-Ad·ams
    syn·drome
sto·ma
    pl sto·mas

stom·ach
stom·ach·ache
sto·mach·ic
sto·mal
sto·ma·ti·tis
    pl sto·ma·tit·i·des
    or sto·ma·ti·tis·es

sto·ma·to·de·um
    pl sto·ma·to·dea

sto·mo·de·al
    or sto·mo·dae·al

sto·mo·de·um
    or sto·mo·dae·um
    pl sto·mo·dea
    or sto·mo·daea
    also sto·mo·de·ums
    or sto·mo·dae·ums

Sto·mox·ys
stone-blind
stone-deaf
sto·rax
stor·es·in
sto·ri·form
stra·bis·mic
stra·bis·mus
strait·jack·et
    or straight·jack·et

stra·mo·ni·um
stran·gle
    stran·gled
    stran·gling
stran·gu·late
    stran·gu·lat·ed
    stran·gu·lat·ing

stran·gu·la·tion
stran·gu·ry
    pl stran·gu·ries

strat·i·fi·ca·tion
strat·i·fied
stra·tig·ra·phy
    pl stra·tig·ra·phies

stra·tum
    pl stra·ta

stra·tum ba·sa·le
    pl stra·ta ba·sa·lia

stra·tum com·pac·
    tum
    pl stra·ta com·pac·ta

stra·tum cor·ne·
    um
    pl stra·ta cor·nea

stra·tum ger·mi·
    na·ti·vum
    pl stra·ta ger·mi·na·ti·
    va

stra·tum gran·u·lo·
    sum
    pl stra·ta gran·u·lo·sa

stra·tum in·ter·me·
    di·um
    pl stra·ta in·ter·me·
    dia

stra·tum lu·ci·dum
    pl stra·ta lu·ci·da

stra·tum spi·no·
    sum
    pl stra·ta spi·no·sa

stra·tum spon·gi·o·
    sum
    pl stra·ta spon·gi·o·sa

straw·ber·ry mark

strep
strepho·sym·bo·lia
strepho·sym·bol·ic
strepo·gen·in
strep·to·ba·cil·lus
  pl strep·to·ba·cil·li
strep·to·coc·cal
  also strep·to·coc·cic
strep·to·coc·cus
  pl step·to·coc·ci
strep·to·dor·nase
strep·to·ki·nase
strep·to·ly·sin
strep·to·my·ces
  pl strep·to·my·ces
Strep·to·my·ce·ta·
  ce·ae
strep·to·my·cete
strep·to·my·cin
strep·to·ni·grin
strep·to·thri·cin
strep·to·thrix
  pl strep·to·thri·ces
strep·to·tri·cho·sis
  also strep·to·thri·cho·
  sis
strep·to·zot·o·cin
stress·or
stretch·er
stretch·er-bear·er
stria
  pl stri·ae
stri·a·tal
stri·ate
stri·at·ed
stria ter·mi·na·lis
stri·a·tion

stri·a·to·ni·gral
stri·a·tum
  pl stri·a·ta
stria vas·cu·la·ris
stric·ture
stri·dor
string·halt
strip·per
stro·bi·la
  pl stro·bi·lae
stro·bi·lar
stro·bi·late
  stro·bi·lat·ed
  stro·bi·lat·ing
stro·bi·la·tion
strob·i·lo·cer·cus
  pl strob·i·lo·cer·ci
stro·ma
  pl stro·ma·ta
stro·mal
stro·ma·tin
strom·uhr
stron·gyle
Stron·gyl·i·dae
stron·gy·li·do·sis
Stron·gy·loi·dea
Stron·gy·loi·des
stron·gy·loi·di·a·sis
  pl stron·gy·loi·di·a·ses
stron·gy·loi·do·sis
stron·gy·lo·sis
Stron·gy·lus
stron·tium
stro·phan·thi·din
stro·phan·thin
stro·phan·thus
struc·tur·al

struc·ture
stru·ma
  pl stru·mae
  or stru·mas
stru·ma lym·pho·
  ma·to·sa
strych·nine
Strych·nos
ST seg·ment
  or S-T seg·ment
Stu·art-Prow·er
  fac·tor
stupe
stu·pe·fy
  stu·pe·fied
  stu·pe·fy·ing
stu·por
stu·por·ose
stu·por·ous
stur·dy
  pl stur·dies
stut·ter
stut·ter·er
stut·ter·ing
Stutt·gart dis·ease
sty
  or stye
  pl sties
  or styes
sty·let
  also sty·lette
sty·lo·glos·sus
  pl sty·lo·glos·si
sty·lo·hy·oid
sty·lo·hy·oi·de·us
  pl sty·lo·hy·oi·dei
sty·loid

sty·lo·man·dib·u·lar

sty·lo·mas·toid

sty·lo·pha·ryn·ge·us
pl sty·lo·pha·ryn·gei

sty·lus
pl sty·li
also sty·lus·es

styp·tic

sty·rax

sty·rene

sty·rol

sub·acro·mi·al

sub·acute

sub·aor·tic

sub·api·cal

sub·apo·neu·rot·ic

sub·arach·noid
also sub·arach·noid·al

sub·atom·ic

sub·cal·lo·sal

sub·cap·su·lar

sub·car·ci·no·gen·ic

sub·cel·lu·lar

sub·chon·dral

sub·class

sub·cla·vi·an

sub·cla·vi·us
pl sub·cla·vii

sub·clin·i·cal

sub·com·mis·sur·al

sub·con·junc·ti·val

sub·con·scious

sub·con·vul·sive

sub·cor·ti·cal

sub·cos·tal

sub·cos·ta·lis
pl sub·cos·ta·les

sub·crep·i·tant

sub·cul·tur·al

sub·cul·ture

sub·cu·ra·tive

sub·cu·ta·ne·ous

sub·cu·tic·u·lar

sub·cu·tis

sub·del·toid

sub·der·mal

sub·di·a·phrag·ma·tic

sub·du·ral

sub·en·do·car·di·al

sub·en·do·the·li·al

sub·epi·der·mal

sub·epi·the·li·al

su·ber·in

sub·fam·i·ly

sub·fas·cial

sub·fer·tile

sub·fer·til·i·ty
pl sub·fer·til·i·ties

sub·gal·late

sub·ge·nus
pl sub·gen·e·ra

sub·gin·gi·val

sub·glot·tic

sub·he·pat·ic

sub·ic·ter·ic

su·bic·u·lar

su·bic·u·lum
pl su·bic·u·la

sub·in·ti·mal

sub·in·vo·lu·tion

sub·ja·cent

sub·ject

sub·jec·tive

sub·jec·tiv·i·ty
pl sub·jec·tiv·i·ties

sub·king·dom

sub·le·thal

sub·leu·ke·mic

sub·li·mate

sub·li·mat·ed

sub·li·mat·ing

sub·li·ma·tion

sub·lime

sub·limed

sub·lim·ing

sub·lim·i·nal

sub·lin·gual

sub·lob·u·lar

sub·lux·at·ed

sub·lux·a·tion

sub·man·dib·u·lar

sub·mar·gin·al

sub·max·il·lary
pl sub·max·il·lar·ies

sub·max·i·mal

sub·men·tal

sub·meta·cen·tric

sub·mi·cron

sub·mi·cro·scop·ic

sub·mi·cro·scop·i·cal·ly

sub·min·i·mal

sub·mis·sive

sub·mi·to·chon·dri·al

sub·mu·co·sa

sub·mu·co·sal

sub·mu·cous
sub·nar·cot·ic
sub·na·sale
sub·ni·trate
sub·nor·mal
sub·nor·mal·i·ty
  pl sub·nor·mal·i·ties
sub·nu·tri·tion
sub·oc·cip·i·tal
sub·op·ti·mal
sub·or·bit·al
sub·or·der
sub·ox·ide
sub·peri·os·te·al
sub·phren·ic
sub·phy·lum
  pl sub·phy·la
sub·pi·al
sub·pleu·ral
sub·pop·u·la·tion
sub·po·ten·cy
  pl sub·po·ten·cies
sub·po·tent
sub·pu·bic
sub·rect·an·gu·lar
sub·ret·i·nal
sub·scap·u·lar
sub·scap·u·lar·is
sub·scrip·tion
sub·se·ro·sa
sub·se·rous
  or sub·se·ro·sal
sub·spe·cial·ty
  pl sub·spe·cial·ties
sub·spe·cies
sub·spe·cif·ic
sub·stage

sub·stan·tia
  pl sub·stan·ti·ae
sub·stan·tia gel·a·ti·no·sa
sub·stan·tia in·nom·i·na·ta
sub·stan·tia ni·gra
  pl sub·stan·ti·ae ni·grae
sub·stan·tia pro·pria
  pl sub·stan·ti·ae pro·pri·ae
sub·ster·nal
sub·stit·u·ent
sub·sti·tute
  sub·sti·tut·ed
  sub·sti·tut·ing
sub·sti·tu·tion
sub·sti·tu·tive
sub·strate
sub·struc·tur·al
sub·struc·ture
sub·ta·lar
sub·ter·tian
sub·te·tan·ic
sub·tha·lam·ic
sub·thal·a·mus
  pl sub·thal·a·mi
sub·thresh·old
sub·ti·lin
sub·til·i·sin
sub·to·tal
sub·tro·chan·ter·ic
sub·type
  sub·typed
  sub·typ·ing

sub·un·gual
sub·unit
sub·val·vu·lar
sub·vi·ral
sub·vo·cal
suc·ce·da·ne·ous
suc·cen·tu·ri·ate
suc·ces·sion·al
suc·ci·nate
suc·cin·ic
suc·cin·i·mide
suc·cin·ox·i·dase
suc·ci·nyl
suc·ci·nyl·cho·line
suc·ci·nyl·sul·fa·thi·a·zole
suc·cus en·ter·i·cus
suck·le
  suck·led
  suck·ling
su·crase
su·crate
su·crose
suc·tion
su·dam·i·na
su·dam·i·nal
Su·dan
su·dan·o·phil·ia
su·dan·o·phil·ic
  also su·dan·o·phil
sud·den in·fant death syn·drome
su·do·mo·tor
su·do·rif·er·ous
su·do·rif·ic
su·do·rip·a·rous
su·et

suf·fo·cate
  suf·fo·cat·ed
  suf·fo·cat·ing
suf·fo·ca·tion
suf·fo·ca·tive
suf·frag·i·nis
suf·fuse
  suf·fused
  suf·fus·ing
suf·fu·sion
sug·ar
sug·gest·ibil·i·ty
  pl sug·gest·ibil·i·ties
sug·gest·ible
sug·ges·tion
sug·gil·la·tion
sui·cid·al
sui·cide
  sui·cid·ed
  sui·cid·ing
sui·cid·ol·o·gist
sui·cid·ol·o·gy
  pl sui·cid·ol·o·gies
sul·cal
sul·cu·lar
sul·cu·lus
  pl sul·cu·li
sul·cus
  pl sul·ci
sul·cus ter·mi·na·lis
  pl sul·ci ter·mi·na·les
sul·fa
sul·fa·cet·a·mide
  also sul·fa·cet·i·mide
sul·fa·di·a·zine
sul·fa·gua·ni·dine

sul·fa·mate
sul·fa·mer·a·zine
sul·fa·meth·a·zine
sul·fa·meth·ox·a·zole
sul·fa·mez·a·thine
sul·fam·ic
sul·fa·nil·amide
sul·fa·nil·ic
sul·fan·i·lyl·gua·ni·dine
sul·fa·pyr·i·dine
sul·fa·qui·nox·a·line
sulf·ars·phen·a·mine
sul·fa·tase
sul·fate
  sul·fat·ed
  sul·fat·ing
sul·fa·thi·a·zole
sul·fa·tide
sulf·he·mo·glo·bin
sulf·he·mo·glo·bi·ne·mia
sulf·hy·dryl
sul·fide
sul·fin·ic
sul·fin·py·ra·zone
sul·fi·nyl
sul·fi·sox·a·zole
sul·fite
sul·fo·bro·mo·phtha·lein
sul·fon·amide

sul·fo·nate
  sul·fo·nat·ed
  sul·fo·nat·ing
sul·fo·na·tion
sul·fone
sul·fon·eth·yl·meth·ane
sul·fon·ic
sul·fo·ni·um
sul·fo·nyl
sul·fo·nyl·urea
sul·fo·sal·i·cyl·ic
sulf·ox·ide
sulf·ox·one
sul·fur
sul·fu·rate
  sul·fu·rat·ed
  sul·fu·rat·ing
sul·fu·ric
sul·fu·rous
su·lin·dac
sul·i·so·ben·zone
su·mac
  also su·mach

sum·bul
sum·mate
  sum·mat·ed
  sum·mat·ing
sum·ma·tion
sun·burn
  sun·burned
  or sun·burnt
  sun·burn·ing
sun·glass·es
sun·lamp
sun·screen
sun·screen·ing

sun·stroke
sun·tan
sun·tanned
su·per·cil·i·ary
su·per·coil
su·per·ego
su·per·fe·cun·da·
tion
su·per·fi·cial
su·per·fu·sate
su·per·fuse
su·per·fused
su·per·fus·ing
su·per·fu·sion
su·per·gene
su·per·he·li·cal
su·per·he·lic·i·ty
pl su·per·he·lic·i·ties
su·per·he·lix
su·per·in·duce
su·per·in·duced
su·per·in·duc·
ing
su·per·in·duc·tion
su·per·in·fect
su·per·in·fec·tion
su·pe·ri·or
su·per·na·tant
su·per·nate
su·per·nor·mal
su·per·nor·mal·i·ty
pl su·per·nor·mal·i·
ties
su·per·nu·mer·ary
su·pero·lat·er·al
su·pero·me·di·al

su·per·ovu·late
su·per·ovu·lat·ed
su·per·ovu·lat·
ing
su·per·ovu·la·tion
su·per·ox·ide
su·per·ox·ide dis·
mu·tase
su·per·po·ten·cy
pl su·per·po·ten·cies
su·per·po·tent
su·per·sat·u·rate
su·per·sat·u·rat·
ed
su·per·sat·u·rat·
ing
su·per·sat·u·ra·tion
su·per·scrip·tion
su·per·sen·si·tive
su·per·sen·si·tiv·i·
ty
pl su·per·sen·si·tiv·i·
ties
su·per·son·ic
su·per·son·i·cal·ly
su·per·vene
su·per·vened
su·per·ven·ing
su·per·volt·age
su·pi·nate
su·pi·nat·ed
su·pi·nat·ing
su·pi·na·tion
su·pi·na·tor
su·pine
sup·ple·ment
sup·ple·men·tal

sup·ple·men·ta·ry
sup·ply
sup·plied
sup·ply·ing
sup·port·er
sup·port·ive
sup·pos·i·to·ry
sup·pos·i·to·ries
sup·press
sup·press·ant
sup·press·ibil·i·ty
pl sup·press·ibil·i·ties
sup·press·ible
sup·pres·sion
sup·pres·sor
sup·pu·rate
sup·pu·rat·ed
sup·pu·rat·ing
sup·pu·ra·tion
sup·pu·ra·tive
su·pra·car·di·nal
su·pra·cer·vi·cal
su·pra·chi·as·mat·
ic
su·pra·cla·vic·u·lar
su·pra·con·dy·lar
su·pra·di·a·phrag·
mat·ic
su·pra·di·a·phrag·
mat·i·cal·ly
su·pra·gin·gi·val
su·pra·glot·tic
also su·pra·glot·tal
su·pra·he·pat·ic
su·pra·hy·oid
su·pra·le·thal
su·pra·lim·i·nal

su·pra·max·i·mal
su·pra·nu·cle·ar
su·pra·oc·cip·i·tal
su·pra·oc·clu·sion
su·pra·op·tic
su·pra·or·bit·al
su·pra·pu·bic
su·pra·pu·bi·cal·ly
  or su·pra·pu·bic·ly

su·pra·re·nal
su·pra·re·nal·ec·to·
  my
  pl su·pra·re·nal·ec·to·
  mies

su·pra·scap·u·lar
su·pra·sel·lar
su·pra·spi·nal
su·pra·spi·na·tus
su·pra·spi·nous
su·pra·ster·nal
su·pra·syl·vi·an
su·pra·ten·to·ri·al
su·pra·thresh·old
su·pra·troch·le·ar
su·pra·vag·i·nal
su·pra·val·vu·lar
su·pra·ven·tric·u·
  lar
su·pra·vi·tal
su·ral
sur·a·min
sur·face-ac·tive
sur·fac·tant
surf·er's knot
sur·geon
sur·geon-in-chief
sur·geon's knot

sur·gery
  pl sur·ger·ies

sur·gi·cal
sur·ra
sur·ro·gate
sur·veil·lance
sur·vive
  sur·vived
  sur·viv·ing

sus·cep·ti·bil·i·ty
  pl sus·cep·ti·bil·i·ties

sus·cep·ti·ble
sus·pen·sion
sus·pen·soid
sus·pen·so·ry
  pl sus·pen·so·ries

sus·ten·tac·u·lar
sus·ten·tac·u·lum
  pl sus·ten·tac·u·la

sus·ten·tac·u·lum
  ta·li

su·tur·al
su·ture
  su·tured
  su·tur·ing

suxa·me·tho·ni·um
sved·berg
swab
  swabbed
  swab·bing

swage
  swaged
  swag·ing

swal·low
Swan-Ganz cath·e·
  ter
sway·back

sway·backed
sweat
  sweat
    or sweat·ed
  sweat·ing

swee·ny
  also swee·ney
  or swin·ney
  pl swee·nies
  also swee·neys
  or swin·neys

swell
  swelled
  swelled
    or swol·len
  swell·ing

Swift's dis·ease
swim·mer's itch
swine·herd's dis·
  ease
sy·co·sis
  pl sy·co·ses
  inflammatory dis-
  ease of the hair folli-
  cles (see psychosis)

sy·co·sis bar·bae
Syd·en·ham's cho·
  rea
syl·vat·ic
Syl·vi·an
sym·bal·lo·phone
sym·bi·ont
sym·bi·on·tic
sym·bi·o·sis
  pl sym·bi·o·ses

sym·bi·ote
sym·bi·ot·ic
  also sym·bi·ot·i·cal

sym·bleph·a·ron
sym·bol
sym·bol·ic
sym·bol·i·cal·ly
sym·bol·ism
sym·bol·iza·tion
sym·bol·ize
  sym·bol·ized
  sym·bol·iz·ing
Syme's am·pu·ta·
  tion
  or Syme am·pu·ta·
    tion

sym·met·ri·cal
  or sym·met·ric

sym·me·try
  pl sym·me·tries

sym·pa·thec·to·
  mized

sym·pa·thec·to·my
  pl sym·pa·thec·to·
    mies

sym·pa·thet·ic
sym·pa·thet·i·cal·ly
sym·pa·thet·i·co·to·
  nia
sym·pa·thet·i·co·
  ton·ic
sym·path·i·co·lyt·ic
sym·path·i·co·to·
  nia
sym·path·i·co·ton·
  ic
sym·path·i·co·trop·
  ic
sym·pa·thin

sym·pa·tho·ad·re·
  nal
sym·pa·tho·go·nia
sym·pa·tho·go·ni·o·
  ma
  pl sym·pa·tho·go·ni·o·
    ma·ta
  or sym·pa·tho·go·ni·o
    ·mas

sym·pa·tho·lyt·ic
sym·pa·tho·mi·
  met·ic
sym·pa·thy
  pl sym·pa·thies

sym·phy·se·al
  also sym·phys·i·al

sym·phys·i·on
sym·phy·si·ot·o·my
  pl sym·phy·si·ot·o·
    mies

sym·phy·sis
  pl sym·phy·ses

sym·phy·sis men·ti
sym·phy·sis pu·bis
symp·tom
symp·tom·at·ic
symp·tom·at·i·cal·
  ly
symp·tom·at·o·log·
  i·cal
  or symp·tom·at·o·log·
    ic

symp·tom·atol·o·gy
  pl symp·tom·atol·o·
    gies

symp·to·mol·o·gy
  pl symp·to·mol·o·gies

sym·pus di·pus

syn·ae·re·sis
  var of syneresis

syn·anas·to·mo·sis
  pl syn·anas·to·mo·ses

syn·an·throp·ic
syn·an·thro·py
  pl syn·an·thro·pies

syn·apse
syn·apsed
syn·aps·ing
syn·ap·sis
  pl syn·ap·ses

syn·ap·tic
syn·ap·ti·cal·ly
syn·ap·to·gen·e·sis
  pl syn·ap·to·gen·e·ses

syn·ap·tol·o·gy
  pl syn·ap·tol·o·gies

syn·ap·to·ne·mal
  com·plex
  or syn·ap·ti·ne·mal
    com·plex

syn·ap·to·som·al
syn·ap·to·some
syn·ar·thro·di·al
syn·ar·thro·sis
  pl syn·ar·thro·ses

syn·cary·on
  var of synkaryon

syn·chon·dro·sis
  pl syn·chon·dro·ses

syn·cho·ri·al
syn·chro·tron
syn·co·pal
syn·co·pe
syn·cy·tial

syrosingopine

syn·cy·tio·tro·pho·
  blast
syn·cy·tium
  pl syn·cy·tia
syn·dac·tyl
syn·dac·tyl·ia
syn·dac·tyl·ism
syn·dac·tyl·ous
syn·dac·ty·ly
  pl syn·dac·ty·lies
syn·des·mo·sis
  pl syn·des·mo·ses
syn·drome
syn·e·chia
  pl syn·e·chiae
syn·eph·rine
syn·ere·sis
  also syn·ae·re·sis
syn·er·get·ic
syn·er·gic
syn·er·gi·cal·ly
syn·er·gism
syn·er·gist
syn·er·gis·tic
syn·er·gis·ti·cal·ly
syn·er·gize
  syn·er·gized
  syn·er·giz·ing
syn·er·gy
  pl syn·er·gies
syn·er·ize
  syn·er·ized
  syn·er·iz·ing
syn·es·the·sia
syn·es·the·te
syn·es·thet·ic
Syn·ga·mus

syn·ga·my
  pl syn·ga·mies
syn·ge·ne·ic
syn·kary·on
  also syn·cary·on
syn·ki·ne·sia
syn·ki·ne·sis
  pl syn·ki·ne·ses
syn·ki·net·ic
syn·onym
syn·onym·i·ty
  pl syn·onym·i·ties
syn·on·y·mize
  syn·on·y·mized
  syn·on·y·miz·ing
syn·on·y·my
  pl syn·on·y·mies
syn·op·to·phore
syn·or·chi·dism
syn·os·to·sis
  pl syn·os·to·ses
syn·o·vec·to·my
  pl syn·o·vec·to·mies
sy·no·via
sy·no·vi·al
syn·ovi·o·ma
  pl syn·ovi·o·mas
  or syn·ovi·o·ma·ta
sy·no·vi·tis
syn·tac·tic
  or syn·tac·ti·cal
syn·tac·tics
syn·ten·ic
syn·te·ny
  pl syn·te·nies
syn·thase

syn·the·sis
  pl syn·the·ses
syn·the·size
  syn·the·sized
  syn·the·siz·ing
syn·the·tase
syn·thet·ic
syn·thet·i·cal·ly
syn·ton·ic
syn·tro·pho·blast
Sy·pha·cia
syph·i·lid
syph·i·lis
syph·i·lit·ic
syph·i·lit·i·cal·ly
syph·i·lo·derm
syph·i·lo·log·ic
syph·i·lol·o·gist
syph·i·lol·o·gy
  pl syph·i·lol·o·gies
syph·i·lo·ma
  pl syph·i·lo·mas
  or syph·i·lo·ma·ta
syph·i·lo·pho·bia
syph·i·lo·ther·a·py
  pl syph·i·lo·ther·a·
  pies
Syr·a·cuse dish
Syr·a·cuse watch
  glass
sy·ringe
  sy·ringed
  sy·ring·ing
sy·rin·go·bul·bia
sy·rin·go·my·elia
sy·rin·go·my·el·ic
syr·o·sin·go·pine

syr·up
  or sir·up

syr·upy
  or sir·upy

sys·tem
sys·tem·at·ic
sys·tem·at·i·cal·ly
sys·tem·at·ics
sys·tem·a·tist
sys·tem·ati·za·tion
sys·tem·atize
  sys·tem·atized
  sys·tem·atiz·ing
sys·tem·ic
sys·tem·i·cal·ly
sys·to·le
sys·tol·ic

T

tab·a·nid
Ta·ban·i·dae
Ta·ba·nus
ta·bar·dil·lo
ta·bes
  pl ta·bes

ta·bes dor·sa·lis
ta·bet·ic
ta·ble
ta·ble·spoon
ta·ble·spoon·ful
  pl ta·ble·spoon·fuls
  also ta·ble·spoons·ful

tab·let

ta·boo
  also ta·bu
  pl ta·boos
  also ta·bus

ta·bo·pa·re·sis
tab tablet
tab·u·lar
ta·bun
tache noire
  pl taches noires

ta·chis·to·scope
ta·chis·to·scop·ic
ta·chis·to·scop·i·cal·ly
tachy·ar·rhyth·mia
tachy·aux·e·sis
  pl tachy·aux·e·ses

tachy·aux·et·ic
tachy·car·dia
  rapid heart action (see bradycardia)

tachy·car·di·ac
tachy·phy·lac·tic
tachy·phy·lax·is
  pl tachy·phy·lax·es

tachy·pnea
tachy·pne·ic
ta·chys·ter·ol
tac·tic
tac·tic·i·ty
  pl tac·tic·i·ties

tac·tile
tac·toid
tac·tual
tae·di·um vi·tae

tae·nia
  also te·nia
  pl tae·nias
  also te·nias
    tapeworm

tae·nia
  or te·nia
  pl tae·ni·ae
  or tae·nias
  or te·ni·ae
  or te·nias
    band of tissue

tae·nia·cid·al
  also te·nia·cid·al

tae·nia·cide
  also te·nia·cide

tae·nia co·li
  or te·nia co·li
  pl tae·ni·ae co·li
  or te·ni·ae co·li

tae·nia·fuge
  also te·nia·fuge

Tae·nia·rhyn·chus
tae·ni·a·sis
  or te·ni·a·sis

tae·ni·id
Tae·ni·idae
tag·a·tose
Ta·ka·ya·su's dis·ease
talc
tal·cum
ta·li
  pl of talus

tali·pes
tali·pes equi·no·var·us
tali·pes val·gus
tali·pes var·us

tegumentary

tal·low
ta·lo·cal·ca·ne·al
ta·lo·cru·ral
ta·lo·na·vic·u·lar
tal·on·id
tal·ose
ta·lo·tib·i·al
ta·lus
  pl ta·li

tam·bour
ta·mox·i·fen
tam·pan
Tam·pi·co jal·ap
tam·pon
tam·pon·ade
  also tam·pon·age

tan·nate
tan·nic
tan·nin
tan·ta·lum
tan·trum
ta·pe·tal
ta·pe·to·ret·i·nal
ta·pe·tum
  pl ta·pe·ta

ta·pe·tum lu·ci·
  dum
tape·worm
ta·pote·ment
tar·an·tism
ta·ran·tu·la
  pl ta·ran·tu·las
  also ta·ran·tu·lae

ta·rax·a·cum
tar·dive

tare
  tared
  tar·ing
tar·get
tar·ry stool
tar·sal
tar·so·meta·tar·sal
tar·sor·rha·phy
  pl tar·sor·rha·phies

tar·sus
  pl tar·si

tar·tar
tar·tar·ic
tar·trate
tar·tra·zine
tat·too
  pl tat·toos

tau·rine
tau·ro·cho·late
tau·ro·cho·lic
tau·ro·dont
tau·to·mer
tau·to·mer·ic
tau·tom·er·ism
tax·is
  pl tax·es

tax·on
  pl taxa
  also tax·ons

tax·o·nom·ic
tax·o·nom·i·cal·ly
tax·on·o·mist
tax·on·o·my
  pl tax·on·o·mies

Tay-Sachs dis·ease
T cell
tea·spoon

tea·spoon·ful
  pl tea·spoon·fuls
  also tea·spoons·ful

teat
tech·ne·tium
tech·nic
tech·ni·cal
tech·ni·cian
tech·nique
tech·no·log·i·cal
  or tech·no·log·ic

tech·nol·o·gist
tech·nol·o·gy
  pl tech·nol·o·gies

tec·tal
tec·to·bul·bar
tec·to·ri·al
tec·to·spi·nal
tec·tum
  pl tec·ta

tec·tum mes·en·
  ceph·a·li
teeth
  pl of tooth
teethe
  teethed
  teeth·ing
teg·men
  pl teg·mi·na

teg·men·tal
teg·men·tum
  pl teg·men·ta

teg·men tym·pa·ni
teg·u·ment
teg·u·men·tal
teg·u·men·ta·ry

Teich·mann's crys·
  tal
tei·cho·ic
te·la
  pl te·lae
te·la cho·roi·dea
  also te·la cho·ri·oi·dea
tel·an·gi·ec·ta·sia
tel·an·gi·ec·ta·sis
  pl tel·an·gi·ec·ta·ses
tel·an·gi·ec·tat·ic
te·la sub·cu·ta·nea
te·la sub·mu·co·sa
tele·bin·oc·u·lar
tele·den·dron
  var of telodendrion
tele·di·ag·no·sis
  pl tele·di·ag·no·ses
te·leg·o·ny
  pl te·leg·o·nies
tele·ki·ne·sis
  pl tele·ki·ne·ses
tele·ki·net·ic
tele·ki·net·i·cal·ly
tele·med·i·cine
tele·me·ter
tele·met·ric
tele·met·ri·cal·ly
te·lem·e·try
  pl te·lem·e·tries
tel·en·ce·phal·ic
tel·en·ceph·a·lon
te·le·o·log·i·cal
  also te·le·o·log·ic
te·le·ol·o·gy
  pl te·le·ol·o·gies
te·le·o·nom·ic

te·le·on·o·my
  pl te·le·on·o·mies
tel·eo·roent·gen·o·
  gram
  or tele·roent·gen·o·
    gram
tel·eo·roent·gen·og·
  ra·phy
  or tele·roent·gen·og·
    ra·phy
  pl tel·eo·roent·gen·og·
    ra·phies
  or tele·roent·gen·og·
    ra·phies
tele·path·ic
tele·path·i·cal·ly
te·lep·a·thy
  pl te·lep·a·thies
tel·es·the·sia
tel·es·thet·ic
tele·ther·a·py
  pl tele·ther·a·pies
tel·lu·ri·um
telo·cen·tric
telo·den·dri·on
  also tele·den·dron
  or telo·den·dron
  pl telo·den·dria
  also tele·den·dra
  or telo·den·dra
te·lo·gen
telo·lec·i·thal
telo·mere
telo·phase
telo·phrag·ma
  pl telo·phrag·ma·ta
Telo·spo·rid·ia
telo·spo·rid·i·an

telo·syn·ap·sis
  pl telo·syn·ap·ses
telo·syn·ap·tic
telo·tax·is
  pl telo·tax·es

tem·per·a·ment
tem·per·ate
tem·per·a·ture
tem·plate
  also tem·plet
tem·ple
tem·po·ral
tem·po·ral·is
tem·po·ro·man·
  dib·u·lar
tem·po·ro·oc·cip·i·
  tal
tem·po·ro·pa·ri·
  etal
te·na·cious
te·nac·u·lum
  pl te·nac·u·la
  or te·nac·u·lums

ten·der
ten·di·ni·tis
  or ten·don·itis
ten·di·nous
  also ten·do·nous
ten·don
ten·don·itis
  var of tendinitis
ten·don of Achil·
  les
ten·don of Zinn
ten·do·nous
  var of tendinous
ten·do·vag·i·ni·tis

te·nes·mus

te·nia
 var of taenia

te·nia·cid·al
 var of tae·nia·cid·al

te·nia·cide
 var of taeniacide

te·nia co·li
 var of tae·nia co·li

te·nia·fuge
 var of taeniafuge

te·ni·a·sis
 var of taeniasis

ten·nis el·bow

te·no·de·sis
 pl te·no·de·ses

te·nol·y·sis
 pl te·nol·y·ses

Te·non's cap·sule

Te·non's space

te·no·plas·ty
 pl te·no·plas·ties

te·nor·rha·phy
 pl te·nor·rha·phies

teno·syn·o·vec·to·my
 pl teno·syn·o·vec·to·mies

teno·syn·o·vi·tis

ten·o·tome

te·not·o·mize
 te·not·o·mized
 te·not·o·miz·ing

te·not·o·my
 pl te·not·o·mies

teno·vag·i·ni·tis

ten·si·om·e·ter

ten·sion

ten·sion·al

ten·sor

ten·sor fas·ci·ae la·tae
 or ten·sor fas·cia la·ta

ten·sor pa·la·ti

ten·sor tym·pa·ni

ten·sor ve·li pa·la·ti·ni

ten·to·ri·al

ten·to·ri·um
 pl ten·to·ria

ten·to·ri·um ce·re·bel·li

te·pa

ter·as
 pl ter·a·ta

te·rato·car·ci·no·ma
 pl te·rato·car·ci·no·mas
 or te·rato·car·ci·no·ma·ta

te·rato·gen

ter·a·to·gen·e·sis
 pl ter·a·to·gen·e·ses

ter·a·to·gen·ic

ter·a·to·ge·nic·i·ty
 pl ter·a·to·ge·nic·i·ties

ter·a·toid

ter·a·to·log·i·cal
 or ter·a·to·log·ic

ter·a·tol·o·gist

ter·a·tol·o·gy
 pl ter·a·tol·o·gies

ter·a·to·ma
 pl ter·a·to·mas
 or ter·a·to·ma·ta

ter·a·to·ma·tous

ter·bi·um

ter·bu·ta·line

ter·e·bene

te·res ma·jor

te·res mi·nor

ter·mi·nal

ter·mi·na·tion

ter·mi·na·tor

ter·mi·nus
 pl ter·mi·ni
 also ter·mi·nus·es

ter·na·ry

Ter·ni·dens

ter·pene

ter·pe·nic

ter·pe·noid

ter·pin

ter·pin·e·ol

ter·tian

ter·tia·ry
 pl ter·tia·ries

ter·tip·a·ra
 pl ter·tip·a·ras
 or ter·tip·a·rae

Te·schen dis·ease

tes·la

test·cross

tes·tes
 pl of testis

tes·ti·cle

tes·tic·u·lar

tes·tis
 pl tes·tes

tes·tos·ter·one

tes·tos·ter·one
  enan·thate

test-tube
  adjective

test tube
  noun

tet·a·nal

te·tan·ic

te·tan·i·cal·ly

tet·a·ni·za·tion

tet·a·nize
  tet·a·nized
  tet·a·niz·ing

tet·a·no·ly·sin

tet·a·no·spas·min

tet·a·nus

tet·a·ny
  pl tet·a·nies

te·tar·ta·no·pia

tet·ra·ben·a·zine

tet·ra·caine

tet·ra·chlo·ride

tet·ra·chlo·ro·eth·
  yl·ene

tet·ra·chlo·ro·
  meth·ane

tet·ra·cy·clic

tet·ra·cy·cline

tet·rad

tet·ra·deca·pep·tide

tet·ra·eth·yl·am·
  mo·ni·um

tet·ra·eth·yl lead

tet·ra·eth·yl·thi·u·
  ram di·sul·fide

tet·ra·hy·drate

tet·ra·hy·drat·ed

tet·ra·hy·dro·can·
  nab·i·nol

tet·ra·hy·dro·fo·
  late

tet·ra·hy·me·na

tet·ra·iodo·phe·nol·
  phtha·lein

te·tral·o·gy of Fal·
  lot

tet·ra·mer

tet·ra·mer·ic

tet·ra·meth·yl·am·
  mo·ni·um

tet·ra·nu·cle·o·tide

tet·ra·pa·ren·tal

tet·ra·pep·tide

Tet·ra·phyl·lid·ea

tet·ra·ple·gia

tet·ra·ploid

tet·ra·ploi·dy
  pl tet·ra·ploi·dies

tet·ra·pyr·role
  also tet·ra·pyr·rol

tet·ra·sac·cha·ride

tet·ra·so·mic

tet·ra·va·lent

tet·ra·zole

tet·ra·zo·li·um

te·tro·do·tox·in

tet·rose

te·trox·ide

Tex·as fe·ver

T-group

tha·lam·ic

thal·a·mo·cor·ti·cal

thal·a·mot·o·my
  pl thal·a·mot·o·mies

thal·a·mus
  pl thal·a·mi

thal·as·se·mia

thal·as·se·mic

tha·las·so·ther·a·py
  pl tha·las·so·ther·a·
  pies

tha·lid·o·mide

thal·li·um

thal·lo·phyt·ic

than·a·to·log·i·cal

than·a·tol·o·gist

than·a·tol·o·gy
  pl than·a·tol·o·gies

than·a·to·pho·ric

Than·a·tos

the·ater
  or the·atre

the·ba·ine

the·ca
  pl the·cae

the·ca ex·ter·na

the·ca fol·lic·u·li

the·ca in·ter·na

the·cal

thei·le·ria
  pl thei·le·ri·ae
  also thei·le·rias

thei·le·ri·al

thei·le·ri·a·sis
  pl thei·le·ri·a·ses

thei·le·ri·o·sis
  pl thei·le·ri·o·ses
  or thei·le·ri·o·sis·es

the·lar·che

The·la·zia
thel·a·zi·a·sis
pl thel·a·zi·a·ses

Thel·a·zi·idae
the·nar
theo·bro·ma oil
theo·bro·mine
the·oph·yl·line
ther·a·peu·sis
pl ther·a·peu·ses

ther·a·peu·tic
ther·a·peu·ti·cal·ly
ther·a·peu·tics
ther·a·peu·tist
the·ra·pia ste·ri·li·sans mag·na
ther·a·pist
ther·a·py
pl ther·a·pies

the·ri·ac
the·ri·a·ca
the·ri·a·ca An·drom·a·chi
Ther·i·di·idae
the·rio·gen·o·log·i·cal
the·rio·ge·nol·o·gist
the·rio·ge·nol·o·gy
pl the·rio·ge·nol·o·gies

therm
ther·mal
therm·is·tor
ther·mo·cau·tery
pl ther·mo·cau·ter·ies

ther·mo·chem·i·cal

ther·mo·chem·is·try
pl ther·mo·chem·is·tries

ther·mo·co·ag·u·la·tion
ther·mo·cou·ple
ther·mo·di·lu·tion
ther·mo·du·ric
ther·mo·dy·nam·ics
ther·mo·gen·e·sis
pl ther·mo·gen·e·ses

ther·mo·gen·ic
ther·mo·gram
ther·mo·graph
ther·mo·graph·ic
ther·mo·graph·i·cal·ly
ther·mog·ra·phy
pl ther·mog·ra·phies

ther·mo·la·bile
ther·mo·la·bil·i·ty
pl ther·mo·la·bil·i·ties

ther·mol·y·sin
ther·mol·y·sis
pl ther·mol·y·ses

ther·mo·lyt·ic
ther·mom·e·ter
ther·mo·met·ric
ther·mom·e·try
pl ther·mom·e·tries

ther·mo·phile
ther·mo·phil·ic
also ther·moph·i·lous

ther·mo·re·cep·tor

ther·mo·reg·u·late
ther·mo·reg·u·lat·ed
ther·mo·reg·u·lat·ing
ther·mo·reg·u·la·tion
ther·mo·reg·u·la·tor
ther·mo·reg·u·la·to·ry
ther·mo·scope
ther·mo·sta·bil·i·ty
pl ther·mo·sta·bil·i·ties

ther·mo·sta·ble
ther·mo·stat
ther·mo·stat·ed
or ther·mo·stat·ted
ther·mo·stat·ing
or ther·mo·stat·ting
ther·mo·stat·ic
ther·mo·stat·i·cal·ly
ther·mo·strom·uhr
ther·mo·tac·tic
ther·mo·tax·is
pl ther·mo·tax·es

ther·mo·ther·a·py
ther·mo·trop·ic
ther·mot·ro·pism
the·sau·ro·sis
pl the·sau·ro·ses
or the·sau·ro·sis·es

the·ta rhythm
the·ve·tin
thia·ben·da·zole

thi·acet·azone
thi·ami·nase
thi·a·mine
  also thi·a·min

Thi·ara
thi·a·zide
thi·a·zine
thi·a·zole
thi·a·zol·i·dine
Thiersch graft
thigh·bone
thig·mo·tac·tic
thig·mo·tax·is
  pl thig·mo·tax·es
thig·mo·trop·ic
thig·mot·ro·pism
thi·mer·o·sal
thin-lay·er chro·
  ma·tog·ra·phy
thio
thio·al·de·hyde
thio·ba·cil·lus
  pl thio·ba·cil·li
thio·bar·bi·tu·ric
thio·car·ba·mide
thio·chrome
thi·oc·tic ac·id
  also 6,8-thi·oc·tic ac·
  id
thio·cy·a·nate
thio·di·phe·nyl·
  amine
thio·es·ter
thio·ether
thio·gly·co·late
  also thio·gly·col·late

thio·gly·col·ic
  also thio·gly·col·lic
thio·gua·nine
thi·ol
thi·o·lic
thio·ne·ine
thi·o·nine
thio·pen·tal
thio·phene
  also thio·phen
thio·rid·a·zine
thio·semi·car·ba·
  zone
thio·sul·fate
thio·sul·fu·ric
thio·te·pa
thio·thix·ene
thio·ura·cil
thio·urea
thio·xan·thene
thi·ram
third-de·gree burn
thixo·tro·pic
thix·ot·ro·py
  pl thix·ot·ro·pies

Thom·as splint
Thom·sen's dis·
  ease
thon·zyl·a·mine
tho·ra·cen·te·sis
  pl tho·ra·cen·te·ses

tho·ra·ces
  pl of thorax

tho·rac·ic
tho·rac·i·cal·ly

tho·ra·co·ab·dom·i·
  nal
  also tho·rac·i·co·ab·
  dom·i·nal

tho·ra·co·acro·mi·
  al
tho·ra·co·cen·te·sis
  pl tho·ra·co·cen·te·ses
tho·ra·co·dor·sal
tho·ra·co·gas·tros·
  chi·sis
  pl tho·ra·co·gas·tros·
  chi·ses
  or tho·ra·co·gas·tros·
  chi·sis·es

tho·ra·co·lum·bar
tho·ra·cop·a·gus
  pl tho·ra·cop·a·gus·es
  or tho·ra·cop·a·gi

tho·ra·co·plas·ty
  pl tho·ra·co·plas·ties

tho·ra·co·scope
tho·ra·co·scop·ic
tho·ra·cos·co·py
  pl tho·ra·cos·co·pies

tho·ra·cos·to·my
  pl tho·ra·cos·to·mies

tho·ra·cot·o·my
  pl tho·ra·cot·o·mies

tho·rax
  pl tho·rax·es
  or tho·ra·ces

tho·ri·um
tho·ron
thor·ough·pin
thread·worm
thready
thre·o·nine

thresh·old

throb
  throbbed
  throb·bing

throm·base

throm·bas·the·nia

throm·bec·to·my
  pl throm·bec·to·mies

throm·bi
  pl of thrombus

throm·bin

throm·bo·an·gi·i·tis
  pl throm·bo·an·gi·it·i·des

throm·bo·an·gi·i·tis ob·lit·er·ans

throm·bo·ar·ter·i·tis

throm·bo·blast

throm·bo·cyte

throm·bo·cyt·ic

throm·bo·cy·top·a·thy
  pl throm·bo·cy·top·a·thies

throm·bo·cy·to·pe·nia

throm·bo·cy·to·pe·nic

throm·bo·cy·to·poi·e·sis
  pl throm·bo·cy·to·poi·e·ses

throm·bo·cy·to·sis
  pl throm·bo·cy·to·ses

throm·bo·em·bol·ic

throm·bo·em·bo·lism

throm·bo·end·ar·te·rec·to·my
  pl throm·bo·end·ar·te·rec·to·mies

throm·bo·gen·ic

throm·bo·ge·nic·i·ty
  pl throm·bo·ge·nic·i·ties

throm·bo·ki·nase

throm·bol·y·sis
  pl throm·bol·y·ses

throm·bo·lyt·ic

throm·bo·pe·nia

throm·bo·pe·nic

throm·bo·phle·bi·tis
  pl throm·bo·phle·bit·i·des

throm·bo·plas·tic

throm·bo·plas·ti·cal·ly

throm·bo·plas·tin

throm·bo·plas·tin·o·gen

throm·bose
  throm·bosed
  throm·bos·ing

throm·bo·sis
  pl throm·bo·ses

throm·bo·sthe·nin

throm·bo·test

throm·bot·ic

throm·box·ane

throm·bus
  pl throm·bi

thrush

thu·jone

thu·li·um

thumb-suck·er

thumb-suck·ing

thumps

thy·mec·to·mize
  thy·mec·to·mized
  thy·mec·to·miz·ing

thy·mec·to·my
  pl thy·mec·to·mies

thy·mic

thy·mi·co·lym·phat·ic

thy·mi·dine

thy·mi·dyl·ic

thy·mine

thy·mo·cyte

thy·mol

thy·mo·lyt·ic

thy·mo·ma
  pl thy·mo·mas
  or thy·mo·ma·ta

thy·mo·nu·cle·ic

thy·mo·poi·et·in

thy·mo·sin

thy·mus

thy·ro·ac·tive

thy·ro·ar·y·te·noid

thy·ro·ar·y·te·noi·de·us

thy·ro·cal·ci·to·nin

thy·ro·cer·vi·cal
thy·ro·epi·glot·tic
thy·ro·gen·ic
thy·ro·glob·u·lin
thy·ro·glos·sal
thy·ro·hy·al
thy·ro·hy·oid
thy·roid
  also thy·roi·dal
  adjective

thy·roid
  noun

thy·roid-bind·ing
  glob·u·lin
thy·roid·ec·to·mize
  thy·roid·ec·to·
    mized
  thy·roid·ec·to·
    miz·ing
thy·roid·ec·to·my
  pl thy·roid·ec·to·mies

thy·roid·itis
thy·roid-stim·u·lat·
  ing hor·mone
thy·ro·nine
thy·ro·para·thy·
  roid·ec·to·mized
thy·ro·para·thy·
  roid·ec·to·my
  pl thy·ro·para·thy·
    roid·ec·to·mies

thy·rot·o·my
  pl thy·rot·o·mies

thy·ro·tox·ic
thy·ro·tox·ic·i·ty
  pl thy·ro·tox·ic·i·ties

thy·ro·tox·i·co·sis
  pl thy·ro·tox·i·co·ses
thy·ro·tro·pic
  also thy·ro·tro·phic
thy·ro·tro·pin
  also thy·ro·tro·phin
thy·ro·tro·pin-re·
  leas·ing hor·
  mone
thy·rox·ine
  or thy·rox·in

thy·rox·ine-bind·
  ing glob·u·lin
Thysa·no·so·ma
tib·ia
  pl tib·i·ae
  also tib·i·as
tib·i·al
tib·i·a·lis
  pl tib·i·a·les
tib·io·fem·o·ral
tib·io·fib·u·lar
tib·io·tar·sal
ti·bric
ti·car·cil·lin
tic dou·lou·reux
tick-borne
tick·icid·al
tick·icide
ti·cryn·a·fen
tid·al
tig·lic
ti·gog·e·nin
ti·go·nin
ti·groid
ti·grol·y·sis
  pl ti·grol·y·ses

ti·ki·ti·ki
tilt·board
tim·bral
tim·bre
  also tim·ber
timed-re·lease
  also time-re·lease
ti·mo·lol
tinc·to·ri·al
tinc·tu·ra
  pl tinc·tu·rae
tinc·ture
tin·ea
tin·ea bar·bae
tin·ea ca·pi·tis
tin·ea cor·po·ris
tin·ea cru·ris
tin·ea pe·dis
tin·ea ver·si·col·or
Ti·nel's sign
Tin·ne·vel·ly sen·
  na
tin·ni·tus
ti·queur
ti·sane
Ti·se·li·us ap·pa·ra·
  tus
tis·sue
tis·su·lar
ti·ta·ni·um
ti·ter
ti·tered
ti·trant
ti·trat·able
ti·trate
  ti·trat·ed
  ti·trat·ing

ti·tra·tion
ti·tra·tor
ti·tri·met·ric
ti·tri·met·ri·cal·ly
ti·trim·e·try
   pl ti·trim·e·tries

tit·u·ba·tion
T lym·pho·cyte
T-maze
toad·stool
to·bac·co
   pl to·bac·cos
to·bra·my·cin
to·co·dy·na·mom·e·ter
   var of tokodynamome·ter
to·col·o·gy
   var of tokology
to·coph·er·ol
toe·nail
to·ga·vi·rus
toi·let
to·ko·dy·na·mom·e·ter
   or to·co·dy·na·mom·e·ter
to·kol·o·gy
   or to·col·o·gy
   pl to·kol·o·gies
   or to·col·o·gies
to·laz·amide
to·laz·o·line
tol·bu·ta·mide
tol·er·ance
tol·er·ant

tol·er·ate
   tol·er·at·ed
   tol·er·at·ing
tol·ero·gen·ic
tol·met·in
tol·naf·tate
to·lo·ni·um
tol·u·ene
to·lu·ic
to·lu·idine
tol·u·ol
tom·a·tine
   or tom·a·tin
Tomes' fi·ber
to·mo·gram
to·mo·graph
to·mo·graph·ic
to·mog·ra·phy
   pl to·mog·ra·phies
tongue
tongue-tie
tongue-tied
ton·ic
ton·i·cal·ly
to·nic·i·ty
   pl to·nic·i·ties
tono·fi·bril
tono·fil·a·ment
to·no·graph·ic
to·nog·ra·phy
   pl to·nog·ra·phies
to·nom·e·ter
to·no·met·ric
to·nom·e·try
   pl to·nom·e·tries
to·no·top·ic
ton·sil

ton·sil·lar
ton·sil·lec·to·my
   pl ton·sil·lec·to·mies
ton·sil·li·tis
ton·sil·lo·phar·yn·gi·tis
   pl ton·sil·lo·phar·yn·git·i·des
ton·sil·lo·tome
to·nus
tooth
   pl teeth
tooth·ache
tooth·brush
tooth·paste
tooth·pick
to·pec·to·my
   pl to·pec·to·mies
to·pha·ceous
to·phus
   pl to·phi
top·i·cal
topo·graph·i·cal
   or topo·graph·ic
to·pog·ra·phy
   pl to·pog·ra·phies
topo·log·i·cal
   also topo·log·ic
to·pol·o·gy
   pl to·pol·o·gies
tor·cu·lar He·roph·i·li
to·ri
   pl of torus
to·ric
tor·pid

tor·pid·i·ty
pl tor·pid·i·ties

tor·por

torque
torqued
torqu·ing

torr
pl torr

tor·sion

tor·sion·al

tor·si·ver·sion

tor·so
pl tor·sos
or tor·si

tor·ti·col·lis

tor·tu·os·i·ty
pl tor·tu·os·i·ties

tor·tu·ous

tor·u·la
pl tor·u·lae
also tor·u·las

Tor·u·lop·sis

tor·u·lo·sis

to·rus
pl to·ri

to·rus tu·ba·ri·us

to·rus ure·ter·i·cus

to·ta·quine
also to·ta·qui·na

to·ti·po·ten·cy
pl to·ti·po·ten·cies

to·ti·po·tent

to·ti·po·ten·tial

to·ti·po·ten·ti·al·i·ty
pl to·ti·po·ten·ti·al·i·ties

Tou·rette syn·drome
or Tou·rette`s syn·drome

tour·ni·quet

tox·a·phene

Tox·as·ca·ris

tox·e·mia

tox·e·mic

tox·ic

tox·i·cant

tox·ic·i·ty
pl tox·ic·i·ties

tox·i·co·den·drol

tox·i·co·der·ma

tox·i·co·der·ma·ti·tis
pl tox·i·co·der·ma·ti·tis·es
or tox·i·co·der·ma·tit·i·des

tox·i·co·gen·ic

tox·i·co·log·i·cal
or tox·i·co·log·ic

tox·i·col·o·gist

tox·i·col·o·gy
pl tox·i·col·o·gies

tox·i·co·ma·nia

tox·i·co·sis
pl tox·i·co·ses

toxi·gen·ic

toxi·ge·nic·i·ty
pl toxi·ge·nic·i·ties

tox·in

tox·in-an·ti·tox·in

toxi·pho·bia

Tox·o·cara

tox·o·ca·ri·a·sis
pl tox·o·ca·ri·a·ses

tox·oid

toxo·phore

toxo·phor·ic
or tox·oph·o·rous

toxo·plasm

toxo·plas·ma
pl toxo·plas·mas
or toxo·plas·ma·ta
also toxo·plas·ma

toxo·plas·mic

toxo·plas·mo·sis
pl toxo·plas·mo·ses

tra·bant

tra·bec·u·la
pl tra·bec·u·lae
also tra·bec·u·las

tra·bec·u·lar

tra·bec·u·la·tion

tra·bec·u·lec·to·my
pl tra·bec·u·lec·to·mies

trac·er

tra·chea
pl tra·che·ae
also tra·che·as

tra·che·al

tra·che·a·lis
pl tra·che·a·les

tra·che·itis

trach·e·lec·to·my
pl trach·e·lec·to·mies

trach·e·lo·mas·toid

trach·e·lo·plas·ty
pl trach·e·lo·plas·ties

trach·e·lor·rha·phy
  pl trach·e·lor·rha·phies

tra·che·o·bron·chi·al

tra·che·o·bron·chi·tis
  pl tra·cheo·bron·chit·i·des

tra·che·o·esoph·a·ge·al

tra·cheo·plas·ty
  pl tra·cheo·plas·ties

tra·che·os·co·py
  pl tra·che·os·co·pies

tra·che·os·to·my
  pl tra·che·os·to·mies

tra·che·ot·o·my
  pl tra·che·ot·o·mies

tra·cho·ma

tra·cho·ma·tous

trac·ing

trac·tion

tract of Gow·ers

tract of Lis·sauer

trac·tor

trac·tot·o·my
  pl trac·tot·o·mies

trac·tus
  pl trac·tus

trac·tus sol·i·ta·ri·us

trag·a·canth

tra·gus
  pl tra·gi

train·able

trance

tran·ex·am·ic

tran·quil·iza·tion

tran·quil·ize
  tran·quil·ized
  tran·quil·iz·ing

tran·quil·iz·er

trans·ab·dom·i·nal

trans·acet·y·lase

trans·ac·tion·al
  anal·y·sis

trans·am·i·nase

trans·am·i·nate
  trans·am·i·nat·ed
  trans·am·i·nat·ing

trans·am·i·na·tion

trans·cal·lo·sal

trans·cap·il·lary

trans·car·ba·myl·ase

trans·cath·e·ter

trans·cor·ti·cal

trans·cor·tin

tran·scribe
  tran·scribed
  tran·scrib·ing

tran·script

tran·scrip·tase

tran·scrip·tion

tran·scrip·tion·al

trans·cu·ta·ne·ous

trans·duce
  trans·duced
  trans·duc·ing

trans·duc·er

trans·duc·tant

trans·duc·tion

trans·duc·tion·al

tran·sect

tran·sec·tion

trans·epi·the·li·al

trans·sep·tal

trans·es·ter·i·fi·ca·tion

trans·fect

trans·fec·tion

trans·fer

trans·fer·ase

trans·fer·ence

trans·fer·rin

trans·form

trans·for·mant

trans·for·ma·tion

trans·fus·able
  or trans·fus·ible

trans·fuse
  trans·fused
  trans·fus·ing

trans·fu·sion

trans·fu·sion·al

trans·fu·sion·ist

trans·glu·co·syl·ase

trans·glu·ta·min·ase

trans·he·pat·ic

tran·sient

trans·il·lu·mi·nate
  trans·il·lu·mi·nat·ed
  trans·il·lu·mi·nat·ing

trans·il·lu·mi·na·tion

tran·sis·tor
tran·si·tion
tran·si·tion·al
trans·late
  trans·lat·ed
  trans·lat·ing
trans·la·tion
trans·la·tion·al
trans·la·to·ry
trans·lo·cate
  trans·lo·cat·ed
  trans·lo·cat·ing
trans·lo·ca·tion
trans·lum·bar
trans·lu·mi·nal
trans·mem·brane
trans·meth·yl·a·tion
trans·mis·si·bil·i·ty
  pl trans·mis·si·bil·i·ties
trans·mis·si·ble
trans·mis·sion
trans·mit
  trans·mit·ted
  trans·mit·ting
trans·mit·ta·ble
trans·mit·tance
trans·mit·ter
trans·mu·ral
trans·mu·ta·tion
trans·neu·ro·nal
trans·or·bit·al
trans·ovar·i·al
trans·ovar·i·an
trans·pep·ti·dase
trans·pep·ti·da·tion

trans·phos·phor·y·lase
trans·phos·phor·y·la·tion
tran·spi·ra·tion
tran·spi·ra·tion·al
trans·pla·cen·tal
trans·plant
trans·plant·abil·i·ty
  pl trans·plant·abil·i·ties
trans·plant·able
trans·plan·ta·tion
trans·pos·able
trans·pos·ase
trans·pose
  trans·posed
  trans·pos·ing
trans·po·si·tion
trans·po·son
trans·py·lor·ic
trans·sex·u·al
trans·sex·u·al·ism
trans·sex·u·al·i·ty
  pl trans·sex·u·al·i·ties
trans·sphe·noi·dal
trans·syn·ap·tic
trans·tho·rac·ic
trans·tho·rac·i·cal·ly
trans·tra·che·al
tran·su·date
tran·su·da·tion
tran·su·da·tive
tran·sude
  tran·sud·ed
  tran·sud·ing

trans·ure·tero·ure·ter·os·to·my
  pl trans·ure·tero·ure·ter·os·to·mies
trans·ure·thral
trans·ve·nous
trans·ver·sa·lis cer·vi·cis
trans·ver·sa·lis fas·cia
trans·verse
trans·ver·sion
trans·ver·sus ab·dom·i·nis
trans·ver·sus pe·rin·ei su·per·fi·ci·a·lis
trans·ver·sus tho·ra·cis
trans·ves·tism
  also trans·ves·tit·ism
trans·ves·tite
tran·yl·cy·pro·mine
tra·pe·zi·um
  pl tra·pe·zi·ums
  or tra·pe·zia
tra·pe·zi·us
trap·e·zoid
trap·e·zoi·de·um
trau·ma
  pl trau·ma·ta
  or trau·mas
trau·mat·ic
trau·mat·i·cal·ly
trau·ma·tism
trau·ma·ti·za·tion

trau·ma·tize
  trau·ma·tized
  trau·ma·tiz·ing
trau·ma·tol·o·gy
  pl trau·ma·tol·o·gies
Trea·cher Col·lins
  syn·drome
trea·cle
tread·mill
treat·abil·i·ty
  pl treat·abil·i·ties
treat·able
treat·ment
tre·ha·lase
tre·ha·lose
Trem·a·to·da
trem·a·to·dan
  or trem·a·to·de·an
trem·a·tode
trem·bles
trem·e·tol
trem·or
trem·or·ine
trem·u·lous
trench foot
trench mouth
Tren·de·len·burg
  po·si·tion
trep·a·na·tion
treph·i·na·tion
tre·phine
  tre·phined
  tre·phin·ing
trep·o·ne·ma
  pl trep·o·ne·ma·ta
  or trep·o·ne·mas
trep·o·ne·mal

Trep·o·ne·ma·ta·
  ce·ae
trepo·ne·ma·to·sis
  pl trepo·ne·ma·to·ses
trepo·neme
trep·o·ne·mi·ci·dal
trep·pe
tri·ac·e·tin
tri·ac·e·tyl·ole·an·
  do·my·cin
tri·ad
tri·ad·ic
tri·age
tri·am·cin·o·lone
tri·am·ter·ene
tri·an·gle
tri·an·gle of Hes·
  sel·bach
tri·an·gu·lar
tri·an·gu·la·ris
  pl tri·an·gu·la·res
tri·at·o·ma
trib·ade
tri·bad·ic
trib·a·dism
tri·ba·sic
tri·bo·lu·mi·nes·
  cence
tri·bo·lu·mi·nes·
  cent
tri·bro·mo·eth·a·
  nol
tri·bro·mo·eth·yl
trib·u·tary
  pl trib·u·tar·ies
tri·bu·tyr·in
tri·car·box·yl·ic

tri·ceps
  pl tri·ceps·es
  also tri·ceps
tri·ceps bra·chii
tri·ceps su·rae
tri·chi·a·sis
tri·chi·na
  pl tri·chi·nae
  also tri·chi·nas
Tri·chi·na
trich·i·nel·la
  pl tri·chi·nel·lae
trich·i·nel·li·a·sis
  pl trich·i·nel·li·a·ses
trich·i·ni·a·sis
  pl trich·i·ni·a·ses
trich·i·nize
  trich·i·nized
  trich·i·niz·ing
trich·i·nosed
trich·i·no·sis
  pl trich·i·no·ses
tri·chi·nous
tri·chlor·fon
  also tri·chlor·phon
tri·chlor·me·thi·a·
  zide
tri·chlo·ro·ace·tic
  also tri·chlor·ace·tic
tri·chlo·ro·eth·y·
  lene
  also tri·chlor·eth·y·
  lene
tri·chlo·ro·meth·
  ane
tri·chlo·ro·phe·nol

tri·chlo·ro·phen·
oxy·ace·tic
tri·chlor·phon
var of trichlorfon
tricho·be·zoar
Tricho·bil·har·zia
tricho·ceph·a·li·a·
sis
pl tricho·ceph·a·li·a·
ses
Tricho·ceph·a·lus
tricho·cyst
Tricho·dec·tes
Tricho·dec·ti·dae
Tricho·der·ma
tricho·epi·the·li·o·
ma
pl tricho·epi·the·li·o·
mas
or tricho·epi·the·li·o·
ma·ta
tri·chol·o·gy
pl tri·chol·o·gies
tricho·mo·na·cid·al
tricho·mo·na·cide
tricho·mo·nad
tricho·mo·nal
Trich·o·mo·nas
tricho·mo·ni·a·sis
pl tricho·mo·ni·a·ses
tricho·my·co·sis
pl tricho·my·co·ses
tricho·phy·tid
tricho·phy·ton
tricho·phy·to·sis
pl tricho·phy·to·ses
Tricho·spo·ron

tricho·stron·gyle
tricho·stron·gy·lid
Tricho·stron·gyl·i·
dae
tricho·stron·gy·lo·
sis
Tricho·stron·gy·lus
tricho·til·lo·ma·nia
tricho·til·lo·man·ic
tri·chro·ism
tri·chro·mat
tri·chro·mat·ic
tri·chro·ma·tism
tri·chrome
trich·u·ri·a·sis
pl trich·u·ri·a·ses
Trich·u·ris
tri·clo·car·ban
tri·cre·sol
tri·cus·pid
tri·cy·clic
tri·di·hex·eth·yl
tri·eth·a·nol·amine
tri·eth·yl·amine
tri·eth·yl·ene·mel·
amine
tri·fa·cial
tri·fluo·per·a·zine
tri·flu·pro·ma·zine
tri·fo·cal
tri·gem·i·nal
tri·glyc·er·ide
tri·gone
also tri·gon
trig·o·nel·line
tri·go·nid
tri·go·ni·tis

tri·go·no·ceph·a·ly
pl tri·go·no·ceph·a·
lies
tri·go·num
pl tri·go·nums
or tri·go·na
tri·go·num ha·ben·
u·lae
tri·go·num ves·i·
cae
tri·hy·brid
tri·hy·drate
tri·hy·dric
tri·hy·droxy
tri·io·dide
tri·io·do·thy·ro·
nine
tri·lam·i·nar
tri·lobed
tri·mep·ra·zine
tri·mer
tri·mer·ic
tri·mer·iza·tion
tri·mes·ter
tri·metha·di·one
tri·meth·a·phan
tri·metho·ben·za·
mide
tri·meth·o·prim
tri·meth·yl
tri·meth·yl·amine
tri·meth·y·lene
tri·mo·lec·u·lar
tri·mor·phic
or tri·mor·phous
tri·mor·phism
tri·ni·trin

tri·ni·tro·glyc·er·in
tri·ni·tro·phe·nol
trin·oc·u·lar
tri·no·mi·al
tri·nu·cle·ate
tri·nu·cle·o·tide
tri·ole·in
tri·or·tho·cre·syl
tri·ose
tri·ox·ide
tri·ox·sa·len
tri·pal·mi·tin
trip·a·ra
tri·par·a·nol
tri·pel·en·na·mine
tri·pep·tide
tri·pha·sic
tri·phe·nyl·meth·ane
tri·phos·pha·tase
tri·phos·phate
tri·phos·pho·pyr·i·dine nu·cle·o·tide
tri·ple·gia
trip·let
trip·lo·blas·tic
trip·loid
trip·loi·dy
    pl trip·loi·dies
tri·que·tral
tri·que·trum
    pl tri·que·tra
tri·ra·di·us
    pl tri·ra·dii
    also tri·ra·di·us·es
tri·sac·cha·ride

tris·kai·deka·pho·bia
tris·mus
tri·so·mic
tri·so·my
    pl tri·so·mies
tri·stea·rin
tri·sub·sti·tut·ed
trit·an·ope
trit·an·opia
trit·an·opic
tri·ter·pene
tri·ter·pe·nic
tri·ter·pe·noid
tri·ti·at·ed
tri·ti·um
tri·tu·ber·cu·lar
trit·u·rate
    trit·u·rat·ed
    trit·u·rat·ing
trit·u·ra·tion
tri·va·lent
tro·car
    also tro·char
tro·chan·ter
tro·chan·ter·ic
tro·che
troch·lea
troch·le·ar
Trog·lo·tre·ma
tro·land
tro·le·an·do·my·cin
trol·ni·trate
Trom·bic·u·la
trom·bic·u·lid
Trom·bi·cu·li·dae
trom·bid·i·id

Trom·bi·di·idae
tro·meth·a·mine
tro·pa·co·caine
tro·pane
tro·pate
tro·pe·ine
troph·ec·to·derm
troph·ede·ma
    pl troph·ede·mas
    or troph·ede·ma·ta
tro·phic
tro·phi·cal·ly
tro·pho·blast
tro·pho·blas·tic
tro·pho·chro·ma·tin
troph·o·derm
tro·phol·o·gy
    pl tro·phol·o·gies
tro·pho·neu·ro·sis
    pl tro·pho·neu·ro·ses
tro·pho·neu·rot·ic
tro·pho·nu·cle·us
tro·pho·zo·ite
tro·pia
tro·pic ac·id
tro·pic·amide
tro·pine
tro·pism
tro·pis·tic
tro·po·col·la·gen
tro·po·my·o·sin
tro·po·nin
troy
trun·cal
trun·cus

trun·cus ar·te·ri·o·sus

trun·cus bra·chio·ce·phal·i·cus

truss

tryp·an blue

try·pano·ci·dal

try·pano·cide

try·pano·so·ma
pl try·pano·so·mas
or try·pano·so·ma·ta

try·pano·so·mal

Try·pano·so·mat·i·dae

try·pano·some

try·pano·so·mi·a·sis
pl try·pano·so·mi·a·ses

try·pan red

tryp·ars·amide

trypo·mas·ti·gote

tryp·sin

tryp·sin·iza·tion

tryp·sin·ize
tryp·sin·ized
tryp·sin·iz·ing

tryp·sin·o·gen

trypt·amine

tryp·tic

tryp·to·phan
also tryp·to·phane

tryp·to·pha·nase

tset·se
pl tset·se
or tset·ses

tsu·tsu·ga·mu·shi

T-tube

tub·al

tu·bec·to·my
pl tu·bec·to·mies

tu·ber

tu·ber ci·ne·re·um

tu·ber·cle

tu·ber·cu·lar

tu·ber·cu·lid
also tu·ber·cu·lide

tu·ber·cu·lin

tu·ber·cu·lo·cid·al

tu·ber·cu·lo·derm

tu·ber·cu·loid

tu·ber·cu·lo·ma
pl tu·ber·cu·lo·mas
also tu·ber·cu·lo·ma·ta

tu·ber·cu·lo·pro·tein

tu·ber·cu·lo·sis
pl tu·ber·cu·lo·ses

tu·ber·cu·lo·stat·ic

tu·ber·cu·lo·stea·ric

tu·ber·cu·lous

tu·ber·cu·lum im·par

tu·ber·os·i·ty
pl tu·ber·os·i·ties

tu·ber·ous

tu·bo·cu·ra·rine

tu·bu·lar

tu·bule

tu·bu·lin

tu·bu·lo·ac·i·nar
or tu·bu·lo·ac·i·nous

tu·bu·lo·al·ve·o·lar

tu·bu·lus
pl tu·bu·li

tu·la·re·mia

tu·la·re·mic

tulle gras

tu·me·fa·cient

tu·me·fac·tion

tu·me·fac·tive

tu·mer·ic
var of turmeric

tu·mes·cence

tu·mes·cent

tu·mid

tu·mid·i·ty
pl tu·mid·i·ties

tu·mor

tu·mor·al

tu·mor·i·cid·al

tu·mori·gen·e·sis
pl tu·mori·gen·e·ses

tu·mor·i·gen·ic

tu·mor·i·ge·nic·i·ty
pl tu·mor·i·ge·nic·i·ties

tu·mor·ous

Tun·ga

tung·sten

tu·nic

tu·ni·ca
pl tu·ni·cae

tu·ni·ca al·bu·gin·ea
pl tu·ni·cae al·bu·gin·e·ae

tu·ni·ca ex·ter·na

tu·ni·ca pro·pria

tu·ni·ca va·gi·na·lis
pl tu·ni·cae va·gi·na·les

tun·nel

tun·nel of Cor·ti

Tur·bel·lar·ia

tur·bel·lar·i·an

tur·bid

tur·bi·dim·e·ter

tur·bi·di·met·ric

tur·bi·di·met·ri·cal·ly

tur·bi·dim·e·try
pl tur·bi·dim·e·tries

tur·bid·i·ty
pl tur·bid·i·ties

tur·bi·nal

tur·bi·nate

tur·bi·nec·to·my
pl tur·bi·nec·to·mies

tur·ges·cence

tur·ges·cent

tur·gid

tur·gid·i·ty
pl tur·gid·i·ties

tur·gor

tu·ris·ta

tur·mer·ic
also tu·mer·ic

Tur·ner's syn·drome

tur·pen·tine

tur·ri·ceph·a·ly
pl tur·ri·ceph·a·lies

tus·sal

tus·sic

tus·sive

T wave

twee·zers

twen·ty-twen·ty
or 20/20

twin

twinge

twin·ning

twin·ship

two-winged fly

ty·ba·mate

ty·lec·to·my
pl ty·lec·to·mies

ty·lo·sin

tym·pan·ic

tym·pa·ni·tes

tym·pa·nit·ic

tym·pa·no·plas·ty
pl tym·pa·no·plas·ties

tym·pa·not·o·my
pl tym·pa·not·o·mies

tym·pa·num
pl tym·pa·na
also tym·pa·nums

tym·pa·ny
pl tym·pa·nies

Tyn·dall ef·fect

type
typed
typ·ing

ty·phoid

ty·phus

ty·po·log·i·cal

ty·pol·o·gy
pl ty·pol·o·gies

ty·ra·mine

ty·ro·ci·dine
also ty·ro·ci·din

Ty·rode so·lu·tion
or Ty·rode's so·lu·tion

ty·ros·i·nase

ty·ro·sine

ty·ro·sin·emia

ty·ro·sin·osis

ty·ro·thri·cin

U

ubi·qui·none

ud·der

ul·cer
ul·cered
ul·cer·ing

ul·cer·ate
ul·cer·at·ed
ul·cer·at·ing

ul·cer·ation

ul·cer·a·tive

ul·cero·gen·ic

ul·cero·glan·du·lar

ul·cero·mem·bra·nous

ul·cer·ous

ule·gy·ria

ul·na
pl ul·nae
or ul·nas

ul·nar

ul·ti·mo·bran·chi·al

ul·tra·cen·trif·u·gal

ul·tra·cen·tri·fu·ga·tion

ul·tra·cen·tri·fuge
  ul·tra·cen·tri·
    fuged
  ul·tra·cen·tri·
    fug·ing
ul·tra·di·an
ul·tra·fil·ter
ul·tra·fil·tra·ble
ul·tra·fil·trate
ul·tra·fil·tra·tion
ul·tra·mi·cro·scope
ul·tra·mi·cro·scop·
  ic
  also ul·tra·mi·cro·
    scop·i·cal
ul·tra·mi·cros·co·
  py
  pl ul·tra·mi·cros·co·
    pies
ul·tra·mi·cro·tome
ul·tra·mi·crot·o·my
  pl ul·tra·mi·crot·o·
    mies
ul·tra·son·ic
ul·tra·sono·gram
ul·tra·so·nog·ra·
  pher
ul·tra·so·no·graph·
  ic
ul·tra·so·nog·ra·
  phy
  pl ul·tra·so·nog·ra·
    phies
ul·tra·sound
ul·tra·struc·tur·al
ul·tra·struc·ture
ul·tra·thin

ul·tra·vi·o·let
ul·tra·vi·rus
um·bel·li·fer
Um·bel·lif·er·ae
um·bel·lif·er·one
um·bi·lec·to·my
  pl um·bi·lec·to·mies
um·bil·i·cal
um·bil·i·cat·ed
um·bil·i·ca·tion
um·bi·li·cus
  pl um·bi·li·ci
  or um·bi·li·cus·es
um·bo
  pl um·bo·nes
  or um·bos
un·anes·the·tized
un·born
un·bro·ken
un·cal
un·cal·ci·fied
un·ci
  pl of uncus
un·ci·form
Un·ci·nar·ia
un·ci·na·ri·a·sis
  pl un·ci·na·ri·a·ses
un·ci·nate
un·cloned
un·com·pen·sat·ed
un·com·pli·cat·ed
un·con·di·tion·al
un·con·di·tioned
un·con·ju·gat·ed
un·con·scious
un·co·or·di·nat·ed
un·cou·pler

un·crossed
unc·tu·ous
un·cus
  pl un·ci
un·deca·pep·tide
un·dec·e·no·ic
un·dec·y·len·ate
un·dec·y·le·nic
un·der·achieve
  un·der·achieved
  un·der·achiev·
    ing
un·der·achiev·er
un·der·ac·tive
un·der·ac·tiv·i·ty
  pl un·der·ac·tiv·i·ties
un·der·arm
un·der·cut
un·der·de·vel·oped
un·der·de·vel·op·
  ment
un·der·feed
  un·der·fed
  un·der·feed·ing
un·der·nour·ished
un·der·nour·ish·
  ment
un·der·nu·tri·tion
un·der·nu·tri·tion·
  al
un·der·sexed
un·der·tak·er
un·der·weight
un·de·scend·ed
un·di·ag·nosed
un·dif·fer·en·ti·at·
  ed

ureterogram

un·du·lant
un·du·la·to·ry
un·erupt·ed
un·guis
   pl un·gues
un·guis in·car·na·tus
un·gu·late
un·healed
un·health·ful
un·health·i·ness
un·healthy
  un·health·i·er
  un·health·i·est
un·hy·gi·en·ic
un·hy·gi·en·i·cal·ly
uni·cel·lu·lar
uni·cel·lu·lar·i·ty
  pl uni·cel·lu·lar·i·ties
uni·cus·pid
uni·fac·to·ri·al
uni·fla·gel·late
uni·fo·cal
uni·la·mel·lar
uni·lat·er·al
uni·loc·u·lar
un·im·mu·nized
uni·ne·phrec·to·mized
uni·ne·phrec·to·my
  pl uni·ne·phrec·to·mies
un·in·fec·ted
uni·nu·cle·ate
  also uni·nu·cle·at·ed
uni·oc·u·lar

uni·ovu·lar
unip·a·ra
  pl unip·a·ras
  or unip·a·rae
uni·pa·ren·tal
uni·pen·nate
uni·po·lar
unip·o·tent
unit·age
uni·va·lent
un·med·ul·lat·ed
un·my·elin·at·ed
Un·na's boot
  or Un·na boot
Un·na's paste boot
un·nil·hex·i·um
un·nil·pen·ti·um
un·nil·qua·di·um
un·of·fi·cial
un·or·ga·nized
un·ox·y·gen·at·ed
un·paired
un·phys·i·o·log·i·cal
  or un·phys·i·o·log·ic
un·re·ac·tive
un·re·sect·able
un·re·spon·sive
un·san·i·tary
un·sa·pon·i·fi·able
un·sat·u·rate
un·sat·u·rat·ed
un·sat·u·ra·tion
un·sex
un·sound
un·sta·ble
un·stri·at·ed

un·struc·tured
un·trans·formed
un·trans·lat·ed
un·treat·able
un·treat·ed
un·vac·ci·nat·ed
un·well
up·take
ura·chal
ura·chus
ura·cil
ura·nin
ura·ni·um
ura·nyl
urate
urat·ic
urea
Urea·plas·ma
ure·ase
ure·ide
ure·mia
ure·mic
ure·om·e·ter
ureo·tel·ic
ureo·te·lism
ure·ter
ure·ter·al
  or ure·ter·ic
ure·ter·ec·to·my
  pl ure·ter·ec·to·mies
ure·ter·o·cele
ure·tero·co·lic
ure·tero·en·ter·os·to·my
  pl ure·tero·en·ter·os·to·mies
ure·ter·o·gram

ure·ter·og·ra·phy
pl ure·ter·og·ra·phies

ure·tero·in·tes·ti·nal

ure·tero·li·thot·o·my
pl ure·tero·li·thot·o·mies

ure·ter·ol·y·sis
pl ure·ter·ol·y·ses

ure·tero·neo·cys·tos·to·my
pl ure·tero·neo·cys·tos·to·mies

ure·tero·plas·ty
pl ure·tero·plas·ties

ure·tero·py·elog·ra·phy
pl ure·tero·py·elog·ra·phies

ure·ter·or·rha·phy
pl ure·ter·or·rha·phies

ure·ter·os·co·py
pl ure·ter·os·co·pies

ure·tero·sig·moid·os·to·my
pl ure·tero·sig·moid·os·to·mies

ure·tero·ste·no·sis
pl ure·tero·ste·no·ses

ure·ter·os·to·my
pl ure·ter·os·to·mies

ure·ter·ot·o·my
pl ure·ter·ot·o·mies

ure·tero·ure·ter·os·to·my
pl ure·tero·ure·ter·os·to·mies

ure·tero·ves·i·cal

ure·thane
also ure·than

ure·thra
pl ure·thras
or ure·thrae

ure·thral

ure·threc·to·my
pl ure·threc·to·mies

ure·thri·tis

ure·thro·cele

ure·thro·cu·ta·ne·ous

ure·thro·cys·tog·ra·phy
pl ure·thro·cys·tog·ra·phies

ure·thro·gram

ure·throg·ra·phy
pl ure·throg·ra·phies

ure·thro·pexy
pl ure·thro·pex·ies

ure·thro·plas·ty
pl ure·thro·plas·ties

ure·thro·rec·tal

ure·thror·rha·phy
pl ure·thror·rha·phies

ure·thro·scope

ure·thro·scop·ic

ure·thros·co·py
pl ure·thros·co·pies

ure·thros·to·my
pl ure·thros·to·mies

ure·thro·tome

ure·throt·o·my
pl ure·throt·o·mies

ure·thro·vag·i·nal

ur·gen·cy
pl ur·gen·cies

ur·gin·ea

uric

uric·ac·i·de·mia

uric·ac·id·uria

uri·case

uri·ce·mia

uri·ce·mic

uri·col·y·sis
pl uri·col·y·ses

uri·co·lyt·ic

uri·co·su·ric

uri·co·tel·ic

uri·co·tel·ism

uri·dine

uri·dyl·ic

uri·nal

uri·nal·y·sis
pl uri·nal·y·ses

uri·nary

uri·nate

uri·nat·ed

uri·nat·ing

uri·na·tion

urine

uri·nif·er·ous

uri·no·gen·i·tal

uri·nom·e·ter

uri·nous

uro·bi·lin

uro·bi·lin·o·gen

uro·ca·nic

uro·chrome
uro·dy·nam·ic
uro·dy·nam·ics
uro·er·y·thrin
uro·gas·trone
uro·gen·i·tal
uro·gram
uro·graph·ic
urog·ra·phy
  pl urog·ra·phies
uro·ki·nase
uro·lag·nia
uro·lith
uro·lith·ia·sis
  pl uro·lith·ia·ses
uro·log·ic
  also uro·log·i·cal
urol·o·gist
urol·o·gy
  pl urol·o·gies
uron·ic
uro·path·ic
urop·a·thy
  pl urop·a·thies
uro·pep·sin
uro·por·phy·rin
uro·por·phy·rin·o·
  gen
uro·ra·dio·log·ic
uro·ra·di·ol·o·gy
  pl uro·ra·di·ol·o·gies
uro·sep·sis
  pl uro·sep·ses
ur·ti·car·ia
ur·ti·car·i·al
ur·ti·car·io·gen·ic

ur·ti·cate
  ur·ti·cat·ed
  ur·ti·cat·ing
ur·ti·ca·tion
uru·shi·ol
us·ti·lag·i·nism
Us·ti·la·go
uta
uter·ec·to·my
  pl uter·ec·to·mies
uteri
  pl of uterus
uter·ine
utero-ovar·ian
utero·pla·cen·tal
utero·sa·cral
utero·sal·pin·gog·
  ra·phy
  pl utero·sal·pin·gog·
  ra·phies
utero·ton·ic
utero·tub·al
utero·vag·i·nal
utero·ves·i·cal
uter·us
  pl uteri
  also uter·us·es
utri·cle
utric·u·lar
utric·u·lo·sac·cu·
  lar
utric·u·lus
  pl utric·u·li
uva·ur·si
uvea
uve·al

uve·itis
  pl uve·it·i·des
uveo·pa·rot·id
uveo·par·oti·tis
uvu·la
  pl uvu·las
  or uvu·lae
uvu·lar
uvu·la ves·i·cae
uvu·lec·to·my
  pl uvu·lec·to·mies
U wave

V

vac·ci·nal
vac·ci·nate
  vac·ci·nat·ed
  vac·ci·nat·ing
vac·ci·na·tion
vac·ci·na·tor
vac·cine
vac·ci·nee
vac·cin·ia
vac·cin·i·al
vac·ci·noid
vac·ci·no·style
vac·u·o·lar
vac·u·o·late
  or vac·u·o·lat·ed
vac·u·o·la·tion
vac·u·ole
vac·u·ol·iza·tion
vac·u·um
  pl vac·u·ums
  or vac·ua

va·gal
va·gi
  pl of vagus
va·gi·na
  pl va·gi·nae
  or va·gi·nas
va·gi·nal
va·gi·na ten·di·nis
vag·i·nec·to·my
  pl vag·i·nec·to·mies
vag·i·nis·mus
vag·i·ni·tis
  pl vag·i·nit·i·des
vag·i·no·plas·ty
  pl vag·i·no·plas·ties
vag·i·no·scope
va·go·lyt·ic
va·got·o·mize
  va·got·o·mized
  va·got·o·miz·ing
va·got·o·my
  pl va·got·o·mies
va·go·to·nia
va·go·ton·ic
va·go·tro·pic
va·gus
  pl va·gi
va·lence
va·len·cy
  pl va·len·cies
va·lent
val·er·ate
va·le·ri·an
va·le·ric ac·id
  also va·le·ri·an·ic ac·
    id
val·e·tu·di·nar·i·an

val·gus
va·line
val·in·o·my·cin
val·late
val·lec·u·la
  pl val·lec·u·lae
val·lec·u·lar
val·pro·ate
val·pro·ic
Val·sal·va ma·neu·
  ver
  also Val·sal·va's ma·
    neu·ver
val·va
  pl val·vae
valve
valve of Has·ner
valve of Hei·ster
val·vot·o·my
  pl val·vot·o·mies
val·vu·la
  pl val·vu·lae
val·vu·la con·ni·
  vens
  pl val·vu·lae con·ni·
    ven·tes
val·vu·lar
val·vu·li·tis
val·vu·lo·plas·ty
  pl val·vu·lo·plas·ties
val·vu·lo·tome
val·vu·lot·o·my
  pl val·vu·lot·o·mies
vam·pire
van·a·date
va·na·dic
va·na·di·um

van·co·my·cin
Van de Graaff gen·
  er·a·tor
van den Bergh test
  also van den Bergh's
    test
van der Waals
  forc·es
va·nil·la
va·nil·late
va·nil·lic
van·il·lin
va·nil·lism
van·il·lyl·man·de·
  lic
van·il·man·de·lic
Van Slyke meth·od
van't Hoff's law
va·por
va·por·iz·able
va·por·iza·tion
va·por·ize
  va·por·ized
  va·por·iz·ing
va·por·iz·er
Va·quez's dis·ease
vari·abil·i·ty
  pl vari·abil·i·ties
vari·able
vari·ant
vari·a·tion
vari·a·tion·al
var·i·ce·al
var·i·cel·la
var·i·cel·la-zos·ter
var·i·cel·li·form

var·i·ces
  pl of varix

var·i·co·cele

var·i·co·cel·ec·to·
  my
  pl var·i·co·cel·ec·to·
    mies

var·i·cog·ra·phy
  pl var·i·cog·ra·phies

var·i·cose
  also var·i·cosed

var·i·co·sis
  pl var·i·co·ses

var·i·cos·i·ty
  pl var·i·cos·i·ties

va·ri·o·la

var·i·o·late
  var·i·o·lat·ed
  var·i·o·lat·ing

var·i·o·la·tion

var·i·ol·i·form

va·ri·o·loid

va·ri·o·lous

var·ix
  pl var·i·ces

var·nish

var·us

vas
  pl va·sa

vas ab·er·rans of
  Hal·ler
  pl va·sa ab·er·ran·tia
    of Hal·ler

va·sa bre·via

va·sa def·er·en·tia
  pl of vas deferens

va·sa ef·fer·en·tia

va·sal

va·sa rec·ta

va·sa va·so·rum

vas·cu·lar

vas·cu·lar·i·ty
  pl vas·cu·lar·i·ties

vas·cu·lar·iza·tion

vas·cu·lar·ize
  vas·cu·lar·ized
  vas·cu·lar·iz·ing

vas·cu·la·ture

vas·cu·lit·ic

vas·cu·li·tis
  pl vas·cu·lit·i·des

vas·cu·lo·gen·e·sis
  pl vas·cu·lo·gen·e·ses

vas·cu·lo·tox·ic

vas def·er·ens
  pl va·sa def·er·en·tia

va·sec·to·mize
  va·sec·to·mized
  va·sec·to·miz·ing

va·sec·to·my
  pl va·sec·to·mies

vas·e·line
  vas·e·lined
  vas·e·lin·ing

va·so·ac·tive

va·so·ac·tiv·i·ty
  pl va·so·ac·tiv·i·ties

va·so·con·stric·tion

va·so·con·stric·tive

va·so·con·stric·tor

va·so·den·tin
  or va·so·den·tine

va·so·de·pres·sor

va·so·di·lat·ing

va·so·di·la·tion
  or va·so·di·la·ta·tion

va·so·di·la·tor

va·so·di·la·to·ry

va·so·for·ma·tive

va·sog·ra·phy
  pl va·sog·ra·phies

va·so·li·ga·tion

va·so·mo·tion

va·so·mo·tor

va·so·pres·sin

va·so·pres·sor

va·so·re·lax·a·tion

va·so·spasm

va·so·spas·tic

va·so·to·cin

va·sot·o·my
  pl va·sot·o·mies

va·so·ton·ic

va·so·va·gal

va·so·va·sos·to·my
  pl va·so·va·sos·to·
    mies

vas·tus ex·ter·nus

vas·tus in·ter·me·
  di·us

vas·tus in·ter·nus

vas·tus lat·er·a·lis

vas·tus me·di·a·lis

vec·tor

vec·tor·car·dio·
  gram

vec·tor·car·dio·
  graph·ic

vec·tor·car·di·og·
ra·phy
pl vec·tor·car·di·og·
ra·phies

vec·to·ri·al

veg·an

veg·an·ism

veg·e·ta·ble

veg·e·tal

veg·e·tar·i·an

veg·e·tar·i·an·ism

veg·e·ta·tion

veg·e·ta·tive

ve·hi·cle

vein of Ga·len

ve·lo·pha·ryn·geal

ve·lum
pl ve·la

ve·na ca·va
pl ve·nae ca·vae

ve·na ca·val

ve·na co·mi·tans
pl ve·nae co·mi·tan·
tes

ve·nae cor·dis min·
i·mae

ve·na vor·ti·co·sa
pl ve·nae vor·ti·co·sae

ven·e·nate
ven·e·nat·ed
ven·e·nat·ing

ven·e·na·tion

ve·ne·punc·ture
var of venipuncture

ve·ne·re·al

ve·ne·re·o·log·i·cal

ve·ne·re·ol·o·gist

ve·ne·re·ol·o·gy
also ven·er·ol·o·gy
pl ve·ne·re·ol·o·gies
also ven·er·ol·o·gies

ven·ery
pl ven·er·ies

vene·sec·tion
also veni·sec·tion

Ven·e·zu·e·lan
equine en·ceph·
a·li·tis

Ven·e·zu·e·lan
equine en·ceph·
a·lo·my·eli·tis

ve·ni·punc·ture
also ve·ne·punc·ture

veni·sec·tion
var of venesection

ve·no·ar·te·ri·al

ve·noc·ly·sis
pl ve·noc·ly·ses

ve·no·con·stric·
tion

ve·no·fi·bro·sis
pl ve·no·fi·bro·ses

ve·no·gram

ve·no·graph·ic

ve·nog·ra·phy
pl ve·nog·ra·phies

ven·om

ven·om·ous

ve·no·pres·sor

ve·nos·i·ty
pl ve·nos·i·ties

ve·nos·ta·sis
pl ve·nos·ta·ses

ve·not·o·my
pl ve·not·o·mies

ve·nous

ven·ter

ven·ti·late
ven·ti·lat·ed
ven·ti·lat·ing

ven·ti·la·tion

ven·ti·la·tor

ven·ti·la·to·ry

ven·tral

ven·tri·cle

ven·tric·u·lar

ven·tric·u·lar·is

ven·tric·u·li·tis

ven·tric·u·lo·atri·al

ven·tric·u·lo·atri·
os·to·my
pl ven·tric·u·lo·atri·
os·to·mies

ven·tric·u·lo·cis·
ter·nos·to·my
pl ven·tric·u·lo·cis·
ter·nos·to·mies

ven·tric·u·lo·gram

ven·tric·u·lo·graph·
ic

ven·tric·u·log·ra·
phy
pl ven·tric·u·log·ra·
phies

ven·tric·u·lo·peri·
to·ne·al

ven·tric·u·los·to·
my
pl ven·tric·u·los·to·
mies

ven·tric·u·lot·o·my
pl ven·tric·u·lot·o·mies

ven·tric·u·lus
pl ven·tric·u·li

ven·tro·lat·er·al

ven·tro·me·di·al

ven·u·lar

ve·nule

Ve·nus·hair

ve·rap·am·il

ve·rat·ri·dine

ver·a·trine

ve·ra·trum

ver·big·er·a·tion

ver·do·glo·bin

ver·do·per·ox·i·dase

ver·gence

Ver·hoeff's stain

ver·mes
pl of vermis

ver·mi·an

ver·mi·ci·dal

ver·mi·cide

ver·mi·form

ver·mif·u·gal

ver·mi·fuge

ver·mil·ion·ec·to·my
pl ver·mil·ion·ec·to·mies

ver·min
pl ver·min

ver·min·osis
pl ver·min·oses

ver·min·ous

ver·mis
pl ver·mes

ver·nal

ver·nix ca·se·o·sa

ver·ru·ca
pl ver·ru·cae

ver·ru·ca acu·mi·na·ta

ver·ru·ca plan·ta·ris

ver·ru·ca vul·ga·ris

ver·ru·cose

ver·ru·cous

ver·ru·ga

ver·ru·ga per·u·a·na
also ver·ru·ga pe·ru·vi·ana

ver·si·col·or

ver·sion

ver·te·bra
pl ver·te·brae
or ver·te·bras

ver·te·bral

ver·te·bra·pro·mi·nens

Ver·te·bra·ta

ver·te·brate

ver·te·bro·ba·si·lar

ver·te·bro·chon·dral

ver·te·bro·ster·nal

ver·tex
pl ver·ti·ces
also ver·tex·es

ver·ti·cal

ver·tig·i·nous

ver·ti·go
pl ver·ti·goes
or ver·ti·gos

ver·u·mon·ta·num

ves·i·cal
adjective
relating to the bladder (see vesicle)

ves·i·cant

ves·i·ca·tion

ves·i·cle
noun
a fluid-filled pouch (see vesical)

ves·i·co·ure·ter·al

ves·i·co·uter·ine

ves·i·co·vag·i·nal

ve·sic·u·lar

ve·sic·u·la·tion

ve·sic·u·lec·to·my
pl ve·sic·u·lec·to·mies

ve·sic·u·lo·bul·lous

ve·sic·u·log·ra·phy
pl ve·sic·u·log·ra·phies

ve·sic·u·lot·o·my
pl ve·sic·u·lot·o·mies

ves·sel

ves·tib·u·lar

ves·ti·bule

ves·tib·u·lo·co·chle·ar

ves·tib·u·lo·spi·nal

ves·tige

ves·tig·ial

vet·er·i·nar·i·an

vet·er·i·nary

vi·a·bil·i·ty
  pl vi·a·bil·i·ties
vi·a·ble
vi·al
Vi an·ti·gen
vi·brate
  vi·brat·ed
  vi·brat·ing
vi·bra·tion
vi·bra·tion·al
vi·bra·tor
vi·bra·to·ry
vib·rio
vib·ri·on
Vib·rio·na·ce·ae
vi·bris·sa
  pl vi·bris·sae
vi·bris·sal
vi·car·i·ous
vid·ar·a·bine
Vid·i·an ar·tery
Vid·i·an ca·nal
Vid·i·an nerve
vig·or
vil·li·ki·nin
vil·lo·nod·u·lar
vil·lous
vil·lus
  pl vil·li
vin·blas·tine
vin·ca
vin·ca·leu·ko·blas·
  tine
Vin·cent's an·gi·na
Vin·cent's dis·ease
Vin·cent's in·fec·
  tion

Vin·cent's or·gan·
  isms
Vin·cent's ul·cer
vin·cris·tine
vin·e·gar
vi·nyl
vi·nyl·ic
vi·o·la·ceous
vi·o·my·cin
vi·os·ter·ol
vi·per
Vi·pera
vi·per·id
Vi·per·i·dae
vi·po·ma
vi·ral
Vir·chow-Ro·bin
  space
vi·re·mia
vi·re·mic
vi·res a ter·go
  pl of vis a tergo
vir·gin
vir·gin·al
Vir·gin·ia snake·
  root
vir·gin·i·ty
  pl vir·gin·i·ties
vir·gin·ium
vi·ri·ci·dal
vi·ri·cide
vir·i·dans
vir·i·din
vir·ile
vir·il·ism
vi·ril·i·ty
  pl vi·ril·i·ties

vir·il·iza·tion
vir·il·ize
  vir·il·ized
  vir·il·iz·ing
vi·ri·on
vi·roid
vi·ro·log·i·cal
  or vi·ro·log·ic
vi·rol·o·gist
vi·rol·o·gy
  pl vi·rol·o·gies
vi·ro·stat·ic
vir·tu·al
vi·ru·cid·al
vi·ru·cide
vir·u·lence
vir·u·lent
vir·u·lif·er·ous
vi·rus
vi·ru·stat·ic
vi·sam·min
vis a ter·go
  pl vi·res a ter·go
vis·cera
  pl of viscus
vis·cer·al
vis·cero·mo·tor
vis·cer·op·to·sis
  pl vis·cer·op·to·ses
vis·cer·op·tot·ic
vis·cero·sen·so·ry
vis·cer·o·to·nia
vis·cer·o·ton·ic
vis·cer·o·trop·ic
vis·cer·ot·ro·pism
vis·cid

vis·cid·i·ty
pl vis·cid·i·ties

vis·co·elas·tic

vis·co·elas·tic·i·ty
pl vis·co·elas·tic·i·ties

vis·com·e·ter

vis·co·met·ric

vis·co·met·ri·cal·ly

vis·com·e·try
pl vis·com·e·tries

vis·co·sim·e·ter

vis·cos·i·met·ric

vis·co·sim·e·try
pl vis·co·sim·e·tries

vis·cos·i·ty
pl vis·cos·i·ties

vis·cous
sticky or not flowing easily

vis·cus
pl vis·cera
internal organ

vis·i·ble

vi·sion

vis·na

vi·su·al

vi·su·al·iza·tion

vi·su·al·ize
vi·su·al·ized
vi·su·al·iz·ing

vi·suo·mo·tor

vi·suo·spa·tial

vi·tal

vi·tal·ism

vi·tal·ist

vi·tal·i·ty
pl vi·tal·i·ties

vi·tals

vi·ta·mer

vi·ta·mer·ic

vi·ta·min
also vi·ta·mine

vi·ta·min·iza·tion

vi·ta·min·ize
vi·ta·min·ized
vi·ta·min·iz·ing

vi·tel·lin
noun
protein in yolk

vi·tel·line
adjective
relating to yolk

vi·tel·lo·gen·e·sis
pl vi·tel·lo·gen·e·ses

vi·tel·lo·gen·ic

vi·tel·lus

vit·i·lig·i·nous

vit·i·li·go

vit·i·li·goid

vit·rec·to·my
pl vit·rec·to·mies

vit·re·ous

vit·ri·ol

vi·var·i·um
pl vi·var·ia
or vi·var·i·ums

vi·vax

vivi·dif·fu·sion

vi·vi·par·i·ty
pl vi·vi·par·i·ties

vi·vip·a·rous

vivi·sect

vivi·sec·tion

vivi·sec·tion·al

vivi·sec·tion·ist

vivi·sec·tor

Vlem·inckx' lo·tion

Vlem·inckx' so·lu·tion

vo·cal

vo·ca·lis

vo·cal·i·ty
pl vo·cal·i·ties

Vo·ges-Pros·kau·er re·ac·tion

Vo·ges-Pros·kau·er test

void

vo·lar

vol·a·tile

vol·a·til·i·ty
pl vol·a·til·i·ties

vol·a·til·iz·able

vol·a·til·iza·tion

vol·a·til·ize
vol·a·til·ized
vol·a·til·iz·ing

vo·li·tion

vo·li·tion·al

Volk·mann's ca·nal

Volk·mann's con·trac·ture
or Volk·mann con·trac·ture

vol·ley
pl vol·leys

vol·sel·la

volt·age

volt-am·pere

volt·me·ter
vol·ume
vol·u·met·ric
vol·u·met·ri·cal·ly
vol·un·tari·ly
vol·un·tary
vo·lu·tin
vol·vu·lus
vo·mer
vom·ero·na·sal
vom·it
vom·i·tu·ri·tion
vom·i·tus
von Hip·pel-Lin·dau dis·ease
von Korff fi·ber
von Reck·ling·hau·sen's dis·ease
von Wil·le·brand's dis·ease
vor·ti·cose
voy·eur
voy·eur·ism
voy·eur·is·tic
voy·eur·is·ti·cal·ly
vul·ner·ary
  pl vul·ner·ar·ies
vul·sel·lum
  pl vul·sel·la
vul·va
  pl vul·vae
vul·val
  or vul·var
vul·vec·to·my
  pl vul·vec·to·mies

vul·vi·tis
vul·vo·vag·i·nal
vul·vo·vag·i·ni·tis
  pl vul·vo·vag·i·nit·i·des

W

wad·ding
wa·fer
waist·line
wake·ful
Wal·den·ström's mac·ro·glob·u·lin·emia
Wal·dey·er's ring
walk·er
walk·ing
Wal·le·ri·an de·gen·er·a·tion
wall·eye
wall-eyed
Wan·gen·steen ap·pa·ra·tus
Wan·gen·steen suc·tion
war·ble
war·bled
War·burg ap·pa·ra·tus
War·burg res·pi·rom·e·ter
war·fa·rin
warm-blood·ed

warm-up
  noun
warm up
  verb
War·thin-Star·ry stain
warty
  war·ti·er
  war·ti·est
wash·ings
wash·out
Was·ser·mann re·ac·tion
Was·ser·mann test
waste
  wast·ed
  wast·ing
wa·ter
wa·ter·borne
wa·ter-ham·mer pulse
Wa·ter·house-Frid·er·ich·sen syn·drome
wa·ter·logged
wa·tery
Wat·son-Crick mod·el
Wat·so·ni·an
  Wat·so·ni·us
watt·age
wave·form
wave·guide
wave·length
waxy
  wax·i·er
  wax·i·est

wean·ling
Web·er-Chris·tian dis·ease
also Web·er-Chris·tian's dis·ease

We·ber-Fech·ner law

We·ber's law

We·ber test
or We·ber's test

Wechs·ler Adult In·tel·li·gence Scale

Wechs·ler-Belle·vue test

weep
wept
weep·ing

weight·less·ness

Weil-Fe·lix re·ac·tion

Weil-Fe·lix test

Weil's dis·ease

Weis·mann·ism

Welch ba·cil·lus

well·ness

Wencke·bach pe·ri·od

Wencke·bach phe·nom·e·non

Werl·hof's dis·ease

Wer·ner's syn·drome

Wer·nick·e's ar·ea

Wer·nick·e's en·ceph·a·lop·a·thy

Wert·heim op·er·a·tion
or Wert·heim's op·er·a·tion

Wes·ter·gren eryth·ro·cyte sed·i·men·ta·tion rate

Wes·ter·gren meth·od

Whar·ton's duct

Whar·ton's jel·ly

wheal

wheat-germ oil

Wheat·stone bridge

wheel·chair

wheeze
wheezed
wheez·ing

whip·lash

Whip·ple's dis·ease

whip·worm

whirl·pool

white·head

Whit·field's oint·ment
also Whit·field oint·ment

whit·low

whoop·ing cough

Wi·dal re·ac·tion
also Wi·dal's re·ac·tion

Wi·dal test
also Wi·dal's test

wide-spec·trum

wild type
noun

wild-type
adjective

Wilms' tu·mor
also Wilms's tu·mor

Wil·son's dis·ease

wind-bro·ken

wind·burn

wind·burned

wind·chill

wind·gall

win·dow

wind·pipe

win·ter·green

Wir·sung's duct

wis·dom tooth

wish-ful·fill·ment

Wis·kott-Al·drich syn·drome

Wis·tar rat

witch ha·zel

with·draw
with·drew
with·drawn
with·draw·ing

with·draw·al

with·ers

Wit·zel·sucht

wohl·fahr·tia

Wolff·ian body

Wolff·ian duct

Wolff-Par·kin·son-White syn·drome

wol·fram

wolfs·bane

womb
wool·sort·er's dis·
  ease
word-as·so·ci·a·
  tion test
word-deaf
work·a·hol·ic
work·a·hol·ism
work·up
  noun
work up
  verb
worm·er
Wor·mi·an bone
worm·seed
worm·wood
Woulff bot·tle
Wright's stain
wrin·kle
  wrin·kled
  wrin·kling
Wris·berg's gan·
  gli·on
wrist·bone
wrist-drop
writ·er's cramp
wry·neck
Wuch·er·e·ria

X

xan·thate
xan·the·las·ma
xan·the·las·ma pal·
  pe·bra·rum
xan·thene

xan·thine
xan·tho·chro·mia
xan·tho·chro·mic
xan·tho·ma
  pl xan·tho·mas
  or xan·tho·ma·ta
xan·tho·ma·to·sis
  pl xan·tho·ma·to·ses
xan·tho·ma·tous
xan·tho·phyll
xan·tho·pro·te·ic
xan·thop·sia
xan·thop·ter·in
xan·tho·sine
xan·tho·tox·in
xanth·uren·ic
xan·thy·drol
X-dis·ease
xe·no·bi·ot·ic
xe·no·di·ag·no·sis
  pl xe·no·di·ag·no·ses
xe·no·di·ag·nos·tic
xe·no·ge·ne·ic
  also xe·no·gen·ic
xe·no·graft
xe·non
xe·no·phobe
xe·no·pho·bia
xe·no·pho·bic
Xen·op·syl·la
Xen·o·pus
xe·no·tro·pic
xe·ro·der·ma
xe·ro·der·ma pig·
  men·to·sum
xe·ro·graph·ic
xe·ro·graph·i·cal·ly

xe·rog·ra·phy
  pl xe·rog·ra·phies
xe·ro·mam·mo·
  gram
xe·ro·mam·mog·ra·
  phy
  pl xe·ro·mam·mog·ra·
  phies
xe·roph·thal·mia
xe·roph·thal·mic
xe·ro·ra·dio·graph·
  ic
xe·ro·ra·di·og·ra·
  phy
  pl xe·ro·ra·di·og·ra·
  phies
xe·ro·sis
  pl xe·ro·ses
xe·ro·sto·mia
xi·phi·ster·num
  pl xi·phi·ster·na
xi·phoid
xi·phop·a·gus
x-ir·ra·di·ate
  x-ir·ra·di·at·ed
  x-ir·ra·di·at·ing
x-ir·ra·di·a·tion
X-linked
x-ra·di·a·tion
x-ray
  verb
X ray
  noun
X-ray
  adjective
xy·lene
xy·le·nol

xy·li·tol

xy·lol

xy·lose

Y

yaws

yeast

yel·low bile

yel·lows

yer·ba san·ta

Yer·sin·ia

yo·gurt
also yo·ghurt

yo·him·bine

Young-Helm·holtz
the·o·ry

yper·ite

yt·ter·bi·um

yt·tri·um

Z

ze·a·xan·thin

Zei·gar·nik ef·fect

ze·in

zeit·ge·ber

Zen·ker's de·gen·
er·a·tion

Zen·ker's flu·id

ze·o·lite

ze·o·lit·ic

ze·ro
pl ze·ros
also ze·roes

Ziehl-Neel·sen
stain

zi·mel·i·dine

zinc

zir·co·ni·um

Zol·ling·er-El·li·
son syn·drome

zo·me·pir·ac

zo·na
pl zo·nae
or zo·nas

zo·na fas·cic·u·la·
ta

zo·na glo·mer·u·lo·
sa

zo·na in·cer·ta

zon·al

zo·na pel·lu·ci·da

zo·na re·tic·u·lar·is

zo·nu·la
pl zo·nu·lae
or zo·nu·las

zo·nu·la cil·i·ar·is

zo·nu·lar

zon·ule

zon·ule of Zinn

zo·o·glea
pl zo·o·gle·as
or zo·o·gle·ae

zo·o·gle·al

zoo·log·i·cal
also zoo·log·ic

zo·ol·o·gist

zo·ol·o·gy
pl zo·ol·o·gies

zoo·no·sis
pl zoo·no·ses

zoo·not·ic

zoo·par·a·site

zoo·par·a·sit·ic

zoo·phil·ia

zoo·phil·ic

zo·oph·i·lism

zo·oph·i·ly
pl zo·oph·i·lies

zoo·phyte

zoo·spore

zoo·spor·ic

zo·os·ter·ol

zoo·tech·ni·cal
also zoo·tech·nic

zoo·tech·nics

zos·ter

zos·ter·i·form

zox·a·zol·amine

Z-plas·ty
pl Z-plas·ties

zwit·ter·ion

zwit·ter·ion·ic

zyg·apoph·y·sis
pl zyg·apoph·y·ses

zy·go·ma
pl zy·go·ma·ta
also zy·go·mas

zy·go·mat·ic

zy·go·mat·i·co·fa·
cial

zy·go·mat·i·co·
max·il·lary

zy·go·mat·i·co·tem·
po·ral

zy·go·mat·i·cus

zy·gos·i·ty
pl zy·gos·i·ties

zy·go·spore
zy·gote
zy·go·tene
zy·got·ic
zy·got·i·cal·ly

zy·mase
zy·mo·gen
zy·mog·e·nous
zy·mo·gram

zy·mo·plas·tic
zy·mo·san
zy·mos·ter·ol
zy·mot·ic

ABBREVIATIONS

Most of these abbreviations have been normalized to one form. In practice, however, there is considerable variation in the use of periods and in capitalization (as in rpm, r.p.m., RPM, R.P.M.), and stylings other than those shown in this section are often acceptable. Chemical symbols (as Na) are included when they can be placed in alphabetical sequence readily without causing confusion.

a about, absent, absolute, absorbency, absorbent, accommodation, acetum, acid, acidity, actin, active, activity, allergist, allergy, alpha, ampere, anode, answer, ante, anterior, aqua, area, artery, asymmetric, asymmetry *

Å angstrom unit

$\overline{\text{aa}}$ *also* **aa** ana (*Latin*, of each)

AA achievement age, Alcoholics Anonymous

AAF ascorbic acid factor

AAL anterior axillary line

A&P anterior and posterior, auscultation and percussion

A&W alive and well

ab abort, abortion, about

AB aid to blind, Artium Baccalaureus (*Latin*, bachelor of arts)

ABC atomic, biological, and chemical

abd abdomen, abdominal

abdom abdomen, abdominal

abs absent, absolute

ABS acute brain syndrome

abt about

ac acute, ante cibum (*Latin*, before meals)

Ac actinium

AC alternating current

acc acceleration, according

AcG accelerator globulin (factor V)

ACh acetylcholine

AChE acetylcholinesterase

ACNM American College of Nurse-Midwives

ACS antireticular cytotoxic serum

ACSW Academy of Certified Social Workers

act active

ACTH adrenocorticotropic hormone

AD average deviation

ADA American Dietetic Association

ADC aid to dependent children

add adduction, adductor

ADH antidiuretic hormone

adj adjunct

ADL activities of daily living

adm administration, administrator, admission, admit

ADP adenosine diphosphate

ae or **aet** or **aetat** aetatis (*Latin,* of age, aged)

AF audio frequency, auricular fibrillation

AFB acid-fast bacillus

AFP alpha-fetoprotein

Ag argentum (*Latin,* silver)

agglut agglutination

agt agent

AHF antihemophilic factor

AHG antihemophilic globulin, antihuman globulin

AI artificial insemination

AID artificial insemination by donor

AIDS acquired immune deficiency syndrome, acquired immunodeficiency syndrome

AIH artificial insemination by husband

AJ ankle jerk

AK above knee

Al aluminum

ALA aminolevulinic acid

alb albumin

alc alcohol

ALG antilymphocyte globulin, antilymphocytic globulin

alk alkaline

ALL acute lymphoblastic leukemia

ALS amyotrophic lateral sclerosis, antilymphocyte serum, antilymphocytic serum

alt alternate, altitude

alv alveolar

am ammeter

Am americium

AM ante meridiem (*Latin,* before noon), Artium Magister (*Medieval Latin,* master of arts)

AMA against medical advice, American Medical Association

amb ambulance, ambulatory

AMI acute myocardial infarction

amp amperage, ampere, ampule, amputation

AMP adenosine monophosphate

amt amount

ana (*Latin,* of each an equal quantity)

ANA American Nurses Association

anal analysis, analytic, analyze

anat anatomic, anatomical, anatomy

anhyd anhydrous

ans answer

ANS autonomic nervous system

ANTU alpha-napthylthiourea

AOB alcohol on breath

AOTA American Occupational Therapy Association

ap apothecaries

AP action potential, alkaline phosphatase, anterior pituitary, anteroposterior, aortic pressure

APC aspirin, phenacetin, and caffeine

APF animal protein factor

app appendix

appl applied

approx approximate, approximately

appt appointment

aq aqua, aqueous

AQ accomplishment quotient, achievement quotient

Ar argon

ARC AIDS-related complex

ARD acute respiratory disease

ARRT American registered respiratory therapist, American Registry of Radiologic Technologists

ART accredited record technician

as astigmatism

As arsenic

AS aortic stenosis, arteriosclerosis

ASA acetylsalicylic acid (aspirin)

ASAP as soon as possible

ASCP American Society of Clinical Pathologists

ASCVD arteriosclerotic cardiovascular disease

ASHD arteriosclerotic heart disease

assn association

asst assistant

as tol as tolerated

at airtight

At astatine

atm atmosphere, atmospheric

ATP adenosine triphosphate

at wt atomic weight

au angstrom unit, antitoxin unit

Au aurum (*Latin*, gold)

aux auxiliary

av average, avoirdupois

AV arteriovenous, atrioventricular

avdp avoirdupois

ax axis

Az azote (*French*, nitrogen)

AZT azidothymidine

b bacillus, barometric, bath, Baumé scale, behavior, bel, born, brother

B boron

Ba barium

BA bronchial asthma

bact bacteria, bacterial, bacteriological, bacteriology, bacterium

BaE *or* **BAE** barium enema

bal balance

BAL British anti-lewisite (dimercaprol)

bar barometer, barometric

baso basophil

BBB bundle branch block

BBT basal body temperature

BC Board certified

BCG bacillus Calmette-Guérin, ballistocardiogram, bromocresol green

b.d. bis die (*Latin*, twice a day)

Bé Baumé

Be beryllium

BE barium enema, below elbow, board eligible

BFP biological false positive

BH bill of health

BHA butylated hydroxyanisole

BHC benzene hexachloride

BHT butylated hydroxytoluene

Bi bismuth

bid bis in die (*Latin*, twice a day)

bili bilirubin

biol biologic, biological, biologist, biology

BJ biceps jerk

Bk berkelium

BK below knee

bld blood

BM Bachelor of Medicine, basal metabolism, bowel movement

BMR basal metabolic rate

BNA Basle Nomina Anatomica

BO body odor

BOD biochemical oxygen demand, biological oxygen demand

bot botanical, botanist, botany, bottle

bp base pair

BP blood pressure, boiling point, British Pharmacopoeia

Br bromine

BRP bathroom privileges

BS bowel sounds, breath sounds

BSN bachelor of science in nursing

BST blood serological test

BT bedtime, brain tumor

Btu British thermal unit

BUdR bromodeoxyuridine

BUN blood urea nitrogen

BW blood Wassermann, body weight

Bx biopsy

BZ — used as an army code word for quinuclidinyl benzilate

c calorie, cathode, centimeter, cervical, clonus, closure, cobalt, cocaine, coefficient, contact, contraction, coulomb, cum (*Latin*, with), curie, cylinder

C Carbon, Celsius, centigrade, complement, congius

Ca calcium

CA cancer, carcinoma, cardiac arrest, chronological age

CABG coronary artery bypass graft

CAC cardiac accelerator center

CAD coronary artery disease

CAI confused artificial insemination

cal small calorie

Cal large calorie

canc canceled

cap capacity, capsule

CAT computed axial tomography, computerized axial tomography

cath cathartic, catheter, cathode

cav cavity

cb centibar

Cb columbium

CB Chirurgiae Baccalaureus (*Latin*, bachelor of surgery)

CBC complete blood count

CBD closed bladder drainage, common bile duct

CBF cerebral blood flow

CBR chemical, bacteriological, and radiological; chemical, biological, and radiological

CBW chemical and biological warfare

cc cubic centimeter

CC chief complaint, commission certified, critical condition, current complaint

CCA chick cell agglutinating

CCI chronic coronary insufficiency

CCK cholecystokinin

CCT chocolate-covered tablet

CCU cardiac care unit

Cd cadmium

CD communicable disease, constant drainage, contagious disease, convulsive disorder, curative dose

CDC calculated date of confinement

cDNA complementary DNA

Ce cerium

CE cardiac enlargement

CEA cardioembryonic antigen

Cel Celsius

cen central

CER conditioned emotional response

cert certificate, certification, certified, certify

cerv cervical

CES central excitatory state

cf confer (*Latin*, compare)

Cf californium

CF complement fixation, cystic fibrosis

CFT complement fixation test

CG chorionic gonadotropin

cgs centimeter-gram-second

ch child, chronic

ChB Chirugiae Baccalaureus (*Latin*, bachelor of surgery)

CHD childhood disease

ChE cholinesterase

chem chemical, chemist, chemistry

CHF congestive heart failure

chg change

chl chloroform

CHO carbohydrate

chol cholesterol

chr chronic

CI chemotherapeutic index

CICU coronary intensive care unit

CK creatine kinase

cl centiliter, clavicle, clinic, closure

Cl chloride, chlorine

CL chest and left arm, corpus luteum, critical list

CLA certified laboratory assistant

clin clinical

CLL chronic lymphocytic leukemia

CLO cod-liver oil

cm centimeter

Cm curium

CM Chirurgiae Magister (*Latin*, master of surgery), circular muscle

CMA certified medical assistant

CMHC Community Mental Health Center

CMV cytomegalovirus
CN chloroacetophenone
CNM certified nurse-mid-wife
CNP continuous negative pressure
CNS central nervous system
Co coenzyme, cobalt
CO carbon monoxide, cardiac output
c/o complains of
coag coagulate, coagulation
COC cathodal opening contraction
COCl cathode opening clonus
coeff *or* **coef** coefficient
COH carbohydrate
col colony, color
coll collect, collection, colloidal, collyrium
comp comparative, compare, composition, compound
conc concentrated, concentration
cond condition
cond ref conditioned reflex
cond resp conditioned response
conf conference
cong congenital, congius
const constant
cont containing, contents, continue, continued
conv convalescent
coord coordination
COPD chronic obstructive pulmonary disease
COPE chronic obstructive pulmonary emphysema
cor corrected

CoR Congo red
cort cortex, cortical
COTA certified occupational therapy assistant
CP capillary pressure, cerebral palsy, chemically pure, compare, constant pressure, cor pulmonale
CPAP continuous positive airway pressure
CPB competitive protein binding
CPC chronic passive congestion
cpd compound
CPE cytopathogenic effects
CPI constitutional psychopathic inferiority
CPK creatine phosphokinase
CPM counts per minute
CPR cardiopulmonary resuscitation
CPZ chlorpromazine
Cr chromium, creatinine
CR cardiorespiratory, chest and right arm, clot retraction, conditioned reflex, conditioned response
CRD chronic respiratory disease
crit critical
CRNA certified registered nurse anesthetist
CRO cathode-ray oscilloscope
CrP creatine phosphate
CRP C-reactive protein
CRT cathode-ray tube, complex reaction time
CRTT certified respiratory therapy technician

cryst crystalline, crystallized

cs case, cesarean section, conditioned stimulus, consciousness, corticosteroid, current strength

Cs cesium

CSF cerebrospinal fluid

CSM cerebrospinal meningitis

CT circulation time, coated tablet, compressed tablet, computed tomography, computerized tomography

CTa catamenia

CTC chlortetracycline

ctr center

CTU centigrade thermal unit

cu cubic

Cu cuprum (*Latin*, copper)

CU clinical unit

CUC chronic ulcerative colitis

cult culture

cur curative, current

CV cardiovascular

CVA cerebrovascular accident

CVP central venous pressure

CVR cardiovascular renal, cardiovascular respiratory, cerebrovascular resistance

CVS clean voided specimen

CW crutch walking

Cy cyanogen

cyl cylinder, cylindrical

cytol cytological, cytology

d date, daughter, day, dead, deceased, deciduous, degree, density, developed, deviation, dexter, diameter, died, diopter, disease, divorced, dorsal, dose, duration

D deuterium

da daughter, day

DA delayed action

DAH disordered action of the heart

D & C dilatation and curettage

DAT delayed action tablet

dau daughter

dbl double

DBP diastolic blood pressure

DBT dry-bulb temperature

DC Dental Corps, diagnostic center, direct current, doctor of chiropractic

DCc double concave

DCR direct critical response

DD developmentally disabled

DDD dichloro-diphenyl-dichloro-ethane

DDS doctor of dental science, doctor of dental surgery

DDT dichloro-diphenyl-trichloro-ethane

DDVP dimethyl-dichloro-vinyl-phosphate (dichlorvos)

dec deceased, decompose

decd deceased

def defecation, deficient, definite

deg degeneration, degree

del delusion

depr depression

derm dermatologist, dermatology

DES diethylstilbestrol

detn detention

devel development

DFP diisopropyl fluorophosphate

dg decigram

DHPG dihydroxy-propoxymethyl guanine

DI diabetes insipidus

dia diameter, diathermy

diam diameter

dil dilute

dilat dilatation

dim diminished

DIP distal interphalangeal

diph diphtheria

dis disabled, disease

disch discharge, discharged

disp dispensary

dissd dissolved

div divide, division, divorced

DJD degenerative joint disease

dkg dekagram

dkl dekaliter

dkm dekameter

dl deciliter

DL danger list

DLE disseminated lupus erythematosus

dm decimeter

DM diabetes mellitus, diastolic murmur

DMD Dentariae Medicinae Doctor (*Latin*, doctor of dental medicine)

DMF decayed, missing, and filled teeth

DMSO dimethylsulfoxide

DMT dimethyltryptamine

DNA deoxyribonucleic acid

DNB dinitrobenzene

DNOC dinitro-*o*-cresol

DO doctor of optometry, doctor of osteopathy

DOA dead on arrival

DOB date of birth

doc document

DOE dyspnea on exertion

DOM dimethoxy methyl

dos dosage

doz dozen

DP doctor of pharmacy, doctor of podiatry

DPA diphemylamine

DPH department of public health, doctor of public health

DPM doctor of podiatric medicine

DPN diphosphopyridine nucleotide

DPT diphtheria-pertussis-tetanus (vaccines)

DQ developmental quotient

dr dram, dressing

Dr doctor

DR delivery room

DRG diagnosis related group

DrPH doctor of public health

DSC doctor of surgical chiropody

DSD dry sterile dressing

DT delirium tremens, distance test, duration of tetany

DTN diphtheria toxin normal

DTP diphtheria, tetanus, pertussis (vaccines)

d.t.'s delirium tremens
DU diagnosis undetermined
dup duplicate
DV dilute volume
DVM doctor of veterinary medicine
DW distilled water
dwt denarius (*Latin*, penny) + weight (pennyweight)
Dx diagnosis
Dy dysprosium

E emmetropia, enema, enzyme, experimenter, eye
ea each
EA educational age
EBV Epstein-Barr virus
ECF extracellular fluid
ECG electrocardiogram
ECT electroconvulsive therapy
ED effective dose, erythema dose
EDB ethylene dibromide
EDR electrodermal response
EDTA ethylenediaminetetraacetic acid
EEE eastern equine encephalomyelitis
EEG electroencephalogram, electroencephalograph
EENT eye, ear, nose, and throat
Eh standard oxidation-reduction potential
EHBF extrahepatic blood flow
EKG electrocardiogram, electrocardiograph
elec electric, electrical, electricity

ELISA enzyme-linked immunosorbent assay
emb embryo, embryology
embryol embryology
EMF electromotive force
EMG electromyogram, electromyography
EMT emergency medical technician
emul emulsion
enl enlarged
ENT ear, nose, and throat
EOG electrooculogram
eos *or* **eosin** eosinophil
epil epilepsy, epileptic
epith epithelial, epithelium
eq equal, equivalent
Er erbium
ER emergency room
ERG electroretinogram
ERPF effective renal plasma flow
Es einsteinium
ESB electrical stimulation of the brain
ESF erythropoietic stimulating factor
ESP extrasensory perception
ESR erythrocyte sedimentation rate
EST electroshock therapy
ESU electrostatic unit
Eu europium
ex examined, example, exercise
exc except, exception
exp experiment, experimental, expired
expt experiment
exptl experimental

ext external, extract, extremity

f farad, faraday, father, female, focal length, foot, formula, function

F Fahrenheit, filial generation, fluorine

FA fatty acid

FACC Fellow of the American College of Cardiology

FACD Fellow of the American College of Dentists

FACOG Fellow of the American College of Obstetricians and Gynecologists

FACP Fellow of the American College of Physicians

FACR Fellow of the American College of Radiology

FACS Fellow of the American College of Surgeons

FAD flavin adenine dinucleotide

Fah *or* **Fahr** Fahrenheit

fam family

FAMA Fellow of the American Medical Association

FAPA Fellow of the American Psychological Association

fasc fasciculus

FD focal distance

FDA Food and Drug Administration

Fe ferrum (*Latin*, iron)

fem female, feminine, femur

FF fat free, filtration fraction

FFA free fatty acids

FHS fetal heart sounds

FHT fetal heart tone

fib fibrillation

FICS Fellow of the International College of Surgeons

fig figure

fl fluid

FL focal length

fl oz fluidounce

Fm fermium

FMN flavin mononucleotide

fp freezing point

FPC fish protein concentrate

fpm feet per minute

fps feet per second

Fr francium

FRCP Fellow of the Royal College of Physicians

FRCS Fellow of the Royal College of Surgeons

freq frequency

FRSC Fellow of the Royal Society of Canada

FSH follicle-stimulating hormone

ft feet, foot

FUO fever of undetermined origin

g acceleration of gravity, gauge, gender, gingival, glucose, grain, gram, gravity

Ga gallium

GABA gamma-aminobutyric acid

gal galactose, gallon

galv galvanic, galvanism, galvanized

GAS general adaptation syndrome

GB gallbladder, sarin (code name)

GC gonococcus

Gd gadolinium
Ge germanium
GE gastroenterology
gen general, genus
GFR glomerular filtration rate
GG gamma globulin
GH growth hormone
GI gastrointestinal
GL greatest length
GLC gas-liquid chromatography
gm gram
GM and S General Medicine and Surgery
GMP guanosine monophosphate
GN graduate nurse
gp group
GP general paresis, general practitioner
gr grain, gravity
GRAS generally recognized as safe
grav gravida
GSH glutathione (reduced form)
G6PD glucose-6-phosphate dehydrogenase
GSR galvanic skin response
GSSG glutathione (oxidized form)
GSW gunshot wound
GTH gonadotropic hormone
GTP guanosine triphosphate
GU genitourinary
GVH graft-versus host
Gy gray
gyn gynecologic, gynecologist, gynecology

h height, hora (*Latin*, hour) — used in writing prescriptions
H heroin, hydrogen
Hb hemoglobin
HBsAg hepatitis B surface antigen
HCG human chorionic gonadotropin
hct hematocrit
HD Hansen's disease, hearing distance
HDL high-density lipoprotein
HDLW distance at which a watch is heard with left ear
HDRW distance at which a watch is heard with right ear
He helium
HEW (Department of) Health, Education, and Welfare
Hf hafnium
hg hectogram
Hg hydrargyrum (*New Latin*, mercury)
Hgb hemoglobin
HGH human growth hormone
HHS (Department of) Health and Human Services
HI hemagglutination inhibition
HIV human immunodeficiency virus
hl hectoliter
HLA *also* **HL-A** human leukocyte antigen
HMD hyaline membrane disease

HMO health maintenance organization

Ho holmium

HOP high oxygen pressure

hosp hospital

HPI history of present illness

HPLC high-performance liquid chromatography

hr hora (*Latin*, hour)

hs hora somni (*Latin*, at bedtime)

HS house surgeon

HSA human serum albumin

HSV herpes simplex virus

ht height

HTLV human T-cell leukemia virus, human T-cell lymphotropic virus

HTLV-III human T-cell leukemia virus type III, human T-cell lymphotropic virus type III

HVL half-value layer

i optically inactive

I iodine

IAA indoleacetic acid

ib *or* **ibid** ibidem (*Latin*, in the same place)

ICN International Council of Nurses

ICSH intestinal-cell stimulating hormone

ICSS intracranial self-stimulation

ICT inflammation of connective tissue, insulin coma therapy

ICU intensive care unit

id idem (*Latin*, the same)

ID identification, inside diameter, internal diameter, intradermal

ID$_{50}$ — used for a dose that produces infection in 50% of the subjects

IDU idoxuridine

IF interferon

IFN interferon

Ig immunoglobulin

IH infectious hepatitis

Il illinium

IM intramuscular, intramuscularly

IMP inosine monophosphate

in inch

In indium

IND investigational new drug

INH isonicotinic acid hydrazide (isoniazid)

inj injection

Io ionium

IP intraperitoneal, intraperitoneally

IPPB intermittent positive pressure breathing

IPSP inhibitory postsynaptic potential

IQ intelligence quotient

Ir iridium

IR infrared

ITP idiopathic thrombocytopenic purpura

IU immunizing unit, international unit

IUCD intrauterine contraceptive device

IUD intrauterine device

IUDR idoxuridine

IV intravenous, intravenously, intraventricular
IVP intravenous pyelogram

J mechanical equivalent of heat
JAMA Journal of the American Medical Association
JCAH Joint Commission on Accreditation of Hospitals
JND just noticeable difference

k kelvin, kilogram
K dissociation constant, ionization constant, kalium (*Latin*, potassium)
ka kathode (*German*, cathode)
kb kilobase
kc kilocycle
kcal kilocalorie, kilogram calorie
kc/s kilocycles per second
kg kilogram
kgm kilogram-meter
KJ knee jerk
kl kiloliter
km kilometer
Kr krypton
KS Kaposi's sarcoma
KUB kidney, ureter, and bladder

L left, levorotatory, light, liquid, liter, lithium, lumbar
La lanthanum
lap laparotomy
laryngol laryngological
LATS long-acting thyroid stimulator

LAV lymphadenopathy-associated virus
lb pound
LC liquid chromatography
LD lethal dose
LDH lactate dehydrogenase, lactic dehydrogenase
LDL low-density lipoprotein
LE lupus erythematosus
Leu leucine
LFD least fatal dose
LH luteinizing hormone
LHRH luteinizing hormone-releasing hormone
Li lithium
liq liquid, liquor
LLQ left lower quadrant
LPN licensed practical nurse
Lr lawrencium
LRCP Licentiate of the Royal College of Physicians
LRCS Licentiate of the Royal College of Surgeons
LRF luteinizing hormone-releasing factor
LSD lysergic acid diethylamide
LTH luteotropic hormone
Lu lutetium
LUQ left upper quadrant
LVN licensed vocational nurse

m Mach, male, married, masculine, mass, meter, mille (*Latin*, thousand), million, minim, minute, molal, molality, molar, molarity, mole, mucoid, muscle
m- meta-
M misce (*Latin*, mix)

ma milliampere
MA mental age
mac macerate
MAC maximum allowable concentration
MAO monoamine oxidase
MAOI monoamine oxidase inhibitor
masc masculine
MASH mobile army surgical hospital
max maximum
MB Medicinae Baccalaureus (*New Latin*, bachelor of medicine
MBD minimal brain dysfunction
mc megacycle, millicurie
MC Magister Chirurgiae (*New Latin*, master of surgery), medical corps
MCAT Medical College Admissions Test
mcg microgram
MCh Magister Chirurgiae (*New Latin*, master of surgery)
MCH mean corpuscular hemoglobin
MCHC mean corpuscular hemoglobin concentration
mCi millicurie
MCV mean corpuscular volume
Md mendelevium
MD medical department, Medicinae Doctor (*New Latin*, doctor of medicine), muscular dystrophy
MDR minimum daily requirement

MDS master of dental surgery
Me methyl
ME medical examiner
med medical
MEDLARS computer data base for medical biographical information
MEDLINE system for accessing medical data base
meg megacycle
mEq milliequivalent
Met methionine
mg milligram
Mg magnesium
mgm milligram
MHC major histocompatibility complex
MHz megahertz
MI mitral incompetence, mitral insufficiency, myocardial infarction
MIC minimal inhibitory concentration, minimum inhibitory concentration
MID minimal infective dose
min minim, minimum, minute
mixt mixture
mks meter-kilogram-second
ml milliliter
MLD median lethal dose, minimum lethal dose
MLT medical laboratory technician
mm millimeter
mmole *also* **mmol** millimole
MMPI Minnesota Multiphasic Personality Inventory
Mn manganese

MN master of nursing
mo month
Mo molybdenum
MO medical officer
MOH medical officer of health
mol molecular, molecule
morph morphological, morphology
mOsm milliosmol
mp melting point
MPC maximum permissible concentration
MPH master of public health
MRI magnetic resonance imaging
mRNA messenger RNA
MS mass spectrometry, master of science, multiple sclerosis
MSc master of science
msec millisecond
MSG monosodium glutamate
MSH melanocyte-stimulating hormone
MSN master of science in nursing
MSW master of social work
MT medical technologist
mv *or* **mV** millivolt
Mv mandelevium
mw milliwatt
Mw megawatt

N nasal, newton, nitrogen, normal
Na natrium (*New Latin,* sodium)

NA Nomina Atomica, numerical aperture, nurse's aide
NAD nicotinamide adenine dinucleotide, no appreciable disease
NADP nicotinamide adenine dinucleotide phosphate
Nb niobium
NB newborn
NBRT National Board for Respiratory Therapy
NCA neurocirculatory asthenia
NCI National Cancer Institute
Nd neodymium
NDT neurodevelopmental treatment
Ne neon
neurol neurological, neurology
NF National Formulary
ng nanogram
NG nasogastric
NGF nerve growth factor
NGU nongonococcal urethritis
NHS National Health Service
Ni nickel
NIH National Institutes of Health
NIMH National Institute of Mental Health
NIOSH National Institute of Occupational Safety and Health
nm nanometer
NMR nuclear magnetic resonance

no number
No nobelium
NOPHN National Organization for Public Health Nursing
Np neptunium
NP neuropsychiatric, neuropsychiatry
NPN nonprotein nitrogen
NPT normal pressure and temperature
nr near
NR no refill
NREM nonrapid eye movement
nsec nanosecond
NSU nonspecific urethritis
NTP normal temperature and pressure

o- orth-, ortho-
O octarius, (*Latin*, pint), opening, oxygen
OB obstetric, obstetrician, obstetrics
OB-GYN obstetrician-gynecologist, obstetrics-gynecology
OBS obstetrician, obstetrics
obstet obstetric, obstetrics
od omnes dies (*Latin*, every day)
OD doctor of optometry, oculus dexter (*Latin*, right eye)
ol oleum
OL oculus laevus (*Latin*, left eye)
OMPA octamethylpyrophosphoramide
OPD outpatient department
opt optician

OR operating room
org organic
Os osmium
OS oculus sinister (*Latin*, left eye)
Osm osmol
ost osteopathic
OT occupational therapist, occupational therapy, old tuberculin
OTC over-the-counter
OTR registered occupational therapist
oz ounce, ounces

P parental, part, percentile, pharmacopeia, phosphorus, pint, pole, population, position, positive, posterior, pressure, pulse, pupil
Pa protactinium
PA pernicious anemia, physician's assistant
PABA para-aminobenzoic acid
PAC physician's assistant, certified
PAF platelet-activating factor
PAH para-aminohippurate, para-aminohippuric acid, polynuclear aromatic hydrocardon
PAS para-aminosalicylic acid, periodic acid-Schiff
PASA para-aminosalicylic acid
pathol pathological, pathologist, pathology
Pb plumbum (*Latin*, lead)
PBB polybrominated biphenyl

PBI protein-bound iodine
PC percent, percentage, post cibos (*Latin*, after meals), professional corporation, purified concentrate
PCB polychlorinated biphenyl
PCP phencyclidine, pentachlorophenol, pneumocystis carinii pneumonia
Pcs preconscious
PCV packed cell volume
PCWP pulmonary capillary wedge pressure
Pd palladium
PD interpupillary distance
PDB paradichlorobenzene
PDR Physicians' Desk Reference
PE physical examination
PEP phosphoenolpyruvate
per period, periodic, person
perf perforated, perforation
PET positron-emission tomography
pf picofarad
pg picogram
PG prostaglandin
PGA pteroylglutamic acid
PGR psychogalvanic reaction, psychogalvanic reflex, psychogalvanic response
PGY postgraduate year
ph pharmacopoeia, phosphor, phot
pH cologarithm of the effective hydrogen-ion concentration or hydrogen-ion activity in gram equivalents per liter
PHA phytohemagglutinin
Phar D doctor of pharmacy

pharm pharmaceutical, pharmacist, pharmacy
Pharm D doctor of pharmacy
PhD doctor of philosophy
PhG graduate in pharmacy
PHN public health nurse
PHS Public Health Service
PID pelvic inflammatory disease
pil pilula (*Latin*, pill)
pK cologarithm of the dissociation constant K or -log K
PK psychokinesis
PKU phenylketonuria
PLSS portable life-support system
Pm promethium
PM post meridiem (*Latin*, afternoon), postmortem
PMN polymorphonuclear neutrophilic leukocyte
pmol *or* **pmole** picomole
PMS premenstrual syndrome
PN psychoneurotic
po per os
Po polonium
pp parts per
PP pellagra preventive
ppb parts per billion
PPD purified protein derivative
PPLO pleuropneumonia-like organism
ppm parts per million
ppt parts per thousand, parts per trillion, precipitate
Pr praesodymium
prn pro re nata (*Latin*, as needed)

ps   picosecond
PSRO   professional standards review organization
psych   psychology
psychol   psychologist, psychology
pt   patient, pint
Pt   platinum
PT   physical therapist, physical therapy
PTA   plasma thromboplastin antecedent
PTC   phenylthiocarbamide, plasma thromboplastin component
PTFE   polytetrafluoro-ethylene
PTH   parathyroid hormone
PTSD   posttraumatic stress disorder
Pu   plutonium
pulv   pulvis (*Latin*, powder)
PUO   pyrexia of unknown origin
PVD   peripheral vascular disease
PVE   prosthetic valve endocarditis
PVP   polyvinylpyrrolidone
pvt   private
Px   pneumothorax, prognosis
PZI   protamine zinc insulin

q   quaque (*Latin*, every)
qd   quaque die (*Latin*, every day)
qh *or* **qhr**   quaque hora (*Latin*, every hour) — often used with a number indicating the hours between

doses ⟨*q4h* — every four hours⟩
qid   quater in die (*Latin*, four times a day)
ql   quantum libet (*Latin*, as much as you please)
qn   quaque nocte (*Latin*, every night)
qp   quantum placet (*Latin*, as much as you please)
qt   quart
qv   quantum vis (*Latin*, as much as you will)

r   roentgen
R   Reaumur, rough
Ra   radium
rad   radix (*Latin*, root)
RAST   radioallergosorbent test
Rb   rubidium
RBC   red blood cell, red blood count
RBE   relative biological effectiveness
rd   rutherford
RD   reaction of degeneration, registered dietitian
RDA   Recommended Daily Allowance
RDS   respiratory distress syndrome
Re   rhenium
rem   roentgen equivalent man
REM   rapid eye movement
rep   repeatur (*Latin*, let it be repeated)
RES   reticuloendothelial system
RF   rheumatic fever

Rh rhesus (blood factor), rhodium

RH relative humidity

RIA radioimmunoassay

RLF retrolental fibroplasia

RLQ right lower quadrant

Rn radon

RN registered nurse

RNA ribonucleic acid

RPh registered pharmacist

RPM revolutions per minute

RPR rapid plasma reagin

RPT registered physical therapist

RQ respiratory quotient

RR recovery room

RRA registered records administrator

RRL registered records librarian

rRNA ribosomal ribonucleic acid

RRT registered respiratory therapist

RSV respiratory syncytial virus, Rous sarcoma virus

RT reaction time, recreational therapist, respiratory therapist

Ru ruthenium

RU rat unit

RUQ right upper quadrant

Rx prescription

S sacral — used with a number to indicate one of the segments of the spinal cord, signa — used to introduce a signature in writing prescriptions, smooth, subject, sulfur, svedberg

s- secondary — used in names of organic compounds

sa secundum artem (*Latin*, according to art — used to introduce a signature in writing prescriptions)

S-A sinoatrial

sat saturated

Sb stibium (*Latin*, antimony)

Sc scandium

ScD doctor of science

SCID severe combined immunodeficiency

ScM master of science

SCM state certified midwife

SDA specific dynamic action

Se selenium

SED skin erythema dose

SEM scanning electron microscope, scanning electron microscopy

sg specific gravity

SGOT serum glutamic-oxaloacetic transaminase

SGPT serum glutamic pyruvic transaminase

SH serum hepatitis

Si silicon

SI Système International d'Unités (*French*, International System of Units)

SIDS sudden infant death syndrome

Sig signa

SK streptokinase

SLE systemic lupus erythematosus

Sm samarium

Sn stannum (*Late Latin*, tin)

SNF skilled nursing facility

SOB short of breath
SOS si opus sit (*Latin*, if occasion requires, if necessary)
SPCA serum prothrombin conversion accelerator, Society for the Prevention of Cruelty to Animals
sp gr specific gravity
Sr strontium
S-R stimulus-response
sRNA soluble RNA (transfer RNA)
SRS-A slow-reacting substance of anaphylaxis
ss semis (*Latin*, one half)
SSPE subacute sclerosing panencephalitis
STD sexually transmitted disease
STH somatotropic hormone
STP standard temperature and pressure
STS serologic test for syphilis
surg surgeon, surgery, surgical

T absolute temperature, tesla, thoracic, tritium
Ta tantalum
TA transactional analysis
tab tablet
T and A tonsillectomy and adenoidectomy
TAT thematic apperception test
Tb terbium
TB tubercle bacillus, tuberculosis

TBG thyroid-binding globulin, thyroxine-binding globulin
Tc technetium
TCDD tetrachlordibenzo-dioxin
TD tardive dyskinesia
tds ter die sumendum (*Latin*, to be taken three times a day)
Te tellurium
TEA tetraethylammonium
tech technician
TEM triethylenemelamine
TEPP tetraethyl pyrophosphate
T-4 thyroxine
Th thorium
THC tetrahydrocannabinol
Ti titanium
TIA transient ischemic attack
tid ter in die (*Latin*, three times a day)
tinct tincture
Tl thallium
TLC tender loving care, thin-layer chromatography
Tm thulium
TM transcendental meditation
TMJ temporomandibular joint
TNT trinitrotoluene
TPI Treponema pallidum immobilization (test)
TPN triphosphopyridine nucleotide
TPP thiamine pyrophosphate
TPR temperature, pulse, respiration

TRF thyrotropin-releasing factor

TRH thyrotropin-releasing hormone

tRNA transfer RNA

Try tryptophan

TSH thyroid-stimulating hormone

TSS toxic shock syndrome

U uranium

UDP uridine diphosphate

UMP uridine monophosphate (uridylic acid)

ung unguentum (*Latin*, ointment)

Unh unnilhexium

Unp unnilpentium

Unq unnilquadium

USAN United States Adopted Names

USP United States Pharmacopeia

UTI urinary tract infection

UTP uridine triphosphate

UV ultraviolet

V vanadium, volt

VAD ventricular assist device

VCG vectorcardiogram

VD venereal disease

VDRL venereal disease research laboratory

vet veterinarian

Vi virulent

VIP vasoactive intestinal peptide

VLDL very low-density lipoprotein

VMA vanillylmandelic acid

VNA Visiting Nurse Association

vol volume

VS vesicular stomatitis

VSD ventricular septal defect

v/v volume per volume

W wolfram (*German*, tungsten)

WAIS Wechsler Adult Intelligence Scale

WBC white blood cell

WEE western equine encephalomyelitis

WHO World Health Organization

ws water-soluble

wt weight

w/v weight in volume

w/w weight in weight

x power of magnification

Xe xenon

xu X unit

Y yttrium

Yb ytterbium

Z atomic number, impedance

Zn zinc

ZPG zero population growth

Zr zirconium

WEIGHTS AND MEASURES

Unit	Abbr or Symbol	Equivalents in Other Units of Same System	Equivalent in Indicated System

length

English system			*metric system*
mile	mi	5280 feet 320 rods 1760 yards	1.609 kilometers
rod	rd	5.50 yards 16.5 feet	5.029 meters
yard	yd	3 feet 36 inches	0.914 meters
foot	ft *or* '	12 inches 0.333 yards	30.480 centimeters
inch	in *or* "	0.083 feet 0.027 yards	2.540 centimeters
metric system			*English system*
myriameter	myr	1×10^4 meters	6.2137 miles
kilometer	km	1000 meters	0.62137 miles
hectometer	hm	100 meters	109.36 yards
dekameter	dkm	10 meters	32.808 feet
meter	m	1 meter	39.370 inches
decimeter	dm	0.1 meters	3.9370 inches
centimeter	cm	0.01 meters	0.39370 inches
millimeter	mm	0.001 meters	0.039370 inches
micron	μ	1×10^{-6} meters	3.9370×10^{-5} inches

weight

avoirdupois weight			*metric system*
ton	tn		
short ton		20 short hundredweight 2000 pounds	0.907 metric tons
long ton		20 long hundredweight 2240 pounds	1.016 metric tons
hundredweight	cwt		
short hundredweight		100 pounds 0.05 short tons	45.359 kilograms
long hundredweight		112 pounds 0.05 long tons	50.802 kilograms
pound	lb *or* lb av	16 ounces 7000 grains	0.453 kilograms
ounce	oz *or* oz av	16 drams 437.5 grains	28.349 grams

| dram | dr *or*
dr av | 27.343 grains
0.0625 ounces | 1.771 grams |
| grain | gr | 0.036 drams
0.002285 ounces | 0.0648 grams |

	troy weight		*metric system*
pound	lb t	12 ounces 240 pennyweight 5760 grains	0.373 kilograms
ounce	oz t	20 pennyweight 480 grains	31.103 grams
pennyweight	dwt *also* pwt	24 grains 0.05 ounces	1.555 grams
grain	gr	0.042 pennyweight 0.002083 ounces	0.0648 grams

	apothecaries' weight		*metric system*
pound	lb ap	12 ounces 5760 grains	0.373 kilograms
ounce	oz ap *or* ℥	8 drams 480 grains	31.103 grams
dram	dr ap *or* ℨ	3 scruples 60 grains	3.887 grams
scruple	s ap *or* ℈	20 grains 0.333 drams	1.295 grams
grain	gr	0.05 scruples 0.002083 ounces 0.0166 drams	0.0648 grams

	metric system		*apothecaries' weight*
metric ton	MT *or* t	1×10^6 grams	2679.2 lbs
quintal	q	1×10^5 grams	267.92 lbs
kilogram	kg	1000 grams	2.6792 lbs
hectogram	hg	100 grams	3.2151 oz
dekagram	dag	10 grams	0.32151 oz
gram	g *or* gm	1 gram	0.032151 oz
decigram	dg	0.10 grams	1.5432 grains
centigram	cg	0.01 grams	0.15432 grains
milligram	mg	0.001 grams	0.015432 grains
microgram	μg	1×10^{-6} grams	1.5432×10^{-5} grains

capacity

	apothecaries' measure		*metric system*
gallon	gal	4 quarts (231 cubic inches)	3.785 liters
quart	qt	2 pints (57.75 cubic inches)	0.946 liters

pint	pt	4 gills (28.875 cubic inches)	0.473 liters
gill	gi	4 fluidounces (7.218 cubic inches)	118.291 milliliters
fluidounce	fl oz or f ℥	8 fluidrams (1.804 cubic inches)	29.573 milliliters
fluidram	fl dr or f ʒ	60 minims (0.225 cubic inches)	3.696 milliliters
minim	min or ♏	1/60 fluidram (0.003759 cubic inch)	0.061610 milliliters

	metric system		*apothecaries' measure*
kiloliter	kl	1000 liters	264.18 gals
hectoliter	hl	100 liters	26.418 gals
dekaliter	dal	10 liters	2.6418 gals
liter	l	1 liter	1.0567 qts
deciliter	dl	0.10 liters	3.3815 fl oz
centiliter	cl	0.01 liters	2.7052 fl dr
milliliter	ml	0.001 liters	16.231 minims
microliter	μl	1×10^{-6} liters	0.016231 minims

SIGNS AND SYMBOLS

apothecaries' measures

℥   ounce
f℥   fluidounce
f℈   fluidram
℟, ℟, ℟,   minim
or min

apothecaries' weights

℔   pound
℥   ounce (as ℥ i *or* ℥ j, one ounce; ℥ ss, half an ounce; ℥ iss *or* jss, one ounce and a half; ℥ ij, two ounces)
℈   dram
℈   scruple

genetics

○   an individual, specif., a female—used chiefly in inheritance charts
□   an individual, specif., a male—used chiefly in inheritance charts
♀   female
♂ *or* ♂   male
×   crossed with; hybrid
+   wild type
F_1 offspring of the first generation
F_2 offspring of the second generation
F_3, F_4, F_5, etc.   offspring of the third, fourth, fifth, etc., generation
N   the haploid or gametic number of chromosomes
2N   the diploid or somatic number of chromosomes

mathematics

+   plus; positive $\langle a + b = c \rangle$—used also to indicate omitted figures or an approximation
−   minus; negative
±   plus or minus (the square root of $4a^2$ is $\pm 2a$)
×   multiplied by; times $\langle 6 \times 4 = 24 \rangle$—also indicated by placing a dot between the factors $\langle 6 \cdot 4 = 24 \rangle$ or by writing factors other than numerals without signs
÷ *or* :   divided by $\langle 24 \div 6 = 4 \rangle$—also indicated by writing the divisor under the dividend with a line between $\langle \frac{24}{6} = 4 \rangle$ or by writing the divisor after the dividend with an oblique line between $\langle 3/8 \rangle$
=   equals $\langle 6 + 2 = 8 \rangle$
>   is greater than $\langle 6 > 5 \rangle$
<   is less than $\langle 3 < 4 \rangle$
:   is to; the ratio of
∞   infinity
√ *or* √   root—used without a figure to indicate a square root $\langle$as in $\sqrt{4} = 2\rangle$ or with an index above the sign to indicate another degree $\langle$as in $\sqrt[3]{3}$, $\sqrt[3]{7}\rangle$; also denoted by a fractional index at the right of a number whose denominator expresses the degree of the root $\langle 3^{1/3} = \sqrt[3]{3} \rangle$

miscellaneous

℞   take—used on prescriptions; prescription; treatment
    poison